**A DISTINGUISHED PHYSICIAN AND SPECIALIST BRINGS YOU
THE MOST COMPLETE HOME HEALTH REFERENCE ON
GYNECOLOGICAL PROBLEMS AND PROCEDURES AVAILABLE TODAY**

Sensitive, accessible, and highly authoritative, this guide to common gynecological conditions answers all the questions women ask about their reproductive system with the most up-to-date medical facts. Filled with personal accounts from women who share their varied gynecological experiences, it covers such disorders as ovarian cysts, menstrual problems, incontinence, endometriosis, cancer, fibroids, pelvic pain, and more.

Unrivaled in its thoroughness, *A Gynecologist's Second Opinion* allows women to intelligently contemplate their options and make informed choices for successful treatment. This extraordinary resource arms women with the knowledge they need to get the best doctors and the best care.

"One of today's best and most sensitive physicians writes a book for all of us. Every woman should read it."
                    —Barbara Kass-Annese, Nurse Practitioner,
                        Los Angeles Regional Family Planning Council

"A clear, understandable, current and accurate summary of gynecologic problems and solutions. This timely reference will become an important resource that will encourage meaningful dialogue between women and their doctors."
                    —Jonathan S. Berek, M.D., Chief of Gynecology and
                        Gynecologic Oncology, UCLA School of Medicine

"Useful advice from a practicing gynecologist at the forefront of his specialty."
                    —Bruce D. Shephard, M.D., co-author of
                        The Complete Guide to Women's Health

D0972905

WILLIAM H. PARKER, M.D., is chairman of obstetrics and gynecology at Santa Monica–UCLA Medical Center and clinical professor of obstetrics and gynecology at UCLA School of Medicine. He maintains an active private practice, is the author of numerous publications in professional journals, and is a board-certified fellow of the American College of Obstetrics and Gynecology. Dr. Parker is listed in *The Best Doctors in America®: Pacific Region.*

RACHEL L. PARKER is a former community health educator and is currently a middle school teacher in Los Angeles.

INGRID A. RODI, M.D., is a board-certified specialist in reproductive endocrinology and infertility and an assistant clinical professor at UCLA School of Medicine.

AMY E. ROSENMAN, M.D., is a board-certified fellow of the American College of Obstetrics and Gynecology and an assistant clinical professor at UCLA School of Medicine, where she specializes in urogynecology.

This book is dedicated to our children,
Aaron, Evan, and Brian,
who bring joy and love to each day.

ACKNOWLEDGMENTS

Many people helped during the writing of this book, and I am enormously grateful to them. First, I would like to thank my partners, Dr. Ingrid Rodi and Dr. Amy Rosenman, for their support to me and their valuable contributions to the book. A number of my teachers, colleagues and friends took the time to review the manuscript and offer their special expertise which proved to be invaluable—Dr. Beth Meyerowitz, Department of Psychology, University of Southern California, Dr. Howard Judd, Department of Obstetrics and Gynecology, Olive View Medical Center, Dr. Jonathan Berek, Department of Obstetrics and Gynecology, UCLA School of Medicine, Dr. John Bornstein, Department of Anesthesiology, Santa Monica-UCLA Medical Center, Barbara Kass-Anesse, NP, Regional Family Planning Center, and Dr. Andrea Rapkin, Department of Obstetrics and Gynecology, UCLA School of Medicine. I would like to express gratitude to our agent, Arielle Eckstut, of James Levine Communications, for her advice and enthusiasm, and our editor, Deborah Brody, for her support and guidance.

I would also like to thank all of my teachers over the years, who have given freely of their time and knowledge, and all of my patients, who have allowed me to care for them and who have taught me so much.

CONTENTS

INTRODUCTION

If you are reading this book, you or someone you care about is probably facing a gynecologic problem. In my practice, I often have the opportunity to see women for a second opinion regarding gynecologic problems. I have always viewed my physician's role as that of an educator. My approach has been to offer each woman all of the medical information available regarding her problem, to be available for all questions and concerns, and to allow the patient to make her own decision as to the best course to follow.

This book was born out of a certain sense of frustration. Over the years it became apparent to me that there were no books for women to read that provide in-depth, compassionate, yet understandable information about the problems I often take care of. The books I found were either encyclopedic, providing only brief descriptions of a large range of women's health care issues, or were focused on one subject, usually hysterectomy, and failed to present information about many of the difficult gynecologic problems that women sometimes face. Other books contained medically incorrect information or lacked the careful analysis of the risks and benefits of treatment that each woman needs to learn in order to make the right medical decision for herself. And some books seemed to have a political agenda and treated the medical facts as a secondary issue.

In order to take an active part in the care you receive, you need an understanding of how your body normally works and an educated idea of what has gone wrong when a problem arises. We have written *A Gynecologist's Second Opinion* to try to fill this need. Arranged in a question-and-answer format, this book provides clear descriptions of common gynecological problems, up-to-date thinking regarding their causes, and state-of-the-art information about treatment. Multiple options for treatment for each problem are outlined; the option of no treatment is discussed when appropriate, treatment with medication, surgery, and current research that may lead to new treatment in the foreseeable future are also discussed. *A Gynecologist's Second Opinion* is filled with the stories of women who have actually had these problems. This makes the medical facts come alive, and allows the reader to experience examples of a search for treatment.

The medical establishment has been questioned about its practice, its research, and its very heart in regards to providing women with care and treatment. However, the beliefs of many physicians and the way medicine in general is practiced are changing dramatically. The days of "automatic" hysterectomies are over. The uterus and ovaries are no longer thought of as non-essential and irrelevant organs once the years of child-bearing have passed. There has been an explosion in knowledge, in new surgical procedures and equipment, and in the attitudes of health practitioners. As a practicing gynecologist, Chairman of the Department of Obstetrics and Gynecology of Santa Monica–UCLA Medical Center, and Clinical Professor of the Department of Obstetrics and Gynecology, UCLA School of Medicine, I have tried to bring you the best medical information available. I have been teaching the new surgical techniques covered in this book for the last ten years as a faculty member for the Houston Laser Institute and the American Association of Gynecologic Laparoscopists. I am a reviewer for the international journals *Obstetrics and Gynecology* and *Journal of the American Association of Gynecologic Laparoscopists* and have published research articles in those journals and others. This experience has permitted me to stay in the forefront of the treatment of gynecologic problems.

A Gynecologist's Second Opinion is not meant to be a substitute for an appointment with a doctor. It is, however, meant to enable you to comfortably gain information and understanding without time constraints or outside pressures. Reading the book may help you to form your questions before you go for a scheduled doctor's appointment. It may empower you to make an appointment you've been avoiding, or it may serve as an educational companion once you have seen your doctor. Your intelligence, your curiosity, and your skepticism are needed in any search for good health care. Any person facing a serious medical problem should be urged to get a second opinion. *A Gynecologist's Second Opinion* is a companion in that quest for answers and good care. We hope this book provides you with a reference to turn to, and we wish you good health.

A
GYNECOLOGIST'S
SECOND OPINION

1

NORMAL BODY, NORMAL EXAM

The human body is a fascinating and complicated creation. The design of a woman's body appears to be intentional and intricate, as evidenced by the changes that accompany monthly hormonal events and pregnancy and childbirth. For example, hormonal changes may heighten a woman's sexual desire around the time of ovulation, the most optimal time for fertilization, thus increasing her odds of conceiving a child by intensifying her desire for sex at the perfect time. Also, the thick mucus produced by the cervix normally hinders the passage of sperm up into the uterus. At the time of ovulation, however, the mucus becomes thin and watery, allowing the sperm easy entry.

It is only over the past one hundred years that the functions of a woman's body have begun to be studied and understood. In medical drawings from the 1700s, the anatomy of a woman's pelvic organs resembles that of the pelvic organs of farm animals. The ignorance behind the anatomists' assumption is understandable because church law prohibited human dissection. As a result, the medical world spent many years working from these incorrect suppositions.

Before the 1900s, the hormonal processes of a woman's body were not recognized at all. Menstruation was believed to result from irritation to the "fallopian tube nerve," a structure that we now know does not exist. Women were thought to bleed because they had more blood than men had, and more than they needed. When an adolescent girl began to menstruate, she was considered susceptible to weakness, lethargy, and disease. The two female hormones, estrogen and progesterone, and the hormonal events that trigger menstruation were not discovered until the 1920s.

In the 1870s, the uterus was believed to be the physical control center of a woman's body, acting through nerve connections to every other organ. Symptoms related to the heart, lungs, liver, and intestines were considered to be the consequence of uterine disease. And one source of uterine disease was assumed to be the reading of romantic novels, which led to the evil of masturbation, which in turn caused problems with the uterus and abnormal periods.

The ovaries were thought to be the main influence on a woman's emotions, and insanity was attributed to disease of the ovaries. "Ovariotomy," removal of the ovaries, was commonly performed for a variety of emotional problems, including overeating and erotic tendencies. The removal of diseased ovaries seemed to produce a "better" woman: one who was more orderly, industrious, and clean.

It is no wonder that doctors were rarely able to diagnose true gynecologic diseases. Pelvic examinations were almost never performed to avoid embarrassing the woman and her doctor. Doctors often made a diagnosis entirely based on reported symptoms sent by the patient via messenger. If the doctor felt an examination was absolutely necessary, the woman was covered entirely by drapes, so that he was unable to see anything. Needless to say, a woman's sense of her own ailment or physical condition was rarely respected.

Although medical research sometimes seems annoyingly slow, there has been a steady march toward our understanding of a woman's reproductive system. With each step, we are able to solve more problems and treat more illnesses.

"Knowledge is power," wrote Francis Bacon in 1597. That statement is particularly true today in regard to your health care. If you understand your own body, you will be in a better position to take care of it in times of sickness as well as health. Staying healthy is always the best medicine. But if you have a medical problem, choosing the right doctor and getting the appropriate treatment will involve making decisions. Put some power into your decisions by being well informed and educated. This chapter will describe what the normal female reproductive system looks like and how it works, as well as what a doctor looks for when he or she examines you. Learning about the normal functionings of the body is a good base from which you can become an informed user of health services and implement preventive health strategies.

What Does the Uterus Look Like?

The uterus, normally about the size of a small pear, is a woman's largest reproductive organ. It is even shaped like an upside-down pear. The uterus extends downward from below the pubic bone to the top of the vagina, where the cervix (the opening of the uterus) attaches (see fig. 1.1). The uterus is a reddish-pink color, much like the color of the inside of your lips. When viewing videotapes or photographs of their uterus, fallopian tubes, and ovaries, most women are surprised to see how attractive these organs actually are. The colors are quite beautiful.

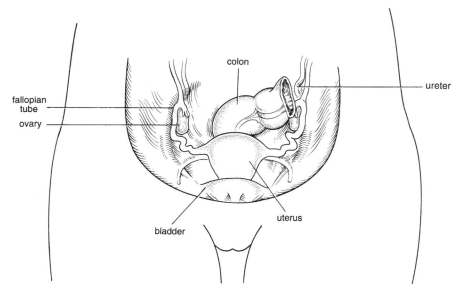

Fig. 1.1.   Position of the uterus, fallopian tubes, and ovaries

How Does the Uterus Work?

The main function of the uterus is to provide a place for a pregnancy to develop, and its ability to grow from its normal size to a size large enough to accommodate a full-term infant is a remarkable achievement. The uterus is composed mostly of muscle, and this muscle has the ability to stretch. In fact, no new muscle cells are added to the uterus during pregnancy. The growth is accomplished entirely by the expansion and stretching of the cells that are already there. As a muscle, the uterus is able to contract and therefore push a baby out during labor and delivery.

Unlike many creatures that are fertile and menstruate only during mating season, women are fertile for a few days every month. The inside lining of the uterus (endometrium) provides the place where the fertilized egg attaches and develops. It is composed of tall cells that are arranged side by side. These cells appear slightly darker and redder than the muscle wall, mostly because the cells are richly supplied with the blood vessels that are designed to provide for the placenta and pregnancy. Under the influence of the hormones produced by the ovaries, the cells all grow together at the same rate. If a woman does not become pregnant, all the cells die and are shed at the same time—the few days of the menstrual period.

What Does the Cervix Look Like?

The cervix is the part of the uterus that can be seen at the top of the vagina (see fig. 1.2). During a pelvic exam, your doctor places a speculum—a duck bill–shaped instrument—in your vagina to inspect your cervix, a raised, pink, doughnut-shaped area. It is firm to the touch and can be moved by mild pressure. In the middle of the cervix is a small opening called the cervical canal, which is the entrance to the uterus.

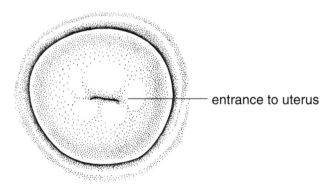

entrance to uterus

Fig. 1.2.   Cervix

Despite being part of the uterus, the cervix has separate functions and develops different conditions and diseases. For example, the virus HPV (see chapter 9) can cause cervical cancer but does not affect other parts of the uterus. And although the Pap smear is an excellent way to detect cervical cancer, it is almost never able to detect uterine cancer. Therefore, while the cervix and uterus are connected, they should be thought of as two separate parts of your reproductive system.

How Does the Cervix Work?

The cervix is the entrance to the uterus and contains cells that regularly make mucus. The mucus is usually thick and helps to keep bacteria and even sperm out of the uterus for most of the month. As the time nears for an egg to leave the ovary (ovulation), hormonal changes cause the mucus to become thin and watery for a few days. While still forming a relatively good barrier against infection, the thinner mucus now allows sperm to enter the uterus. Within a day or two after ovulation the mucus is once again thick and resists the passage of the sperm. This precise timing permits the sperm access to the egg only at the time when the egg is most receptive to being fertilized.

What Do the Fallopian Tubes Look Like?

The fallopian tubes are flexible, soft wands of pink tissue that extend from the top of the uterus outward and toward the ovaries on either side (see fig. 1.3). The tube is open at the end near the ovary, where feathery, short tentacles are responsible for picking up the egg at the time of ovulation. The tubes are loosely attached to the uterus all along their course by thin, soft tissue that allows them to move back and forth.

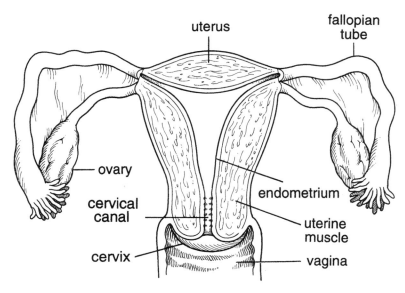

Fig. 1.3.   Reproductive System

How Do the Fallopian Tubes Work?

The freedom of the tubes to move is a necessary design. Just at the time of ovulation, when the egg is released from the ovary, muscles in the attachments between the tube and ovary pull the tube closer to the ovary. The tube then drapes its feathery tentacles over the ovary so that the egg is captured. This movement of the tube toward the ovary is an incredible sight that has been caught on film.

Once captured, the egg can begin its journey through this passageway to the uterus. The cells that line the inside of the tube have tiny hairlike extensions that actively push the egg down the tube. Fertilization by sperm takes place in the middle of the tube, and the tubal cells continue to push the fertilized egg into the uterus. The egg's journey down to the uterus takes about six days.

What Do the Ovaries Look Like?

The ovaries are small, walnut-sized, off-white lumps of tissue that are about one inch away from the top of the uterus on either side. In young girls and adolescents, they are smooth, but after the onset of menstruation, the ovaries begin to go through a series of events that leads to a change in their appearance.

Just prior to ovulation, a small (one-half inch), clear collection of fluid forms around the developing egg and becomes visible below the surface of the ovary. This combination of the fluid, hormone-producing cells, and egg is called a *follicle*. During ovulation, the surface of the ovary bursts open, and the egg is carried away in a surge of fluid. The surface cells of the ovary heal quickly, leaving behind a yellowish pocket of cells called the corpus luteum. The corpus luteum produces the hormone progesterone until the developing placenta takes over; if no pregnancy occurs, it disappears shortly after the menstrual period. As time goes on, the surface of the ovary becomes pitted and irregular, evidence of many ovulations and subsequent healings. After menopause, the monthly formation of follicles and ovulation cease. The ovaries decrease in size to that of an almond and become pale white.

How Do the Ovaries Work?

At the start of a normal menstrual cycle, the pituitary gland, situated at the base of the brain, releases a hormone called follicle-stimulating hormone (FSH) into the bloodstream. When FSH reaches the ovary, it stimulates an egg and the cells around that egg (the follicle) to develop. The follicular cells surrounding the egg then begin to produce estrogen, the main female hormone.

Around the middle of the cycle, the pituitary gland produces luteinizing hormone (LH). LH causes the cells on the surface of the ovary to break open and release the egg. After the egg is released, the ovary begins to produce progesterone, another female hormone, in addition to estrogen. If you become pregnant, the ovary continues to make these hormones for about three months, until the placenta is able to take over hormone production for both itself and the developing fetus.

If you don't become pregnant, the ovary stops making both estrogen and progesterone about two weeks after ovulation. Without these hormones, the uterine-lining cells cannot survive; they die and are shed as the menstrual flow. Then the cycle starts all over again. These finely balanced hormonal events are crucial to controlling the changes you associate with your menstrual cycle and the normal pattern of bleeding that you expect.

Although the ovary produces eggs and estrogen to enable a pregnancy to take place, it also produces estrogen as a necessary supporting hormone for many other parts of your body. Estrogen affects a vast array of tissues. Your bones, heart, bladder, vagina, breasts, and skin all need estrogen in order to stay strong and healthy.

What Does the Doctor Feel When Your Pelvic Examination Is Performed?

The manual part of the pelvic examination allows the doctor to feel the size and shape of the uterus, fallopian tubes, and ovaries. During this part of the examination, the doctor pushes the cervix upward from the inside of the vagina. This moves the top of the uterus closer to your abdominal wall, where the size and shape of the uterus can be felt between the doctor's two hands (see fig. 1.4). Thus, the doctor should be able to detect conditions such as fibroids that increase the size of the uterus.

Prior to menopause, normal ovaries are about the size of a small walnut and can be felt on either side of the uterus during the examination. Abnormally large ovaries usually indicate the presence of cysts, benign tumors, or, very rarely, cancer. The fallopian tubes are so soft and mobile that they are not able to be felt during the examination. Tenderness in the area of the tubes sometimes indicates infection. Endometriosis (see chapter 6) or scar tissue from previous infection or surgery present near the tubes also can lead to tenderness during the examination.

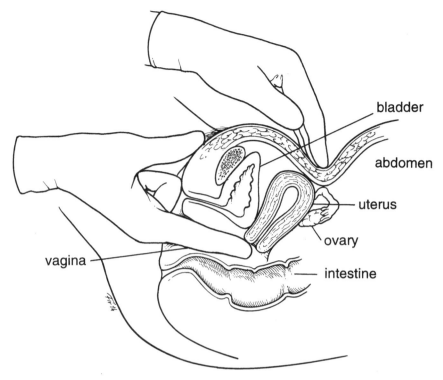

Fig. 1.4.   Performing the manual exam

How Often Should You Have a Pelvic Examination?

The pelvic examination should be performed yearly, starting at the time a woman becomes sexually active or by the age of eighteen. This will allow for the early detection of uterine abnormalities such as fibroids and ovarian abnormalities such as cysts or tumors. The Pap smear is performed at the same time. Pelvic pain, abnormal bleeding, or abnormal vaginal discharge are reasons to see the doctor for a pelvic examination at any time.

How Often Should You Have a Pap Smear?

The Pap smear is used to find cervical abnormalities long before they are actually a threat to your well-being. The major cause of cervical cancer appears to be human papillomavirus (HPV), a virus that is transmitted sexually. Therefore, once you become sexually active you should start having Pap smears. Beginning at the age of eighteen, you should have an annual Pap smear and pelvic examination, even if you are not sexually active.

Cervical cancer starts as dysplasia, a precancerous phase that is detectable on the Pap smear (see chapter 9). The progression of dysplasia into cancer usually takes many years; therefore, *yearly* Pap smears should detect changes in the cells long before they become cancerous, while the abnormal cells are easily treatable.

After three normal annual Pap smears, you and your doctor may discuss the possibility of having the test every two or three years. Since dysplasia is usually a slowly progressive disease, it is unlikely that cancer would develop within a three-year period. Although that is the official policy of the American College of Obstetricians and Gynecologists, I still recommend annual Pap smears to my patients. Cervical dysplasia and even cancer can develop rapidly on occasion. Since these changes are easy to detect, an annual Pap smear will usually allow early discovery and treatment.

How Is the Pap Smear Performed?

The cervix is the opening of the uterus, and it can be seen at the upper end of the vagina. Your doctor uses a speculum for this part of the examination. When opened, the speculum spreads apart the walls of the vagina, and the cervix is visible at the top of the vagina. This examination should be performed gently and should not hurt.

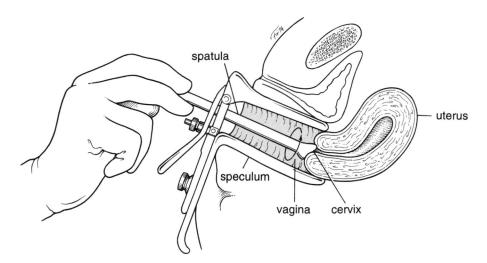

Fig. 1.5a. Performing the Pap smear

Using a small plastic or wood spatula shaped like a Popsicle stick, your doctor carefully scrapes the surface of the cervix to remove some skin cells (see fig. 1.5a). The doctor inserts a small, soft brush just inside the cervix to sample cells from that area. All the cells are spread on a glass slide and sprayed with a solution to preserve them (see fig. 1.5b). The slide is sent to a lab where a pathologist or specially trained technician examines the cells under a microscope for any abnormalities.

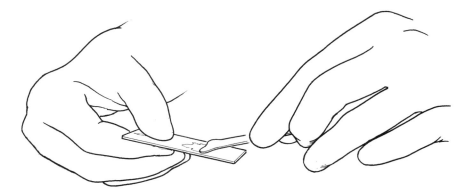

Fig. 1.5b.   Preparing the Pap smear

Can the Pap Smear Detect Ovarian Cancer or Uterine Cancer?

The Pap smear is performed by scraping cells off the cervix in order to examine them under a microscope. Although there is a continuous channel from the ovary, down through the fallopian tubes, into the uterus, and out the cervix, cells from the ovary never make it down that channel to the cervix. Therefore, the diagnosis of ovarian cancer cannot be made from the Pap smear.

The uterine-lining cells are high up inside the uterus; consequently, they are not removed during the Pap smear. On occasion, uterine-lining cells may fall through the cervix, and the pathologist will see them on the Pap smear. If these cells appear abnormal on the Pap smear, a D&C (see chapter 10) should be performed to evaluate whether uterine precancer or cancer is present. However, it is uncommon to find any cells other than cervical cells on the Pap smear, and the test is basically designed for the detection of cervical dysplasia and cervical cancer.

How Is the Breast Examination Performed?

A breast examination should be performed by your physician at the time of your annual exam. There are many ways to do this, each one designed to insure that all areas of the breast are examined. During the breast exam, you will be sitting or lying down with your arms over your head to make your breast tissue easier to feel. I start the examination by feeling, with the flat part of my fingers, the area of the breast closest to the armpit. Breast cancers most commonly occur in the upper, outer part of the breast. I then move my fingers across the breast in a straight line until I feel the breastbone. Then I position my fingers down an inch or so and move them across the breast in the opposite direction. I follow this back-and-forth pattern until all of the breast tissue has been examined.

What Does Breast Cancer Feel Like?

Many women get nervous when they feel a slight lump or irregularity in their breast and assume it is cancer. However, most lumps are not cancer. Breast cancer is usually not a subtle finding: It feels obviously different from your normal breast tissue. Prior to menopause, normal breast tissue is soft but often has irregular, firm, lumpy areas. In addition, since your breasts are influenced by hormonal changes, they may feel more irregular, firmer, and more tender just before and during your menstrual periods. After menopause, breast glands are replaced somewhat by fat, and the breasts feel less firm and less irregular. This accounts for the change in the appearance of the breasts that women note after menopause.

Breast cancer usually feels like a distinct and hard lump. More often than not, breast cancer is not tender to the touch and if pushed will not move within the breast. However, new lumps that persist for more than a cycle should be reported to your doctor, even if they are not tender and move when pushed. Since cyclical changes in the breast don't occur after menopause, postmenopausal women should report *any* new lump. Many women will detect a breast lump at some time in their lives, and nearly all of these lumps will be benign. But if a new lump is causing you anxiety, see your physician, so you can end the worry and know for sure that you are all right. Further evaluation by mammogram and biopsy will be recommended for any suspicious lump that may be cancerous (see page 14).

Should You Perform a Monthly Breast Self-Examination?

It is a good idea for you to perform a breast self-examination every month. Although the idea of self-examination makes some women uncomfortable, doing it will allow you to get familiar with the normal appearance and feel of your breasts. If any changes occur in your breast, you will be aware of them. Your breasts change as you age and will feel different as the years go by. Self-examination will keep you aware of these subtle changes.

Your doctor will examine your breasts only once or twice a year and may examine a few hundred women between your visits. For even the most attentive doctor, remembering exactly what *your* breasts felt like a year ago is difficult. However, you are examining one person, and you're doing the examination twelve times a year. You are much more likely to know if a lump has always been present and is, therefore, not worrisome. Or, if a significant change occurs, you will be aware of it and can discuss it with your doctor. However, if breast self-examination is difficult for you or causes anxiety, you may choose to see your doctor every three or four months for a breast exam.

When and How Should You Do a Breast Self-Examination?

It is probably best to do a breast self-examination after your period is over, when your breasts are less likely to be tender or lumpy. If you are postmenopausal and are taking hormones, it may be best to do the exam right after the hormonally induced monthly bleeding stops. If you are taking both estrogen and progesterone every day, so that no bleeding is expected, or if you do not take hormones, then plan to do the self-examination around the same time every month.

There is no magic way to examine your breasts. The important thing is to get a solid sense of how your breasts usually look and feel. If you are familiar with your own body, you'll know if it has changed. It is a good idea to start by looking at your breasts in a mirror, first with your hands at your sides, then with your hands behind your head. Look for any lumps or dimples in the skin and gently squeeze the nipples to look for any discharge. The second part of the examination involves feeling your breasts for any lumps or irregularities. Some women prefer to check their breasts while standing in the shower, some while sitting in a chair, some while lying down. Some women examine their breasts in a circular motion; others use an up-and-down technique as seen in fig. 1.6. In general, breast cancer feels like an obvious lump and is often firm, irregular, and nontender. However, if you are premenopausal, any lump that *persists* for a cycle or two should be reported to your doctor. If you are postmenopausal, *any* lump should be reported right away.

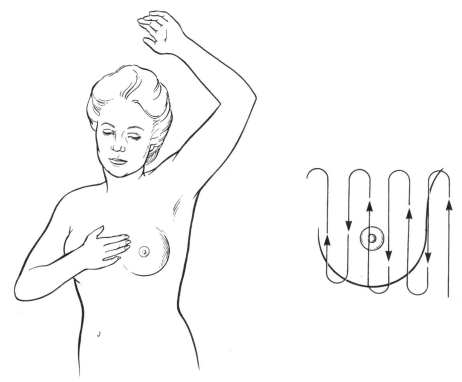

Fig 1.6.   Breast self-examination

How Often Should You Have a Mammogram?

The mammogram is an X ray of the breast designed to detect breast cancer at an early stage, often before it can be felt by the patient or the doctor. Early detection of breast cancer with screening mammography appears to improve chances for a cure. The recommendations regarding the frequency of mammogram screening seem to change every year or two. Without question, the techniques and X-ray machines used for mammograms are more accurate and much safer than they were years ago. Today the X-ray dose you get from one mammogram is less than the radiation you would get flying in an airplane from coast to coast. The risk to your health from the radiation exposure during one mammogram is equivalent to the risk of smoking *one cigarette* in your lifetime.

The accuracy of the mammogram differs in pre- and postmenopausal women. The mammogram is less accurate before menopause because your breasts tend to be fuller and more dense. This texture sometimes makes interpretation of the mammogram more difficult. This means a cancer may not be as easily detected in some premenopausal women, and in others the normal dense tissue may actually look suspicious. After menopause, the breast tissue becomes less dense, and it allows X rays to pass more easily, which results in a better picture. So, if breast cancer is present in a postmenopausal woman, the mammogram will find it 90 percent of the time. This is true even if you are taking estrogen replacement therapy.

Having said all that, what are the current recommendations? The American College of Obstetricians and Gynecologists recommends that women between the ages of forty and fifty have a mammogram every one or two years. The mammogram should be performed every year after the age of fifty. If you have a mother or sister who has had breast cancer, you should consider having yearly mammograms starting a few years before the age at which your relative was diagnosed with the disease.

Some women avoid mammograms because of the discomfort involved. Most women report that they don't feel any pain, but they do find the procedure to be awkward and briefly uncomfortable because of the pressure that is applied to the breast by the plates of the mammography apparatus. In addition, the plates are frequently cold, and the pose you are expected to hold is undeniably awkward. But most women find that the good feeling of relief they get once they are told "all is well, see you next year" is worth the cold squeeze for a few unpleasant moments. Think of the long-term gain, not the short-term discomfort.

What Happens If a Suspicious Breast Lump Is Detected?

If a suspicious area is detected in the breast by either examination or mammogram, further evaluation will be recommended. Gynecologists and family doctors usually are not trained to manage these problems beyond the initial examination, and you should be referred to a general surgeon for the detailed evaluation.

Based on the surgeon's examination and evaluation of your mammogram, cells from the suspicious area may need to be removed (biopsied) and examined under the microscope in order to determine if cancer is present. There are many different ways to get these cells, and the type of technique used will depend on the size of the abnormal area and the degree of suspicion of cancer. The technology for these procedures is changing, so you should discuss which type of biopsy is most appropriate for your situation. One technique uses a fine needle attached to a syringe to draw out cells from the area. This *fine-needle aspiration* is performed with local anesthesia in the doctor's office. However, the aspirated cells are sometimes difficult for the pathologist to interpret. If the cells look like cancer, then the test is usually accurate. If the test is negative, you may need a larger biopsy to be sure that cancer is not present.

A *stereotactic core biopsy* uses a larger needle placed with the guidance of a special mammography machine. This biopsy is performed in the radiologist's office with local anesthesia. The machine uses a computer to guide the needle directly into the area that looks suspicious. The larger needle is able to remove more tissue, making it easier for the pathologist to interpret. An *excisional biopsy* is performed by a surgeon. If the area to be removed is small, local anesthesia can be used, and the procedure may be performed in the doctor's office or outpatient area of the hospital. Using a scalpel, the surgeon removes the entire suspicious area of the breast. Larger areas may need to be removed under general anesthesia in the hospital. The incisions are small, and the stitches dissolve by themselves. If cancer is diagnosed by any of these techniques, other tests will be performed to determine appropriate treatment. See the books referenced at the end of this chapter for a discussion of the complex issues involved in the treatment of breast cancer.

Do You Really Need a Rectal Examination?

For most women, the rectal examination is their least favorite part of a visit to the gynecologist. But the rectal examination is important because it enables the physician to detect signs of precancerous and cancerous polyps of the rectum and colon. In the intestines, unlike the uterus, polyps can lead to cancer. Colon cancer can be prevented if polyps are found and removed in the precancerous stage.

A rectal examination should be performed *yearly*, after the age of forty, at the time of your annual examination. The doctor places a gloved finger inside the rectum in order to feel for any hard areas that might represent a tumor. The stool that remains on the examining glove is then spread on a chemically treated pice of paper and tested for the presence of blood. Colon cancer causes tissue to become fragile and bleed. The blood can become mixed with stool and may not be visible to you. This chemical test on specially treated paper, however, can detect even small amounts of blood. Sometimes the test may detect blood from food you have eaten or blood from common hemorrhoids; therefore, a positive test should not be alarming but should be further evaluated by your doctor.

How Often Should You Have a Sigmoidoscopy?

Cancer of the colon is a *preventable* disease. Virtually all colon cancers start in polyps present in the colon. These polyps can be visibly detected by your doctor, who places a flexible telescope into your rectum and passes it up into your lower intestines. This test is called a sigmoidoscopy, and it is performed in your doctor's office in about thirty minutes. A sigmoidoscopy is another test most of us would prefer to avoid, and the process of preparing for it is not appealing. For a day prior to the test, you must clean out your intestines by drinking a medication that causes diarrhea. Needless to say, that day of preparation is no one's idea of fun.

Following the guidelines for screening with sigmoidoscopy can drastically reduce the incidence of colon cancer. The current recommendations suggest that the test be performed every three to five years after the age of fifty. If you have a history of colon cancer in your family, your doctor will recommend how frequently you should have a sigmoidoscopy. This diagnostic test has saved many lives and should not be avoided simply because it is unpleasant. Comfort yourself during that day of preparation by knowing that for most people the preparation is the worst part. Think of something fun for yourself to do once it is over and you've gotten a clean bill of health. Celebrate your good judgment and good health.

How Often Should You Have a Pelvic Sonogram?

A sonogram may be a useful test if a doctor thinks he or she feels something abnormal during your pelvic examination. The sonogram can confirm the presence of an abnormality and can determine its size and composition. For example, ovarian cysts and fibroids can be accurately diagnosed with this test.

However, as discussed fully in chapter 8, the regular use of pelvic sonograms for *healthy* women is *not indicated*. This test often will suggest that something is wrong, when, in fact, no cancer is present. Any abnormal finding may then lead to unnecessary surgery, as well as to unnecessary anxiety. The use of yearly sonograms is being tested on women who are at high risk for developing ovarian cancer—women with a mother or sister, or both, who have had ovarian cancer (see chapter 8). Even for these high-risk women, the results have not been very encouraging. Some women at high risk have developed ovarian cancer despite a normal sonogram, and others with abnormal tests have been found to have a benign ovarian cyst at the time of surgery.

It is clear that a test for the early detection of ovarian cancer is imperative in order to reduce mortality from this frightening disease. Even though much time and research money are being invested in this search, annual pelvic examinations by your doctor are still the best way to early diagnosis.

How Often Should You Have Your Blood Tested?

Your blood can be tested for an almost infinite number of biochemicals and hormones. Obviously, if you have any medical conditions, your doctor will check your blood periodically, depending on the particular condition and its severity. However, even if you are well, you should probably have your cholesterol checked every five years. This test measures the biochemical that carries fat in your blood. A high cholesterol level increases your risk of heart disease, the leading killer of women today, and stroke. If your cholesterol level is elevated, exercise and dietary changes may be in order to lower it. Medications may also be used if you have a very high cholesterol level that is resistant to diet and exercise regimens.

What Else Can You Do for Your Health?

We all want to lead long, healthy lives and then die peacefully in our sleep when old but not yet declining. You and I both know that, at present, there are no ways to guarantee such an end for ourselves. But keeping our bodies strong and healthy is something that we do have some control over. People feel better, both mentally and physically, when their bodies are fit. But getting there is sometimes a struggle. We are blessed with a wealth of food in this country, but much of it is too high in fat, sugar, salt, and calories. We are also blessed with the finest health care services in the world, but some of us are unable or unwilling to use them.

I can only urge you to do the very best you possibly can for yourself. If you hate exercising, just make sure you walk around a bit. Even walking for thirty minutes a few times a week can be beneficial to your health. Pick up the pace if you're strolling through the mall or in your neighborhood. Take the stairs occasionally instead of the elevator. Lift some one- or three-pound weights while watching your favorite television program. Every little bit helps, and once you get started you may find that you actually enjoy the exercise.

If you smoke, try to stop. This is the most significant thing you can do for your health! In addition to its well-known effects—lung cancer, respiratory disease, and heart attacks—smoking increases your risk of cervical cancer (see page 224).

If you have trouble keeping the fat and calories to a minimum in your diet, begin with small steps toward healthier eating. Have fruits and vegetables with your meals each day. Switch to low-fat milk and cheeses. Try whole grains. Hold the mayo. There are many great foods out there that are healthy and truly delicious. We all can't look, eat, or work out like the latest celebrity with an exercise video. But we can do a little better for ourselves than we do now, and it wouldn't take that much effort. When the small changes in exercise and diet start to make a difference in the way you feel or look, you may do more. Don't strive for perfection, just strive for improvement.

While we know that there are limits to our control over our health, we can do our best to stay healthy. For a woman, a Pap smear, mammogram, and annual pelvic and breast examinations can go a long way toward gynecologic health. If you have questions or problems, be sure to get answers. Be informed. This book will provide you with the foundation to help you make decisions about your health. Use preventive health strategies and seek the best care possible when you need it. Here's to your good health!

REFERENCES

Love, Susan. 1990. *Dr. Susan Love's Breast Book.* [1995-Second Edition] Reading, Mass.: Addison-Wesley.

Morra, M., and E. Potts. 1994. *Choices: The New, Most Up-to-Date Sourcebook for Cancer Information.* New York: Avon.

National Institutes of Health. *What You Need to Know About Breast Cancer.* Call 1-800-4-CANCER [422-6237] for a free copy.

Bettman, O. 1956. *A Pictorial History of Medicine.* Springfield, Ill.: Charles C. Thomas.

Singer, C. 1962. *A Short History of Medicine.* Oxford: Oxford University Press.

2

IF YOU HAVE FIBROIDS

What Are Fibroids?

Fibroids are noncancerous (benign) growths of the muscle wall of the uterus. They are probably responsible for more unnecessary gynecologic surgery than any other condition. *Every year*, a staggering *600,000* American women have a hysterectomy. And about 30 percent of those hysterectomies, 180,000 in all, are performed because of fibroids. For many years these growths have been surgically removed, often because of fear of the problems they might cause in the future. Those problems are often overstated. While approximately 30 percent of all women will have fibroids during their lifetime, the vast majority of these women will *never* have symptoms and will *never* require treatment. And there are many sound and effective options available for the rare patient who does have a problem. Hysterectomy should be the solution of last resort.

What Causes Fibroids?

While there is much we don't know about fibroids, we do know that each individual fibroid starts from a single cell growing the wrong way. But, despite ongoing research, the reason why this one cell grows to cause a fibroid remains a mystery. Does something genetic prompt these individual cells to change? Are there environmental causes? We simply do not know. What we do know is that the female hormone estrogen is necessary for fibroid growth. Fibroids do not occur before puberty, when estrogen production begins, and if a woman has a fibroid, it will shrink after menopause, when estrogen production ceases. Recent evidence suggests that progesterone, the hormone produced for two weeks following ovulation, may also be necessary for the growth of fibroids. It appears that fibroids may start from a single cell mutation, but the growth of a fibroid requires the complex interaction of estrogen, progesterone, and cell growth factors.

Surprisingly, even though the body greatly increases estrogen production at puberty, fibroids usually do not develop until much later, generally between ages twenty-five and thirty-five. You might expect that women with fibroids are making too much estrogen, which causes the fibroids to grow. However, women with fibroids have *absolutely normal* amounts of estrogen in their blood. It appears that the muscle cells in the uterus undergo a change that causes them to use up, or *metabolize*, more of the estrogen in the blood than usual. As a result, the cells are stimulated to overgrow, causing a round swelling of the uterine muscular wall. Importantly, this change in the metabolism of estrogen does not appear to affect any other area of the body. Women with fibroids are not more prone to "fibrocystic" changes in the breast, a totally different and unrelated condition. And they are *not* more prone to develop any other benign or cancerous conditions.

Do Birth Control Pills Cause Fibroids?

At one time it was suspected that if a woman took birth control pills, she faced an increased risk of developing fibroids. Since the pills contain estrogen and progesterone, it made some sense that they might cause this problem. However, recent studies have convincingly shown that women who take birth control pills are no more likely to develop fibroids than women who have never taken the pill. Another study demonstrated that most women who already have fibroids can take the pill without any increased growth of the fibroids.

What Are the Different Types of Fibroids?

All fibroids begin as a growth somewhere within the uterine muscular wall. The symptoms caused by fibroids depend on where they grow in the wall (see fig. 2.1). Fibroids that grow and bulge toward the outside of the uterus, called *subserosal* fibroids, can press on the organs surrounding the uterus, such as the bladder or rectum. Sometimes, they may grow large enough to push outward and cause a noticeable swelling in the abdomen.

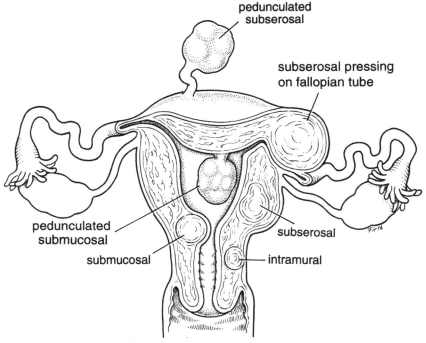

Fig. 2.1. Types of fibroids

Fibroids that grow and bulge toward the inside of the uterus are called *submucosal* fibroids. These grow directly below the lining cells of the uterus and may interfere with the cells that are shed during the menstrual period. As a result, submucosal fibroids may lead to heavy or irregular bleeding. Fibroids that stay mostly embedded within the middle of the wall of the uterus are called *intramural* fibroids. If they grow closer to the outside of the uterus, they can cause pressure, and if they grow closer to the inside, they can cause bleeding. Some fibroids may form on stalks that connect them to the uterus. These are called *pedunculated* fibroids and can be either submucosal or subserosal.

Can Fibroids Cause Bleeding Problems?

It is not uncommon for fibroids to cause an increase in the amount of menstrual bleeding. There are a number of theories as to why this happens. At the time of the menstrual period, when the uterine lining is shed, the inside of the uterus is raw and bleeding. The uterus has two basic ways to stop itself from bleeding. The first is the normal blood-clotting mechanism that works throughout the body by forming plugs in the blood vessels. However, because the uterus is a muscle, it also has the unique ability to contract and squeeze the bleeding vessels. Much like stepping on a hose, this action prevents more blood loss. These contractions are what you may feel as menstrual cramps. Now imagine the fibroid as a marble and picture the uterus filled with these marbles while it tries to contract. The fibroids don't allow the uterus to squeeze down properly, and it can't stop the flow of blood from the vessels. The blood vessels in the uterus stay open longer, and you lose more blood.

While heavy bleeding is most often associated with fibroids, bleeding between periods can also occur. Other medical conditions may cause heavy bleeding or bleeding between periods. For example, hormonal changes, polyps, overgrowth of the uterine lining, and, rarely, even precancer or cancer of the uterus can all result in abnormal bleeding. Therefore, any abnormal bleeding should be reported to your physician, and you should get a thorough examination.

When heavy menstrual bleeding persists over time, your body may not be able to make new blood cells fast enough to replace those that have been lost. In mild cases, this deficiency may be easy to correct by taking iron pills. But some women find iron pills difficult to tolerate because they can upset the stomach or cause constipation. The pills are less bothersome if taken with food. An increase in fluids and vegetables in the diet will alleviate the constipation. Some women with fibroids find that the bleeding is so severe that even iron pills cannot correct the problem, and anemia develops. Anemia results in weakness, fatigue, and, if severe, light-headedness. If you have these symptoms, treatment beyond iron pills is indicated.

Emily's Abnormal Bleeding and Myomectomy

Emily, a new patient to my practice, came bounding angrily into my office. Her regular gynecologist had recommended a hysterectomy for fibroids, but Emily was resistant to that idea. As far as she was concerned, her fibroids had taken too much time out of her life already. She was hoping for another solution and would only consider major surgery as a last resort. After she explained her circumstances to me, I understood more why she didn't want to lose anymore time. Emily, a forty-five-year-old mother of two grown children, had been injured in an automobile accident seven years before. The accident had been quite serious, and Emily had had to endure many months of pain and treatment. As part of her rehabilitation, she had begun to lift weights. She had never been the least bit athletic or even interested in fitness prior to this time. Much to her delight and to the shock of her family, Emily loved weight lifting and began to crave her daily workout. She found she loved to sweat and just loved the way this sport made her feel. From the original emphasis on rehabilitating her injured body, Emily began to train seriously. The "cuts" of her muscles became an enormous new source of pride and self-esteem for this full-time mother and homemaker. In her second year of bodybuilding Emily started competing at bodybuilding events.

For a year she had been having heavy and irregular bleeding. By the time she saw her gynecologist, she was changing menstrual pads every hour for four of the seven days of her period. The bleeding was sapping her strength; she was often exhausted. When her gynecologist diagnosed fibroids, he recommended a hysterectomy. Although she realized that a hysterectomy would provide a permanent solution to her problem, having to stop training for two months while recovering from major surgery wasn't acceptable. She came to my office seeking a second opinion.

After examining her, I noted that she had small fibroids, all together about the size of a lemon. Although she came to me requesting a laparoscopic hysterectomy (a hysterectomy done through small incisions with the aid of a small telescope), I also discussed other procedures that might alleviate her symptoms with even less risk and less time for recovery.

First, a simple procedure called hysteroscopy was performed in my office, which revealed a small fibroid protruding into the cavity of her uterus. Based on this information and Emily's desire for a rapid recovery, I recommended a procedure called hysteroscopic myomectomy and endometrial ablation (see pages 51 and 78). I performed the procedure on Emily as an outpatient in the hospital. I inserted a small telescope through Emily's vagina into her uterus, and the fibroid was removed without any incisions. I also removed the lining cells of the uterus so that her periods would decrease or stop altogether. Emily spent less than four hours in the hospital. She was back lifting weights in two days and was able to successfully compete in her next bodybuilding competition.

Can Fibroids Cause Pain or Pressure?

Your uterus lies below the pubic bone, well down in the pelvis (see fig. 1.1 on page 3). It is just under the bladder, just above the rectum, and surrounded by the intestines. Since it is so near to these organs, growth of the uterus from fibroids may cause pressure or, rarely, pain in the pelvis. The normal uterus is about the size of a small pear and weighs less than one-quarter pound. With fibroids, the uterus may enlarge to the size of a small watermelon and weigh one or two pounds or more. Just the change in the size and weight of the uterus can cause an awareness of fullness or pressure that was previously not apparent. If the fibroids grow toward your back, pressure on your rectum can cause constipation (see fig. 2.2). You may also feel pressure or pain in the lower back or discomfort with activity or intercourse.

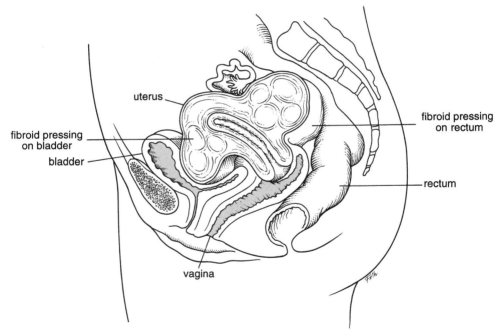

Fig. 2.2.   Fibroids may cause pressure

If the uterus grows as large as a cantaloupe, it may be seen as a noticeable swelling in the lower abdomen, perhaps even making a woman appear pregnant. While not dangerous, the enlarged uterus may cause enough discomfort or enough visible change to warrant treatment.

Sybil's Abdominal Pressure

Sybil is a forty-two-year-old woman who has been coming to my office for routine gynecologic care for about ten years. She had no health problems until two years ago when I noted that her uterus was beginning to enlarge from fibroids. The enlargement was only moderate; her uterus was then the size of a large apple. Since she was feeling well, no treatment was needed, and I examined her every four months in order to keep track of the fibroids.

Sybil's fibroids continued to slowly enlarge, which is unusual and not at all what we had hoped for. Sybil assumed she was just putting on weight, and had to switch to long overblouses and pants with elastic waists. At the time of her next scheduled exam, she looked about five months pregnant. I could feel the fibroids reaching up to her navel. She was increasingly uncomfortable from the pressure of the fibroids on her bladder and back.

The combination of discomfort, change in her appearance, and fear about just how big these fibroids were getting galvanized Sybil's desire to begin some kind of treatment. But she was reluctant to have surgery. Sybil was fearful of anesthesia and had long ago promised herself to have surgery only if her life depended on it. While she hated her current condition, we both knew that her life was in no danger.

We discussed the possibility of using medication, Lupron or Synarel (see page 36), to temporarily shrink the fibroids, relieve her symptoms, and allow her time to consider surgery. She agreed and about six weeks after beginning the medication, she felt a decrease in the pressure in her abdomen. When examined, her uterus was clearly shrinking. After three months, her uterus was about half the size it had been, and her symptoms of pressure and discomfort disappeared. Although bothered by the common side effects of hot flashes and insomnia that the medication often causes, Sybil felt much better, and her negative feelings about surgery resurfaced. She asked if we could put off her surgery for a while, allowing her time to come to grips with an operation.

I agreed and we began to give Sybil low doses of estrogen and progesterone pills to protect her from osteoporosis. Lupron temporarily turns off the ovaries so that no estrogen is produced. Since estrogen is needed to help absorb calcium from the diet, prolonged use of the medication will lead to osteoporosis. Therefore, estrogen in small doses can help prevent this bone loss.

Unfortunately, after about six months on this combination of medication and estrogen, her uterus began to grow again. At this point, we had tried the simple solutions and had failed. She now wanted to have surgery. We planned to perform a myomectomy, removing just the fibroid. But because of the large size of the fibroid, we also needed to discuss the possibility of a hysterectomy.

I told her I would make every effort to avoid hysterectomy unless the fibroids had replaced so much of the healthy muscle that little remained to reconstruct into a functioning uterus. We also spent a great deal of time talking about anesthesia, which had been so frightening to her. We arranged for her to meet her anesthesiologist prior to surgery for reassurance about the minimal risk and her likelihood of a safe surgery.

At the time of the operation, we found a single large subserosal fibroid. We were able to remove the fibroid and easily reconstruct her uterus. In the recovery room, Sybil was able to smile in relief; her fibroid was gone, and her worst fears had not come true. At her six-week postoperative visit, the pressure, discomfort, and "pregnant" appearance were gone, and she felt like herself again.

Can Fibroids Cause Sudden Pain?

As living tissue, fibroids need blood and oxygen to survive. If a fibroid grows quickly, blood vessels feeding it may not be able to grow fast enough to supply the new tissue with enough blood and oxygen to keep it alive. If this happens, the fibroid undergoes a process called *degeneration*, or cell death. As the cells in the fibroid die, chemical substances are released that cause pain and swelling in the uterus. This pain may be severe but usually is not associated with any serious problems. If these chemicals reach the bloodstream, they may cause a low fever. As some of the fibroid dies, the blood supply to the rest of it will be enough to keep it alive and healthy. At this point, the pain will go away. When a woman with fibroids develops pain, examination by a physician is important to help figure out the source of the problem. If you have a degenerating fibroid, a heating pad on your abdomen will be comforting, and pain medication should provide relief for a few days until the pain naturally begins to subside.

In rare instances, a *pedunculated fibroid* can twist around on its stalk so that *no* blood can get through the stalk to the fibroid. If that happens, the *entire* fibroid begins to die, and the pain becomes very severe. Surgery is usually necessary to remove the dying tissue.

Can Fibroids Cause Urinary Problems?

The uterus lies directly behind the bladder, and they are partially attached at one point. If a fibroid begins to grow forward, it may squeeze the bladder so that it cannot fill properly with urine (see fig. 2.2). You may notice that your bladder often feels full and you need to urinate more often. When you laugh, cough, or sneeze, the fibroid may push against the bladder and cause you to lose urine. This is called *stress incontinence*. While this may be only a minor inconvenience for some women with fibroids, others may be so bothered by the incontinence that they limit their activity to avoid embarrassment. There are other causes of incontinence, so it's important to get a careful examination (see chapter 5). A number of treatments other than surgery are available for many of the causes of incontinence. Stress incontinence is not something you "just have to live with."

Denise's Frequent Urination

Denise is a forty-year-old woman who had a myomectomy three years before being seen in our office. New fibroids had recently grown, and she noticed that she needed to urinate all the time. She had been advised to have a hysterectomy and came to us requesting a second opinion. Denise could no longer sit through a two-hour movie and sometimes had to leave the theater twice to go to the bathroom. At work, she was frequently getting up from her desk and felt that these trips to the bathroom were breaking her concentration and making her less productive.

A pelvic examination revealed a four-inch fibroid on the outside of her uterus (subserosal), pushing right against the bladder. We discussed her options, which included follow-up with frequent exams, myomectomy, and hysterectomy as a last resort. After a full discussion of all of her options, she chose to be followed closely with frequent pelvic exams. Denise also began to see a homeopathic doctor and began homeopathic remedies for her fibroids.

The fibroid remained unchanged for a year and a half, but then on her routine exam it was noted to have grown to about five inches, and a new three-inch fibroid was also felt. She was beginning to feel more unhappy about the frequent trips to the bathroom, feeling that they were part of the reason why she was passed over for a promotion at work. Her homeopathic physician could offer nothing new. Denise was glad she had given homeopathy a chance, but at this point, frustrated with her symptoms, she requested surgery. She knew that she did not want children and certainly did not want to have surgery for fibroids again. She felt the time had come for a hysterectomy. The surgery went well, and she has no regrets. She feels that she gave her body every opportunity to get better and that finally surgery had been necessary.

Can Fibroids Cause Infertility?

Fibroids are *not* usually a cause of infertility. In a published study of infertility patients, only 9 percent of these women had fibroids as the sole cause of their infertility. In order to cause infertility, the fibroids must be near the opening of the fallopian tubes and actually block the passage of the egg as it enters the uterus. Both tubes must be obstructed, since only one open tube is needed for pregnancy to occur.

Can Fibroids Cause Miscarriage?

Fibroids rarely cause repeated miscarriages. The fertilized egg comes down the tube and takes hold in the lining of the uterus. If a submucosal fibroid happens to be nearby, it often thins out the lining and decreases the blood supply to the developing embryo. The fetus cannot develop properly, and miscarriage may result. However, it is very unlikely that the egg will settle in exactly the same location for the next pregnancy. Therefore, it is unusual for fibroids to cause repeated miscarriages. Only fibroids that are within the uterine cavity and have been associated with two or more miscarriages should be considered for removal.

Sara's Miscarriages

Sara is a thirty-two-year-old woman who had been trying to have a baby but had had two miscarriages in the past year. She also realized that her periods were getting heavier. Her gynecologist had performed a number of tests and had been reassuring, but a recent ultrasound had shown a small fibroid. I recommended that a hysteroscopy be performed to see if the fibroid was in the uterine cavity and perhaps responsible for her problems. The hysteroscopy revealed a small submucosal fibroid that was bulging into the uterine cavity. Because of her history of repeated miscarriages and abnormal bleeding, removal of the fibroid seemed indicated. Sara was admitted to the hospital, and a hysteroscopic resection of the fibroid (see page 51) was performed without any difficulty. She left the hospital a few hours later and was back to work in two days. The outcome was excellent: Sara got pregnant four months after surgery and had a healthy baby boy.

Can Fibroids Cause Problems During Pregnancy?

The vast majority of women who are pregnant and have fibroids encounter no problems. They have full-term, healthy babies without difficulty. Fibroids most often occur in women in their late thirties and forties, at a time when many women have already completed their families. As a result, fibroids are present in only about 3 percent of all pregnancies.

During pregnancy, large amounts of estrogen are made by the placenta. These high levels of estrogen often will cause any fibroids already present to grow larger. If the fibroids grow too quickly, the blood vessels supplying them may not be able to get enough oxygen to the tissue, and the fibroid cells will die. This process of degeneration usually resolves itself in a few days without treatment, just as it does in nonpregnant women, and without harm to the baby. Some women may have mild contractions during this time, but it is extremely rare for premature labor to actually begin. However, a pregnant woman with fibroids *must* see her physician if she experiences pain or contractions in order to make sure everything is all right. Bedrest, heat, and pain medication will usually be prescribed, and medications to inhibit premature labor may sometimes be needed.

Do Fibroids Mean You Need a Cesarean Section?

Rarely, a fibroid may grow in the lowest portion of the uterus, near the cervix, during the pregnancy. In this position, the fibroid may get in the way and prevent the baby from coming through the birth canal. This problem is not dangerous for the baby and can often be diagnosed by a sonogram before labor begins. Sometimes this problem is discovered during labor, because the baby does not come down the birth canal. A cesarean section is performed, and the fibroid is seen in the birth canal when the baby is delivered. Because of the large amount of blood supplying the uterus during pregnancy, removal of a fibroid at the time of a cesarean section is associated with excessive blood loss and is not recommended. What I have just described is actually unusual. Most women with fibroids deliver their babies without any problems.

Do Growing Fibroids Mean Cancer?

Fibroids, by definition, are *benign* uterine growths. However, a *leiomyosarcoma*, an extremely rare form of malignant tumor of the uterine muscle, also causes enlargement of the uterus. But only two out of every thousand women admitted to a hospital for surgery because of fibroids will be found to have a sarcoma. And since 80 percent of women with fibroids are never admitted to a hospital for surgery, the incidence of sarcoma in all women with fibroids is extraordinarily low. The average age of women who develop fibroids is thirty-eight. And although sarcoma can occur in young women, the average age of a woman who develops a sarcoma is fifty-eight. So, if you have fibroids, there is not much reason to worry about sarcoma.

Most gynecologic textbooks teach physicians that if a woman has a rapidly growing uterus, she should have surgery to determine whether she has a uterine sarcoma. Surgery is needed to remove tissue for microscopic analysis, since no other available tests can make the diagnosis of sarcoma. However, during the course of my training and years in practice, I have never seen a "rapidly growing fibroid" actually turn out to be a sarcoma. And, when I review all the medical information available on this subject, it appears that while this statement about rapid growth and sarcoma is often made, there is no evidence to support it.

Although often presented as fact, the science and art of medicine includes both carefully studied principles and other assumptions based on unstudied observation. Unfortunately, the enormous amount of information absorbed during medical education often blurs the lines between fact and assumption. This appears to have been the case with sarcomas. Gynecologists have assumed that rapid growth means sarcoma, but that fact has never been proved.

In order to look into this assumption, I began a clinical study at the two hospitals where I practice. I reviewed the charts of 1,330 women admitted for surgery because of uterine fibroids. Interestingly, only three women (0.2 percent) were found to have a sarcoma. In addition, of the

370 patients admitted because of rapidly growing fibroids, only one (0.2 percent) had a sarcoma. This study showed that the risk of developing a sarcoma is extremely low, even if your fibroids are rapidly growing.

If you have a growing fibroid, it is perfectly reasonable to have a pelvic examination every one to three months. If the fibroid begins to cause bothersome symptoms, then surgery may be considered. If the fibroid continues to grow very rapidly, doubling in size in a few weeks or months, then surgery may be indicated. However, because of the rarity of sarcomas (especially in women younger than fifty), we found no justification for assuming that growth in a fibroid means that cancer is developing; therefore, surgery is not usually indicated.

If you are a woman in her fifties or sixties, the issue of growth of fibroids is a little different. Published reports show that sarcomas most often occur in women in their fifties and sixties. If you are *postmenopausal* and *not* on estrogen replacement therapy, your body will lack the estrogen that fibroids need for growth; therefore, any growth in your uterus is cause for concern. Since there are no tests at the present time that can diagnose sarcoma, surgery is needed to remove the growing fibroid. A microscopic examination can then be done by a pathologist to conclusively show if cancer is present.

Interestingly, in our study, we found that in the small number of postmenopausal women who were taking estrogen and were noted to have growing fibroids, none was found to have a sarcoma. A reasonable option for these women would be to discontinue taking estrogen and see if the uterus shrinks back to its previous size. If the fibroid does shrink (because estrogen is no longer present), then you would need to consider the following options. You could stay off estrogen and avoid surgery. Or, if estrogen is necessary for bothersome menopausal symptoms or because of your risk for heart disease or osteoporosis, you can restart the estrogen with the knowledge that surgery will probably be necessary if the fibroids grow again. If you stop taking estrogen and your uterus does not shrink, or especially if it continues to grow, then surgery should be performed because of the possibility of uterine sarcoma.

Laura's Fibroids Grow Rapidly

Laura is a twenty-four-year-old single woman who saw her gynecologist because of a feeling of pressure and discomfort in her lower abdomen. Her mother had been assuring her that her symptoms were "just gas" and were caused by her fast-food diet.

Laura had tried changing her eating habits, but the symptoms remained. She fearfully realized that what she was feeling in no way resembled the sensation of gas, and it was time to see her family doctor.

On examination she was noted to have a very enlarged uterus, the size of a large grapefruit. This concerned her doctor because her uterus had felt normal during her last examination one year ago. The doctor questioned whether this rapid growth might represent cancer of the uterine muscle and suggested that immediate exploratory surgery was necessary. Laura was referred to me by her family physician, and at the time she was very anxious about the rapid change in her body and the possibility of cancer. Laura's mother accompanied her to the office, feeling extremely anxious and guilty about the advice she had given her daughter.

After the examination, we discussed the *extremely rare* possibility of Laura having cancer. Most patients with a rapidly growing uterus have benign fibroids, and most patients with sarcoma are fifty to sixty years old. I felt Laura had two options: close observation or surgery. Observation would require frequent pelvic examinations, perhaps every month, until we were certain there was no further growth. Following that, exams every three months would be recommended to monitor any change in symptoms or growth of the uterus. If further growth was noted, we would reconsider surgery.

Laura was so worried she requested immediate surgery. The goal of surgery would be the removal of the fibroid (myomectomy) and repair of the uterus. A hysterectomy would be performed only if obvious cancer was found. At surgery, a bikini incision was made, and we found what appeared to be a benign fibroid. We removed the fibroid and repaired the uterus without difficulty. The next day the pathology report came back disclosing a benign fibroid and no evidence of cancer. Laura was greatly relieved and then recovered without problems. She and her mother came for her follow-up visit feeling very grateful for Laura's good health.

What If You Have Large Fibroids?

Gynecologists are often taught that a uterus enlarged because of bulky fibroids should always be removed. Doctors measure the size of a uterus containing fibroids by comparing it to the size of a pregnant uterus, according to the number of weeks of pregnancy. Uterine size is often expressed by comparing it to common items such as fruits. Talking about fibroids in relation to lemons and grapefruits, while not exactly scientific, helps doctor and patient to visualize their size more easily.

Doctors have been taught that if a woman was walking around with fibroids about the size of a large grapefruit (or a twelve-week pregnant uterus), she would be at risk for other health problems; even if she felt perfectly fine, eventually she would begin to feel discomfort because of her large fibroids. This reason—the future possibility of problems—simply does not make sense to me. If you have a large fibroid and you are feeling fine, I see no need to undergo surgery. It is actually likely that your large fibroid will never cause you any bothersome symptoms.

Doctors also feel that large fibroids make it difficult for them to perform a thorough pelvic examination. In chapter 1 it was noted that a pelvic exam is done so that the doctor can feel for the size, texture, and presence of any abnormalities of the ovaries, fallopian tubes, and uterus. A large fibroid can get in the way, and doctors fear that a less-than-optimum pelvic examination can result in missing an early diagnosis of ovarian cancer.

Unfortunately, ovarian cancer is extremely difficult to diagnose in the early stages, even with the most sophisticated and expensive testing, whether or not fibroids are present (see chapter 8). This is a frustrating and difficult reality for physicians. Usually, by the time a gynecologist can feel an abnormality on exam, the disease has already spread. And, unfortunately, no study has ever shown that removal of a uterus enlarged with fibroids will make any difference in the early detection of ovarian cancer.

Another argument proposed for the aggressive removal of a fibroid uterus is that the ability to detect leiomyosarcoma, a rare cancer of the muscle wall of the uterus (see page 30), is difficult if the uterus is too large. The risk of sarcoma among patients with fibroids is extremely low (0.23 percent); therefore, justifying surgery for everyone on this basis doesn't make any sense.

Another argument for aggressive surgery is the belief that the risks and complications of surgery are greater if the surgery is delayed and the uterus grows larger. Based on my fifteen years of performing these surgeries and discussions with my colleagues, it is my observation that the risks and complications for a woman with a large uterus who has a hysterectomy are not greater. As shown in a recent study by Dr. Robert Reiter of the University of Iowa, College of Medicine, the complication rate for women who have hysterectomies for large fibroids is no different from that for women with small fibroids.

Surgery is reasonable only if you have symptoms that truly warrant the risk, time, stress, and cost that an operation entails. Remember, *most patients with uterine fibroids need no treatment.* If you have fibroids, the odds are you will not need to do anything about them.

Can My Fibroids Just Be Watched?

Although 30 percent of all women will have fibroids during their lifetime, only a small number of them will ever need treatment. The vast majority of women with fibroids are unaware of them until their doctor feels them at the time of a routine exam. Some women have very minor symptoms, which are not bothersome. If that is the case for you, then no treatment is necessary. I consider careful observation to be the primary treatment option.

The cause of the growth of fibroids is not well understood, and their rate of growth is unpredictable. Most fibroids never grow; others grow gradually over the course of many years; and some seem to go through growth spurts and then may stop growing altogether. The only way to know what is happening is to have a regular pelvic examination. I usually examine women with fibroids every three to six months. If the fibroid grows during that period, the growth will be discovered early, and a number of options, short of hysterectomy, should still be available. If the fibroid seems to be growing, I usually do exams more frequently, generally every month, until the growth stops. Ultrasonography, a simple test that uses sound waves to make a picture, may also be used to determine the size of the fibroids. Although expensive, it is an accurate way to measure both the number and the size of the fibroids present, and is sometimes necessary to give your doctor more information about the fibroids and your uterus.

On the other hand, some fibroids may grow large enough to cause constant discomfort, pressure, and even pain (see page 32). The discomfort, though not dangerous, may lead you to choose surgery as a treatment for fibroids.

TREATMENT FOR UTERINE FIBROIDS

What Are the Treatment Options for Fibroids?

If you need treatment for fibroids, there are a number of options available to you. The choices regarding treatment of uterine fibroids are guided by the medical problems the fibroids are causing, your desire to have children, and your feelings and thoughts about surgery. I think it is helpful for you to know all of the options available. At the time of the consultation, I usually begin with an overview of all the treatment options. Even if some of the treatments do not apply at the current time, your condition or symptoms may change. If you understand the potential for future symptoms and problems, as well as the alternative means of treatment available, much of the mystery of fibroids will disappear. Once the unknown is discussed, some of your anxiety will diminish. Fibroids almost never need urgent or immediate treatment. For the vast majority of women, there is plenty of time for careful thought and planning.

Can You Take Medication for Fibroids?

A variety of medications have been used in an attempt to treat the symptom of fibroids. Unfortunately, there are no medications that *prevent* the formation of fibroids or *permanently* shrink them once they are present. Medications are used to buy time or reduce symptoms. For some women, a reduction in discomfort is enough to indefinitely postpone surgery. Medications allow some women to take their time to prepare emotionally and physically for an inevitable surgery. By temporarily reducing the size of the fibroids enough to allow for a less invasive surgery, medications can promote a quicker recovery. For some women who are approaching menopause, this extra time may lead them right into menopause, when the natural loss of estrogen shrinks the fibroids. Once again, hysterectomy is the choice of last resort.

Are There Any New Medications for Fibroids?

In the mid-1980s a number of new medications were developed based on the hormone that regulates the menstrual cycle. The hormone, produced in the brain, is called GnRH, short for *Gon*adotropin-*R*eleasing *H*ormone. By slightly altering parts of this hormone and by changing the length of time it could last in the bloodstream, scientists were able to completely change the effect of the hormone on the menstrual cycle. Usually, the release of this hormone in the brain causes the cyclic release of estrogen and progesterone from the ovaries. These cyclic hormonal changes then lead to the monthly menstrual period. But the new medications work by *temporarily* shutting off the ovaries' ability to make estrogen and progesterone, and menstrual periods temporarily cease. Since estrogen and probably progesterone are also necessary for fibroids to grow, the lack of hormones causes fibroids to shrink.

Lupron and Synarel are two of the GnRH–based medications most often used to shrink fibroids. Because these medications are destroyed by the fluids in the stomach, they must be taken in a nonpill form. Lupron is given by injection and works for an entire month. Synarel is administered by nasal spray. The nasal spray, used twice a day, coats the thin nasal tissue with medication, and it is absorbed directly by the blood vessels. The advantage of the nasal spray is convenience: The patient can give herself the medication and avoid the extra trips to the doctor for injections. Lupron's advantage is that it is administered only once a month. Their effectiveness is virtually identical, so the choice of medication should be up to the patient.

In about two weeks the medications begin to shrink the fibroids, and the full effect is seen after three months. Most fibroids will decrease in size by about 50 percent of their volume. The shrinking effect is maintained for as long as you use the medication, but there is rarely any further shrinkage after the third month of treatment. Unfortunately, if the medication is stopped, the ovaries begin to produce hormones again and the fibroids return to their original size within three months. The medication has no permanent effect and is primarily used to reduce symptoms and provide time to plan surgery. In addition, long-term use of these medications is limited by their side effects.

What Are the Side Effects of Lupron and Synarel?

Like most medications, Lupron and Synarel cause side effects. Your brain needs estrogen to regulate your body temperature. Since the medications stop the ovaries' production of estrogen, minor temperature changes can occur that you feel as hot flashes, which may be bothersome during the day and may disturb your sleep. The lack of restful sleep can lead to irritability or mood changes. One of my patients told me that Lupron affected her husband as much as it did her; her restless nights kept him sleep-deprived as well. Progesterone pills taken at the same time can help the hot flashes and promote more restful sleep. However, their use during the first three months of therapy prevents the shrinkage of the fibroids. If you are planning to be on Lupron or Synarel for longer than three months, low doses of progesterone can be added after the fibroids have shrunk. Another medication, Bellergal, may also relieve hot flashes. It has a mild sedative effect on some women, but if used before bedtime it often helps you get a good night's sleep.

The lack of estrogen may also cause a decrease in normal vaginal secretions, leading to vaginal dryness and discomfort during intercourse. Infrequently, patients experience headaches when using these medications. Some women using Synarel have reported nasal irritation that may cause them to discontinue the medication. You may experience an initial episode of menstrual bleeding two weeks after you start the medication. Following that, periods should cease until after you stop the medication. When you discontinue the medication, periods resume within a few weeks. These medications have absolutely no effect on a woman's fertility. In fact, they are also used to treat some infertility patients in order to enhance the effectiveness of fertility drugs.

The maximum benefit from Synarel or Lupron occurs after three months' use, and surgery is usually scheduled at that time. If these medications are used alone for longer than six months, the resulting low levels of estrogen may prevent your body from absorbing calcium from the foods you eat. Prolonged use may put you at risk for developing osteoporosis, or thinning of the bones.

Osteoporosis can be a serious problem, and research efforts are under way to prevent the side effects that may result from prolonged use of these medications. Recent studies have shown that after the initial shrinking of the fibroids, you may take small doses of estrogen and progesterone while you continue to use Lupron or Synarel. Remember, these medications stop the normal supply of estrogen from the ovaries that is necessary for the growth of fibroids. But a small dose of estrogen, the same dose used for postmenopausal women, seems to be too low to allow the fibroids to flourish. And these small doses of estrogen are enough to prevent the development of osteoporosis. Perhaps there will come a time when a medication is developed that permanently shrinks fibroids, but none is on the horizon.

Another disadvantage of using these medications is cost: nearly $300 per month for Lupron or Synarel. The dose of Lupron needed to shrink fibroids is half of that contained in one bottle, so to control the expense, we split a bottle of Lupron between two patients. Once opened, the medication needs to be used within twenty-four hours or it becomes inactive. It takes a fair amount of time for our nurses to coordinate two women on the same schedule, but the savings for the patient are worth the effort.

Here's what to expect when taking Lupron or Synarel: mild hot flashes that can disrupt sleep; moderate bleeding within a few weeks after beginning the medication, which is generally not heavy and lasts less than a week; cessation of menstrual periods; about 50 percent shrinkage of fibroids at the end of three months. Fortunately, the medication is given for only a few months, so most women can tolerate the side effects fairly well during this relatively short period of time.

When Should Lupron or Synarel Be Used?

Lupron or Synarel is most often used prior to anticipated surgery. For women who have experienced heavy bleeding because of fibroids, cessation of the bleeding that results from taking the medication is a major benefit. It allows you to rebuild your blood supply and regain energy and strength prior to surgery. When your blood count returns to normal, you can then donate your own blood, which will be frozen and used if a transfusion is necessary (*autologous blood*) after surgery.

After the fibroids decrease in size, it may sometimes be feasible to remove the fibroids by laparoscopic surgery, with a few small incisions (see page 42). A few studies have shown that the use of these medications reduces blood loss from surgery. However, the need for blood transfusions is no lower in women treated with Lupron or Synarel so that the decrease in blood loss may not be significant.

A woman with fibroids who is approaching menopause can use Lupron or Synarel until menopause begins. Then the natural supply of estrogen will cease, and the fibroids will remain small without any medication. However, because the exact age of natural menopause is unpredictable, this treatment can turn into an expensive proposition— $2,000 per year—and usually is not covered by medical insurance.

What About Danocrine?

Danocrine was once the treatment of choice to reduce fibroid size. But since the development of Lupron and Synarel, I no longer use Danocrine in my practice. Danocrine may cause a great deal of unpleasant side effects. If your doctor has suggested treatment with Danocrine, please consider the following information.

Danocrine (danazol) is a hormonal medication derived from the male hormone testosterone. It stops the process of ovulation, which results in very low levels of estrogen, and menstruation ceases. Danocrine also works on a cellular level to inhibit the action of estrogen, so abnormal bleeding, one of the major problems caused by fibroids, can be effectively treated with Danocrine. However, shrinkage of fibroids with Danocrine has not been well documented, and the drug causes a number of male hormone side effects that may be bothersome and/or unacceptable to many women. Weight gain, bloating, oily skin, acne, mood changes, and facial hair growth can all occur. Because of these side effects, I do not prescribe Danocrine.

Can Progesterone Be Used to Treat Fibroids?

Progesterone was one of the first medications used to treat women who developed symptoms from fibroids. In certain areas of the body progesterone has the opposite effect of estrogen. Since estrogen makes fibroids grow, it only seemed reasonable that progesterone would make fibroids shrink. Unfortunately, this does not happen, and recent studies have found that progesterone may increase the growth of fibroids. In addition, progesterone has a number of bothersome side effects. It can cause emotional changes or even depression, which abate after the medication is stopped. Mild water retention is another side effect that disappears after the medication is finished. Although not effective for shrinking fibroids, progesterone's thinning effect on the lining cells of the uterus may decrease vaginal bleeding. However, I do not prescribe progesterone for treating fibroids because of its possible detrimental growth effect.

Are Holistic Remedies Effective for Treating Fibroids?

After practicing medicine for eighteen years, it is apparent to me that Western medicine does not have all the answers. A number of my patients have tried holistic therapy for fibroids while under my observation. My overall impression has been that these remedies have not been effective. The growth of fibroids is unpredictable, often ceasing even when no treatment has been given. Therefore, claims that holistic remedies have been successful may be no more than coincidence. The only way we have of assessing the value of a treatment is to give a large number of women one treatment and another large group no treatment and compare the results. If the group of people given the treatment does better, then the therapy is felt to have some value. Unfortunately, holistic practitioners have not performed scientific studies to determine the effectiveness of their therapy.

On the other hand, what really matters is how *you* feel after treatment. Therefore, I am comfortable with patients seeking alternative remedies for fibroids. A number of my patients have tried vegetarian diets, eliminating meat that might contain estrogen used in animal feed.

Others have tried various vitamin supplements. Although none of these remedies or diets has been shown to be effective, I have never seen a patient harmed by these treatments. I do feel it's important for a woman exploring holistic alternatives to be closely monitored by a physician, so that any change in the fibroids or symptoms can be evaluated.

Do You Need Surgery for Fibroids?

There are three main reasons why surgery may be required for fibroids: uncontrollable bleeding, a concern that the fibroids may be causing kidney damage, or a concern that cancer might be present.

What If You Have Uncontrollable Bleeding?

Surgery is indicated if you experience heavy, persistent bleeding that leads to severe anemia. Anemia can lead to chronic exhaustion and light-headedness and will eventually lower your body's resistance. We can measure the amount of blood that you have in your body by two tests: the hemoglobin and hematocrit. The hemoglobin is a measure of the weight of the number of molecules present in the blood that carry oxygen. Normal amounts are about 12 to 14 grams per liter (quart) of blood. The blood is made up of many components, but the two largest components are the fluid that carried the blood cells, the *plasma*, and the red blood cells that carry oxygen. The normal percentage of red blood cells in the blood is about 40 percent; 60 percent of the blood is plasma. The *hematocrit* measures the percentage of the blood that is red blood cells, and high numbers are best.

If your fibroids cause heavy bleeding and if your hemoglobin is less than 10 grams (or your hematocrit is less than 30 percent), you have a fairly significant anemia and probably will need treatment. Resectoscope myomectomy and/or endometrial ablation are very effective for most patients with this problem (see pages 51 and 78). Other women may choose to have a myomectomy (see page 42), and others with severe or unrelenting symptoms may choose to have a hysterectomy.

What If You Are at Risk for Kidney Damage?

Another indication for surgery for fibroids relates to your kidneys. The ureters are thin tubes that connect the kidneys (which are below the shoulder blades) to the bladder, which is in front of the uterus. In the pelvis, the ureters are about one-half inch away from the uterus. In some women, fibroids may grow sideways and press against the ureters, slow-ing or stopping the flow of urine out of the kidney. If urine cannot flow freely from the kidney, pressure builds up. This pressure damages the cells that clean the blood of impurities and can be dangerous. This process is slow and usually produces no symptoms. It is also *extremely rare*. If you are being closely followed by a physician, it is very unlikely that any damage will occur to your kidneys. On examination, a doctor can feel if the fibroids are too near the ureters. Some action would then be recommended before the slow process of damage to the kidneys begins.

Blockage of the ureter can be detected by an X ray called an *intravenous pyelogram*, or *IVP*. During this X ray, a special iodine dye is injected into a vein of the arm. The dye then collects in the kidneys and flows down the ureters. The X ray shows the path of the dye, and abnormalities of the kidneys or ureters can be detected. In eighteen years of practice, I have never seen a woman suffer kidney damage from fibroids. Surgery is indicated if the IVP shows a risk to the kidneys. Either myomectomy or hysterectomy can reestablish the normal flow of urine and prevent permanent damage to a vital organ.

What If There Is Concern That the Fibroids Might Be Cancer?

As discussed on page 30, surgery is often performed when a woman is found to have rapidly growing fibroids because of the fear of cancer. However, uterine sarcoma is extremely rare, occurring in less than two patients per thousand who have surgery for fibroids. And since 80 percent of women with fibroids never even have surgery, the incidence of this cancer is extraordinarily low. Most patients determined to have sarcomas are postmenopausal women in their fifties and sixties, whereas most patients with fibroids are in their thirties and forties. Virtually all premenopausal women with growing fibroids have benign uterine fibroids. Therefore, most patients with rapidly growing fibroids may be followed with frequent pelvic examinations. However, if you are postmenopausal and do not take estrogen, any growth of the uterus is an indication for surgery.

TYPES OF SURGERY FOR FIBROIDS

What Is a Myomectomy?

Myomectomy is the surgical removal of just the fibroid, with reconstruction and repair of the uterus. Through an abdominal incision, a vaginal excision, a laparoscopy, and a hysteroscopy are the ways a myomectomy may be performed. These procedures are described in the following sections. General considerations regarding surgery are discussed in chapter 12.

What Is an Abdominal Myomectomy?

First performed about ninety years ago, abdominal myomectomy is excellent for women who wish to maintain their ability to have children, or who just prefer to avoid removal of the uterus. The standard method of performing a myomectomy is by *laparotomy*: A four-to-six-inch "bikini" incision is made just below the pubic hair line. The intestines and bladder are pushed out of the way so that the uterus can be seen in the pelvic cavity.

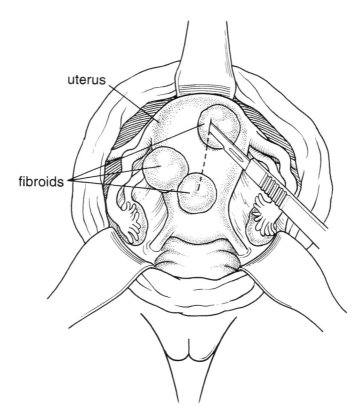

Fig. 2.3a.   Abdominal myomectomy: incision in the uterus

After inspection to determine the number and position of the fibroids, the uterus is injected with pitressin, a solution that slows bleeding during the surgery. The covering of the uterus overlying the fibroids is then cut, and the fibroids are separated from the normal uterine muscle. The remaining normal uterine muscle is then sewn back together (see fig. 2.3a–c). This procedure takes about one to two hours depending on the number and position of the fibroids. The intestines often take a few days to recover from all the pushing and irritation. Eating too soon after surgery can lead to nausea and vomiting. For this reason, and because of the moderate discomfort associated with the incision, a woman who has an abdominal myomectomy may need to stay in the hospital for three to four days.

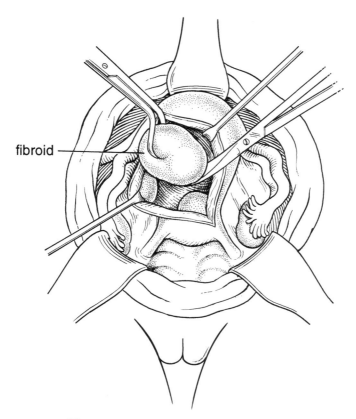

fibroid

Fig. 2.3b.   Removing the fibroids

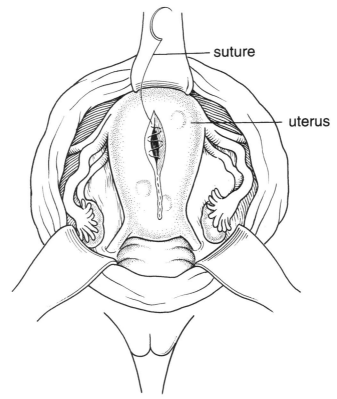

Fig. 2.3c. Repairing the uterus

What Is a Laparoscopic Myomectomy?

Laparoscopic myomectomy is another way to surgically remove fibroids. This method was developed in the early 1980s by Dr. Kurt Semm in Kiel, Germany. Laparoscopic surgery is usually performed as outpatient surgery under general anesthesia. It has revolutionized gynecologic surgery because of the short hospital stay and quick recovery. The technique continues to evolve as new instruments are developed. Because of the small size of the incisions and the level of surgical skill required, this procedure is actually harder for a physician to perform than abdominal myomectomy.

The laparoscope is a slender telescope that is inserted through the navel to view the pelvic and abdominal organs. Two or three small, half-inch incisions are made below the pubic hair line. Instruments are passed through these small incisions to perform the surgery. For laparoscopic myomectomy, a small scissors or a laser is used to open the thin covering of the uterus. The fibroid is found underneath this covering, grasped, and freed from its attachments to the normal uterine muscle (see fig. 2.4). The deeper the fibroid is embedded within the muscle wall of the uterus, the more difficult the procedure.

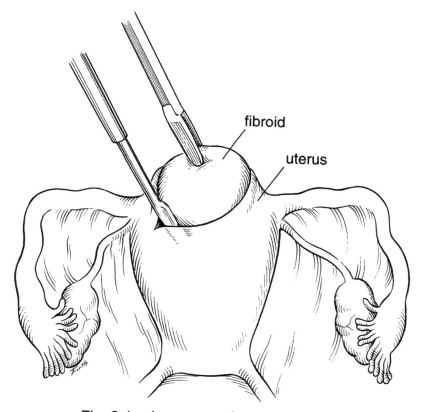

Fig. 2.4.   Laparoscopic myomectomy

After the fibroid is separated from the uterus, it must be removed from the abdominal cavity. The fibroid is cut into small pieces (*morcellation*), and the pieces are removed through the small incisions. This process is time consuming. Specially designed laparoscopic suture holders and grasping instruments are then used to suture closed the opening in the uterus. The procedure can take one to three hours, depending on the number, size, and depth of the fibroids within the muscle wall.

Following laparoscopic myomectomy, some women are able to

leave the hospital the same day as surgery. For more extensive surgery, a one- or two-day stay may be necessary. Because the incisions are small, recuperation is usually associated with minimal discomfort. Since the abdominal cavity is not opened, bacteria are less likely to reach the area of surgery, and the risk of infection is low. The intestines are not exposed to the drying effect of air or the irritating effects of the sterile gauze sponges used to hold the bowel out of the way during abdominal surgery. As a result, the intestines usually begin to work normally again immediately after laparoscopic surgery. This avoids the one- or two-day delay before a person is able to eat that follows regular abdominal surgery. After laparoscopic myomectomy, women usually return to normal activity, work, and exercise within two weeks (see page 308).

The use of laparoscopic myomectomy for women who desire to have children is controversial. There is concern about how well the uterus will be able to withstand the stress of labor after having been cut and repaired with laparoscopic techniques. The uterine scar appears to heal as securely as it does following myomectomy done by laparotomy, but the number of women who have gone through labor and vaginal delivery after laparoscopic myomectomy is still somewhat limited. Many physicians recommend cesarean section for delivery after laparascopic myomectomy in order to avoid the stress of labor on the uterus. A comparison study of the effects of laparoscopic myomectomy and standard myomectomy on fertility and the outcome of pregnancy has not yet been undertaken.

Unfortunately, the ability to perform laparoscopic myomectomy has led to its overuse and abuse, partly because small fibroids that are seen during laparoscopy are removed when this may not be necessary. The indications for laparoscopic myomectomy should be the same as for myomectomy by laparotomy. Small fibroids less than two inches almost never cause bothersome symptoms and usually do not need to be removed. Any surgery has some risk. As discussed on page 49, myomectomy may cause the formation of scar tissue, which can lead to infertility or pain. Therefore, as with all surgery, laparoscopic myomectomy should be performed only if appropriate indications exist. And since it is technically difficult surgery, your physician should have the extra training and experience that it requires. When talking to your doctor or interviewing a gynecologic surgeon, it is your right to ask questions: How were you trained to do this surgery? How many of these operations have you performed for women with a situation like mine? Have you had any complications?

Mary Jane's Pelvic Pressure

Mary Jane is a thirty-five-year-old woman who had been diagnosed with fibroids two years ago. She had been examined regularly, and the fibroids had not grown since that time. However, at her most recent checkup, her doctor had noted that the fibroids had enlarged to the size of a very large grapefruit. Her doctor had recommended careful follow-up with frequent exams. At the time I saw her, the fibroid extended two inches higher than her pubic bone and could be felt by pressing on her abdomen.

We discussed her options, which included frequent exams versus surgical removal of the fibroid. Mary Jane was married and had three children. She was tired of the increased pelvic pressure she was feeling but was sure she did not want a hysterectomy unless absolutely necessary. She found herself worrying about the fibroid constantly and imagining that we were missing something, that the fibroid could, in fact, be malignant. The worry and anxiety made her feel as if her life was at a standstill. She very much wanted to have the fibroid removed. She had heard of other women having fibroids removed laparoscopically and knew that this would mean a shorter recovery period. Mary Jane requested laparoscopic surgery.

Although the fibroids were large, I advised her that laparoscopy might be feasible under two conditions. First, she would need to take the medication Lupron (see page 35) to help to temporarily shrink the fibroids. Second, we would need to perform an MRI prior to the surgery. This test, which I rarely recommend because it is expensive, uses a large magnet to make a detailed picture of the inside of the body. It can accurately differentiate normal uterine muscle from fibroid tissue and determine if fibroids are deep within the uterine wall or near the surface, where they are easier to remove. If they are near the surface, laparoscopic surgery is often possible. In most women, an ultrasonogram can provide similar information, but because of the size and position of Mary Jane's fibroid, I thought the MRI would be more accurate.

She agreed to this plan and received her first dose of Lupron to shrink the fibroid. During the three months of treatment, she experienced the typical side effects of hot flashes, sleeplessness, and vaginal dryness. The MRI was performed prior to surgery and showed that the fibroid was actually attached to the outside of the uterus by a small stalk. Since the fibroid did not invade the wall of the uterus, no repair of the uterus would be necessary and the surgery would be easier to accomplish. This mean that Mary Jane was a perfect candidate for laparoscopic surgery.

At the time of surgery, removal of the fibroid was quickly and easily accomplished by cutting the thin stalk to the uterus. Removal of the fibroid from the abdomen was more difficult because of its size. After two hours of cutting the fibroid into small pieces and removing it through the small incisions, the surgery was completed. Mary Jane recovered well and was back to normal activity in about two weeks.

Can Lasers Be Used for Myomectomy?

Lasers have been used to perform gynecologic surgery since 1982. By concentrating very-high-energy light in a very small area, lasers are able to cut through tissue quickly and accurately. Traditionally, surgery has been performed with a scalpel or with instruments that use electricity to create heat that cuts through tissue. At first, lasers were thought to cause less damage to the tissue during surgery. However, recent studies have not found a significant difference between the results of surgery performed with a laser versus that done by electrosurgery or with a scalpel.

Some studies have reported that the use of a laser decreases the amount of blood lost during surgery by a small amount, but there is not enough difference to make this an important advantage. In fact, the transfusion rate is the same whether a laser, electrosurgery, or a scalpel is used. Lasers cost a medical facility approximately $100,000, and the use of a laser during a surgical procedure adds about $800 to the hospital bill. Also, a surgeon requires a substantial amount of specialized training and experience before he or she is truly competent to use a laser. Since scientific studies have not shown that the results of surgery depend on the use of lasers, you physician should use whatever instrument he or she is most comfortable with. Don't be fooled because an instrument or technique is new—it may not be any better or any safer.

Laparoscopic myomectomy can be performed with either electrosurgery or laser surgery. Both are equally effective and safe. My own preference for laparoscopic myomectomy is the KTP/YAG laser, which is available at both of the hospitals where I operate. This combination laser performs both cutting and coagulation (stops bleeding) quickly and accurately. However, new electric instruments have been developed that are safe and provide similar accuracy at less expense.

Can Myomectomy Lead to Scar Tissue?

Any surgery can lead to the formation of scar tissue. Your body makes new tissue as part of the healing process to help paste things back together. This new tissue is called scar tissue or adhesions. The inside of your body can scar from what it perceives to be an injury, just as the skin on your knee forms a scar after a bad cut. Unfortunately, this natural defense can work against us when it occurs internally after surgery, because scar tissue may stick to the normal tissue around it, pulling on it and causing pain. Myomectomy performed by either laparotomy or laparoscopy may lead to the formation of scar tissue near the uterus, fallopian tubes, or ovaries. This new tissue is sometimes thin and flimsy, but it can be thick and inelastic. Scar tissue near the tubes or ovaries may decrease fertility by making it difficult for the egg to travel to the fallopian tube.

One of the major benefits of laparoscopic surgery is that, in some cases, it has been shown to cause fewer adhesions than laparotomy; however, laparoscopic myomectomy has not been studied. Therefore, at the present time, you need to carefully consider which type of surgery is best for you.

What Is Vaginal Myomectomy?

In rare instances, a fibroid growing within the uterus on a stalk is pushed by contractions of the uterus out through the cervix. This process is usually associated with cramps and vaginal bleeding. When a speculum is placed in the vagina, the fibroid can be seen coming out, or *prolapsing*, through the cervix. Because of the bleeding and discomfort, removal of the fibroid is necessary.

Vaginal myomectomy is an outpatient procedure. The doctor places a speculum in the vagina, cuts the stalk of the fibroid, and removes the entire fibroid. To see if any other fibroids are inside the cavity, the doctor views the inside of the uterus with a telescope (hysteroscopy). If the fibroids are small and appear to be easy to remove, a small wire attachment to the telescope, called a resectoscope, can cut through the fibroids and remove them (see page 51). If the fibroids are large, they may need to be removed at a later time after shrinking them with a medication such as Lupron.

What Is Myoma Coagulation?

Myoma coagulation, sometimes called myolysis, is a fairly new surgical procedure developed to shrink fibroids without removing them. The procedure is performed through a laparoscope and uses either a laser or electrical needle that is passed directly into the fibroid. When the instrument is activated, it delivers high-temperature energy to the tissue and destroys both the fibroid tissue and the blood vessels feeding it. The procedure takes less time than either abdominal or laparoscopic myomectomy because no tissue is removed and no suturing of the uterus is necessary. At the present time, myoma coagulation is not recommended for women who want to have children. Two potential problems exist. First, some women may form scar tissue around the uterus after myoma coagulation, and this might impair future fertility. Second, the effect of myoma coagulation on the strength of the uterine wall is not known. Because of the potential risk of the uterus tearing during labor, we advise that women do not attempt to get pregnant after they have had myoma coagulation.

Although myoma coagulation has been performed on a few hundred women throughout the world with very good results, it is still too early to know what its long-term effects will be. I am presently conducting a multicenter study to compare myoma coagulation to abdominal and laparoscopic myomectomy.

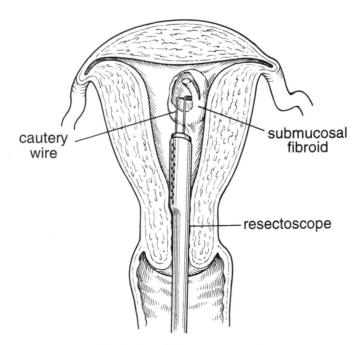

cautery
wire

submucosal
fibroid

resectoscope

Fig. 2.5.   Myoma resection

What Is a Resectoscope Myomectomy?

Resectoscope or hysteroscopic myomectomy is a technique that can be performed only if the fibroids causing the symptoms are within the uterine cavity (*submucosal*). This procedure is performed as outpatient surgery without any incisions (see fig. 2.5). Anesthesia is needed because the surgery may take one to two hours and would otherwise be uncomfortable. Your doctor passes the resectoscope, a small telescope, through the cervix, and the internal uterine cavity is seen. A small camera is attached to the telescope and the view is projected on a video monitor. This magnifies the picture and allows your physician to perform the surgery while sitting in a comfortable position. The surgery can then proceed more rapidly.

Electricity passes through the thin wire attachment of the telescope, allowing the instrument to cut through the fibroid like a hot knife through butter. As the fibroid is shaved from within the uterine cavity, the heat from the instrument sears blood vessels so that blood loss is usually minimal. Patients go home the same day and recovery is remarkably fast. Most women are able to go back to normal activity in one or two days.

Pregnancy rates following resectoscope myomectomy are about 50 percent when fibroids are the cause of infertility. Nearly 90 percent of patients who experienced heavy bleeding return to normal menstrual flow. Only a few years ago, treatment for fibroids in the cavity of the uterus involved major surgery—an abdominal incision and either cutting open the entire uterus to remove the fibroid or performing a hysterectomy. Resectoscope myomectomy is a major advance in the treatment of women who have submucosal fibroids.

Should I Consider Endometrial Ablation?

Endometrial ablation is an outpatient procedure used to stop or decrease bleeding from the uterus. It is described in detail on page 78. Endometrial ablation can be very effective in treating women who experience bleeding from fibroids and who do not want to have children. The procedure may be performed at the same time as a resectoscope myomectomy. However, endometrial ablation has not been as successful in women who have a fibroid uterus larger than a fourteen-week pregnancy. Physicians are not exactly sure why this is the case, but the difficulty in reaching and treating all of the lining cells in the uterus may be the reason. Therefore, myomectomy or hysterectomy may be a better option for these women.

Do I Need a Hysterectomy for Fibroids?

I believe hysterectomy for uterine fibroids should be performed as a last resort. The issues concerning hysterectomy are fully discussed in chapter 11. Hysterectomy is a major operation and carries with it the risk of infection, injury to other organs, anesthesia complications, and blood loss that can sometimes result in the need for transfusion. Complications are uncommon, but they should not be taken lightly. Recovery from abdominal hysterectomy takes four to six weeks, and recovery from vaginal hysterectomy may take as long as four weeks. That's a large chunk out of your life. Surgery is expensive, including doctor's fees, anesthesia fees, hospital charges, and operating room charges. It is preferable to avoid major surgery if possible.

Hysterectomy has two positive attributes as treatment for fibroids. First, the surgery has been shown to cause less blood loss than abdominal myomectomy. However, if you are able to give your own blood prior to surgery, then transfusion should probably not be considered as a major risk factor. Second, since the entire uterus is removed, the possibility of new fibroids is eliminated. Hysterectomy is removal of only the uterus, not the ovaries and fallopian tubes. The medical term for removal of the ovaries and tubes is salpingo-oophorectomy (see fig. 11.1c on page 267). Whether your ovaries should be removed is discussed in chapter 11.

Removal of the uterus should be discussed as an option for a woman who has symptoms from fibroids that *require* her to have surgery and who does not wish any, or any more, children. Hysterectomy may be appropriate for a woman who has multiple fibroids or very large fibroids and who does not want to take a chance that another surgery may be needed at a later time. Hysterectomy can be an option for women who have fibroids, but only when fertility is not an issue, only when other options have been tried, only when they are emotionally prepared, only as a last resort.

ADENOMYOSIS

Adenomyosis is a noncancerous condition of the uterus that can mimic many of the signs and symptoms of fibroids. This condition results when the lining cells of the uterus grow directly into the muscle wall. When the lining cells of the uterus bleed at menstruation, these misplaced cells in the muscle bleed as well, causing pain. As the blood accumulates, the surrounding muscle swells and forms fibrous tissue in response to the irritation. This swollen area within the uterine muscle wall, called an adenomyoma, feels very much like a fibroid on examination and is often confused with a fibroid on a sonogram. Adenomyosis is present in about 10 percent of women and, therefore, is less common than fibroids.

What Are the Symptoms of Adenomyosis?

Adenomyosis may be mild and cause no symptoms at all; in more severe forms, it may lead to heavy bleeding and severe cramping during menstrual periods. If you experience heavy bleeding and severe cramping with your periods, adenomyosis is one of the conditions that your doctor may consider as the cause of your symptoms.

How Is the Diagnosis of Adenomyosis Made?

Adenomyosis is suspected if the uterus is enlarged and tender to the touch on pelvic examination. However, a diagnosis of adenomyosis based on these findings is often inaccurate, and other causes—fibroids, endometriosis, or polyps—are often found to be the cause for the bleeding or discomfort. The diagnosis may be suggested by the appearance of the uterus on a sonogram, although it is often difficult to tell the difference between adenomyosis and fibroids by using sonography. MRI is somewhat better at detecting adenomyosis, but the test is very expensive and is rarely used for this purpose. Unfortunately, surgery is the only way to establish the diagnosis of adenomyosis with certainty. Once removed, the tissue can be examined under a microscope, and the uterine lining cells can be seen within the muscle wall.

What Is the Treatment for Adenomyosis?

The medications Lupron and Synarel (see page 36) can stop the bleeding and associated menstrual cramping and even lead to shrinkage of the swelling associated with adenomyosis. However, the effect is temporary; when the medication is discontinued, the symptoms return. At the present time, the only treatment for adenomyosis is surgery. If adenomyosis is confined to isolated areas in the muscle wall, an attempt may be made to surgically remove these areas and repair the rest of the uterus. If the majority of the uterus is affected, hysterectomy may be the only choice.

REFERENCES

Dubuisson, M., L. Mandelbrot, F. Lecuru, F. Aubriot, H. Foulot, and M. Mouly. 1991. Myomectomy by laparoscopy: a preliminary report of 43 cases. *Fertility and Sterility* 56:827–30.

Friedman, A., and S. Haas. 1993. Should uterine size be an indication for surgical intervention in women with myomas? *American Journal of Obstetrics and Gynecology* 168:751–55.

Friedman, A., and P. Thomas. 1995. Does low-dose combination oral contraceptive use affect uterine size or menstrual flow in premenopausal women with leiomyomas? *Obstetrics and Gynecology* 85:631–35.

Parker, W., and I. Rodi. 1994. Patient selection for laparoscopic myomectomy. *Journal of The American Association of Gynecologic Laparoscopists* 2:23–27.

Parker, W., Y. Fu, and J. Berek. 1994. Uterine sarcomas in patients operated on for presumed leiomyoma and rapidly growing leiomyoma. *Obstetrics and Gynecology* 83:414–18.

Rein, M., R. Barbieri, and A. Friedman. 1995. Progesterone: a critical role in the pathogenesis of uterine myomas. *American Journal of Obstetrics and Gynecology* 172:14–18.

Reiter, R., P. Wagner, and J. Gambone. 1992. Routine hysterectomy for large asymptomatic uterine lyomyomata: a reappraisal. *Obstetrics and Gynecology* 79:481–84.

Stoval, T., F. Ling, L. Henry, and M. Woodruff. 1991. A randomized trial evaluating leuprolide acetata before hysterectomy as treatment for leiomyomas. *American Journal of Obstetrics and Gynecology* 164:1420–25.

3

PROBLEMS WITH YOUR PERIOD

Throughout history, menstruation has been associated with myth and superstition. Menstrual blood was used to cure leprosy, warts, birthmarks, gout, worms, and epilepsy, and to ward off demons and evil spirits. Menstruating women have been separated from their tribes in order to prevent a bad influence on the crops or the hunt. As recently as 1930, an undue exposure to cold or wet just prior to the beginning of a woman's period was considered to be the cause of abnormal menstrual bleeding. "Excess" or "immoderate" sexual intercourse was thought to induce profuse menstruation. Treatment for abnormal periods included avoiding thin shoes that exposed the feet to undue cold, taking warm baths, drinking syrup made from mashed cooked beets, and, not surprisingly, stopping intercourse altogether, or at least decreasing its frequency.

In modern times we have learned that menstruation is the end of the monthly cycle a woman's body goes through if conception has not occurred to allow the uterine lining to regenerate for the next cycle. We have made a quantum leap toward understanding the role menstruation plays in preparing a woman's body for reproduction. And we have learned a great deal about the treatment of many of the problems of abnormal periods. Science has thankfully dispelled the myths and superstitions that surrounded menstruation and sexuality, but the mystery and wonder of these processes is still with us.

Since the days when I studied the female hormone system in medical school, new research has revealed an astonishingly complex system of hormones and nerve transmitter proteins that interplay to regulate the monthly menstrual cycle. The system is balanced, but it is easily upset in certain situations, such as times of stress, when body weight changes, or when taking medications. Once the balance is upset, bleeding can occur that is outside of the normal pattern. Also, cells that form abnormal growths within the uterine lining—polyps, hyperplasia, cancer—can cause bleeding as they develop. The first part of this chapter will deal with the circumstances and solutions for problems with bleeding. The second part of the chapter will deal with painful periods and the new ideas and treatments for this common, bothersome, and sometimes incapacitating problem.

What Kind of Period Is Normal?

The onset of menstrual periods occurs between the ages of nine and seventeen; the average age is thirteen. Adolescents tend to have periods that are far apart and then establish more regularity over the subsequent few years. Most adult women will have a menstrual cycle measured from the first day of any bleeding to the next episode of bleeding, about every twenty-one to thirty-five days. Although women expect to bleed every twenty-eight days, only 15 percent of women actually have cycles that length. Bleeding usually lasts four to six days, but some women bleed a few days more or less. Most women lose about six teaspoons of blood each month. Interestingly, the number of days between periods changes over time, with periods becoming further apart as women reach their forties.

What Makes Your Cycle Regular?

The lining cells of the uterus go through a series of changes every month in response to the hormones made by your ovaries. These cells grow, mature, break down, and finally are shed during your menstrual period. The changes these cells undergo are so predictable that a pathologist can determine how many days it has been since your last period just by looking at the size and shape of the lining cells under a microscope.

The first signal to start your monthly cycle comes from an area in the middle of your brain called the hypothalamus. The hypothalamus releases a hormone called GnRH (gonadotropin-releasing hormone) that is transported to your pituitary gland at the base of the brain. If you touch your tongue to the roof of your mouth as far back as it will go, you will be touching directly below the site of the pituitary gland.

When GnRH reaches the pituitary gland, it provokes the release of follicle-stimulating hormone (FSH). This hormone causes the cells around an egg (the follicle) to develop. The follicular cells then begin to produce estrogen, the main female hormone. When estrogen reaches the uterus by way of the bloodstream, it stimulates the lining cells to grow.

Near the middle of your cycle, the pituitary gland produces luteinizing hormone (LH). LH causes the cells surrounding the egg to break open and release the egg (ovulation). After ovulation, the ovary begins to produce progesterone in addition to estrogen. Progesterone causes the uterine-lining cells to stop growing, and they begin to secrete nutrients that encourage the implantation of a fertilized egg.

If you don't become pregnant, the ovary stops making both estrogen and progesterone. Without these hormones to support their growth, the uterine-lining cells die and are shed as the menstrual flow, and the cycle starts all over again. These hormonal events are crucial to controlling the normal pattern of bleeding that you expect.

Keep in mind that this whole system is designed to get you pregnant. Interestingly, at the time of ovulation the ovary increases its production of androgens, or male hormone. These hormones boost libido, and it is probably no accident that they increase at the time a woman is fertile. The cycle is designed to intensify your desire for sex at the time of the month in which you are most likely to conceive. The complex design inherent in this process is truly remarkable.

When Is Bleeding Abnormal?

Bleeding is abnormal when you have a period more often than every twenty-one days or less often than every thirty-five days, or when you bleed or spot between periods. Very heavy bleeding, saturating a pad or tampon every hour or two for more than a few hours, is also abnormal. There are a number of causes of abnormal bleeding, and the good news is that almost all of them are benign and easily treatable. The most common causes are hormonal changes, ovarian cysts, uterine or cervical polyps, overgrowth of the uterine-lining cells (hyperplasia), fibroids, and, rarely, precancer or cancer of the uterus. The following sections will explain each of these problems in detail.

HORMONAL PROBLEMS

Are Adolescents Prone to Abnormal Bleeding?

When you are an adolescent and begin having periods, it may take a year or two to fully establish the normal balance of hormones. Most young women will not ovulate more than a few times during the first one or two years of their cycles. The estrogen that is produced by the ovaries causes the lining of the uterus to grow, but without ovulation and the resulting production of progesterone, this growth is not controlled. These overgrown cells become fragile and start to bleed on their own. If the time between periods stretches out over a few months, the overgrown cells can accumulate, so that when bleeding finally does occur, it can be extremely heavy. It is therefore *common* for young women to have irregular and very unpredictable cycles until all of the hormones come into balance, and ovulation occurs on a regular basis. If an adolescent has very heavy bleeding, she should contact her doctor. Treatment with the hormone progesterone can usually stop the bleeding within a day or two.

Kinesha's Heavy Bleeding

Kinesha is a fourteen-year-old who I initially saw in the emergency room because she was having a very heavy menstrual period. She had not had her period for four months, and this period had started off fairly heavy. Now, four days later, she needed to change her menstrual pad every fifteen or twenty minutes. The examination showed that she was still bleeding. She was also starting to feel exhausted. Her blood count indicated that she had lost about one-third of her red blood cells. We began to give her high doses of progesterone pills, and within two days the bleeding had stopped. We gave her the progesterone for seven days during each of the next three months, and her periods returned to normal.

Unfortunately, after a few more months of normal periods, her periods became irregular again. The next time I saw Kinesha, she was bleeding very heavily and needed another treatment with progesterone pills. Even though she was not sexually active, we discussed starting her on birth control pills to help regulate her periods. The pill contains high doses of progesterone and tends to thin out the lining cells of the uterus over time. The thinner the lining, the less severe the bleeding. Also, the pill supplies the body with steady levels of both estrogen and progesterone. Kinesha's ovaries had been making irregular amounts. Kinesha and her mother agreed she should start taking the pill, and within two months she was having regular and light periods. Her blood count returned to normal, and her strength and energy returned. She felt better than she had in a year. We stopped the pills after a year to see if her system had straightened out and found that she had begun to have regular periods of normal flow, which have continued to this day.

Can Stress Interfere with Your Period?

Today's scientists are only beginning to understand the relationship between stress and the functioning of the human body. We do conclusively know, however, that stress can affect the secretion of chemicals in the brain and the release of hormones from the pituitary gland. The sensitivity of the brain to stress is evidenced by the fact that about 20 percent of all female college freshmen will experience abnormal periods during that first year of academic and social pressure. The finely balanced symphony of events we referred to earlier, which is required for each menstrual cycle, can be upset by stress.

Sara's Abnormal Periods

Sara, a twenty-four-year-old woman, came to the office because she had been experiencing spotting for the past few months between her normally regular periods. While not excessive, the bleeding was becoming a nuisance. She had recently begun a new job and was preoccupied with her responsibilities. She was not sexually active, so she wasn't worried about pregnancy, but now she began to worry that something might be wrong.

The examination of her uterus, fallopian tubes, and ovaries was entirely normal. This was immediately reassuring to Sara, since she secretly suspected that something might be growing inside her. During our conversation, it became obvious that she was under a fair amount of stress at her new job. The demands of learning the job, getting along with the other employees, and pleasing her new boss were taking up a considerable amount of energy. Because of her young age, the possibility of cancer, polyps, or fibroids was small. With a normal examination, the most likely diagnosis was a hormonal imbalance as a result of her stress. Because these imbalances are almost always temporary, she and I discussed doing nothing for a while to see if the irregular bleeding would stop by itself. I asked her to call me if the bleeding became heavier or more frequent, or if the problem persisted after two months. Sara called three months later to say that the abnormal bleeding had resolved itself, and she was feeling at home in her new job.

Can Your Weight Affect Your Period?

The fat cells in your body take up hormones made by the adrenal gland and actually change the chemical structure of these hormones into estrogen. Women who are overweight have more fat cells and therefore change more adrenal hormone into more estrogen. Normally, your ovaries make lower levels of estrogen at the end of the menstrual cycle. These low levels act as a trigger to signal the brain to begin a new cycle. If the levels of estrogen never go down because of the extra estrogen from fat cells, then a new menstrual cycle won't begin. In this way, being overweight can interfere with the menstrual cycle.

In addition, weight loss can interfere with your menstrual cycles. It appears that women need a minimum percentage of body fat to maintain menstrual function. A loss of weight to 10 to 15 percent below the normal weight for your height may lead to loss of your menstrual periods. In one study of 170 women who had missed periods, 25 percent had lost weight prior to missing their periods.

While missed periods are not dangerous, avoiding the disruption of your hormones is one reason why slow and moderate weight loss is better for your body than rapid and drastic weight reduction. Slow, moderate weight loss allows your body to make the proper adjustments to keep your hormones at normal levels. If you miss your period while on a diet, you should see your doctor just to be sure no other problem exists.

Can Changes in the Amount of Exercise You Do Cause Abnormal Bleeding?

Serious athletes who train vigorously sometimes will notice that their cycles are irregular. Some even stop menstruating altogether. Abnormal periods occur in about 20 percent of women runners and 50 to 75 percent of women ballet dancers. The reason for this is not totally understood, and a number of factors may be at work.

Exercise and weight loss result in low levels of body fat. It appears that these low levels of body fat cause the body to change normal estrogen into another form of estrogen that is inactive. This inactive estrogen fails to give the proper signals to the brain and menstrual function ceases. Strenuous athletic training associated with weight loss is also stressful to your body. It has been proposed that the body shuts down menstrual function during stressful times in order to prevent pregnancy at times of apprehension or turmoil.

Exercise also increases the levels of brain endorphins, the body's natural sedative. Interestingly, endorphins have about ten times the relaxant effect on the brain than does pure morphine. This may be the explanation for "runner's high," the feeling of relaxation and well-being that follows strenuous exercise. High levels of these endorphins can interfere with both the production of your normal brain hormones and your menstrual cycle. One or all of these factors can be responsible for a decrease in estrogen production, the halting of ovulation, and the cessation of periods.

The lack of bleeding in and of itself is not dangerous. However, a low level of estrogen over a period of six months or longer can cause calcium loss from the bones and lead to the beginnings of osteoporosis. If very prolonged, it could lead to fractured bones, even in an otherwise healthy woman. Within a few months of ending high levels of exercise, weight loss, or stress, most women will return to normal cycles. If caught early, the beginnings of osteoporosis may be reversible with a return to normal cycles. And happily, these women are also perfectly capable of getting pregnant once their normal cycles return.

Shawn Exercises Too Much

Shawn is a thirty-four-year-old woman who recently decided to get back into the shape she was in when she was twenty. She began to run before work every morning. She was soon looking forward to this exercise and the "high" that she got after her run and morning shower. As the months went by, Shawn increased her run from the initial twenty minutes to an hour of vigorous, full-out running. Shawn was not only in the best shape of her life, but she was "hooked" on running. Each week she kept trying to increase her time and distance. She soon noticed that her periods were becoming lighter, usually just spotting, and some months she missed them entirely. After missing two months in a row, she made an appointment to see what was wrong.

Shawn's examination was entirely normal. She was in superb condition and had lost twenty pounds since her appointment a year before. We discussed her exercise schedule and the fact that this amount of exercise can often lead to a decrease in the level of estrogen in the body, causing less growth of the uterine-lining cells and less bleeding. Also, if her body continued to produce low levels of estrogen over a period of six months or longer, she was at high risk for osteoporosis.

We discussed two options. The first was for Shawn to decrease her exercise to a more moderate level, which would allow her estrogen levels to rise back to normal and lead to a return of monthly periods. The second option was to continue her rigorous exercise schedule but to also take supplemental estrogen in pill form in order to replace what her body was not able to make. The idea of taking supplemental estrogen did not appeal to Shawn, so she chose to decrease her exercise to running only forty-five minutes four times a week. Within three months her periods returned to normal, and she has done very well since.

Can Anorexia Nervosa Interfere with Your Period?

Anorexia nervosa is a serious eating disorder that is associated with extreme weight loss. It also causes the cessation of menstrual periods. The majority of female sufferers are between the ages of ten and thirty. Anorexia appears to have deep psychological roots. It usually affects young women from achievement-oriented families who feel pressure to perform and be perfect. The initial loss of weight may be a way for the young woman to gain some sense of control in a life that may not be to her liking.

Our culture may also contribute to the onset of this illness by placing a high value on young women being thin. Advertisements featuring women who in past decades would have been considered undernourished have set the contemporary standard of beauty. Many young women work very hard at achieving a thinness that may actually be detrimental to their health. Bulimia may also be a part of the disease of anorexia, involving cycles of binge eating followed by self-induced vomiting, which leads to further weight loss.

Because of the weight loss associated with anorexia, the brain shuts down the normal hormonal secretions associated with the control of the menstrual cycle. In effect, the brain returns to a prepubertal state. In an apparent effort by the body to conserve energy, other functions are also affected, resulting in low blood pressure, slow heart rate, constipation, and low body temperature. Anorexia is a serious and tragic disease. Between 5 and 15 percent of its sufferers virtually starve themselves to death. Psychiatric help is essential, and early intervention may prevent the problem from reaching its full extent. If you know someone with this problem, or if you think you suffer from it yourself, seeking help from a qualified psychiatrist is critical to defeating this disease. Under proper treatment, a return to normal eating habits is associated with a return to normal weight and body functions.

Can Any Medications Interfere with the Menstrual Cycle?

Most medications used to treat medical illnesses do not interfere with menstrual function. However, sleeping pills, tranquilizers, and antidepressants can all change your cycle by affecting the area of your brain that regulates the flow of hormones. Taking these medications often results in missed periods, although frequent and irregular bleeding can occur. These missed periods are not medically worrisome but may be emotionally worrisome, adding to the stress you already feel. It may not be clear whether the source of your missed periods is the stress or the medication you are taking to help you cope with the stress. A discussion between your gynecologist and the doctor or therapist prescribing your medication can help clarify which medication might be best for you, and for how long it should be taken.

Can Narcotic Use Cause Abnormal Periods?

Drug use, particularly narcotic use, affects the area of the brain that controls your menstrual cycle. This often leads to missed periods or more frequent bleeding. If you use drugs, you should inform your doctor. This information will be kept confidential, but will be factored into your medical evaluation and treatment. Abnormalities of your period related to drug use should go away a few months after you stop taking the drug.

Can Problems with Your Thyroid Gland Interfere with Your Period?

For unknown reasons, thyroid problems are much more common in women than in men. The thyroid gland, found at the base of your neck, produces the hormone that controls the production of energy in all the cells in your body. Sometimes the symptoms of thyroid disease are obvious. An overactive thyroid can cause weight loss despite a normal or increased appetite. It may make you feel nervous or "hyper" and cause your heart to beat rapidly. You may feel warm at times when others around you are comfortable or even cold. An underactive thyroid can cause weight gain and make you feel sluggish or cold. However, subtle changes in thyroid function may only be detectable by measuring thyroid hormone in your blood.

Abnormalities of the thyroid gland can cause abnormal bleeding, usually resulting in less frequent periods. Therefore, thyroid hormone blood tests will often be checked if your periods become less frequent. Problems with the thyroid gland are usually easy to treat with medication, and your periods should return to normal shortly after treatment.

Can Other Hormonal Problems Interfere with Your Period?

Prolactin is another hormone that is produced in the pituitary gland. After childbirth, it is produced in large amounts and is responsible for stimulating your breasts to produce milk. For unknown reasons, in a small number of women prolactin production may increase when a woman has not recently given birth. Higher than normal levels of this hormone can interfere with the production of other female hormones, causing missed periods. The high level of prolactin may also lead to a little milky discharge from your breasts. After childbirth, breast feeding maintains high levels of prolactin, which usually suppress menstrual periods for at least a few months. This is why nursing sometimes works as a form of birth control, but it is not reliable.

An elevated amount of prolactin can be detected by a simple blood test. An elevated level usually does not need to be treated and is not worrisome. Infrequently, the prolactin level is extremely high, signifying a substantial but benign overgrowth of the cells that produce prolactin in the pituitary gland. Very rarely, this *benign* tumor can press on nearby areas of the brain and cause headaches or loss of peripheral vision. When the tumor causes these symptoms, it needs to be treated. A medication can be effectively used to shrink the cells and relieve symptoms and restore menstrual function. In very rare cases, when the medication has been ineffective, surgery on the pituitary gland may be needed to remove the tumor.

Can Ovarian Cysts Cause Irregular Periods?

As an ovarian cyst develops, it often will interfere with the production of hormones from the normal ovarian tissue. As a result of this abnormal hormone production, the lining cells of the uterus start to break down and are shed irregularly, resulting in irregular bleeding. The cyst can lead to more frequent and lighter bleeding than normal, or it can be associated with missed periods followed by heavy bleeding. Ovarian cysts and the problems associated with them are discussed fully in chapter 4.

Can Missing Periods Lead to Any Other Problems?

Missing periods over four to six months as a result of weight loss, stress, or too much exercise can be associated with a chronically low level of estrogen. Estrogen is needed in order to keep the calcium in your bones. Without estrogen, your bones start to lose calcium, and osteoporosis may result. While we know that exercise actually strengthens your bones, the benefit from exercise is totally negated by low levels of estrogen that result in decreased calcium absorption. Therefore, you can't rely on exercise to protect you from bone loss if you are not having periods. The amount of bone lost, about 1 to 2 percent per year, may not sound like very much, but over time it can add up. The overall effect of six or more missed periods in a row may be the start of the loss of bone strength. Osteoporosis resulting from missed periods can happen at any age!

What Is the Treatment for Abnormal Periods?

The first line of treatment for abnormal bleeding related to hormonal problems is the correction of the primary cause. Relief of stress, correction of weight gain or loss, changes in exercise patterns, or adjustments in medication use will often correct the abnormal bleeding. If a hormonal cause is fairly certain and these solutions fail, and if the bleeding is bothersome or persistent, then treatment with hormones can be undertaken.

If you are regularly missing periods, you should consider taking estrogen pills in order to prevent osteoporosis. Taking estrogen will prevent the loss of calcium from your bones and keep them from becoming brittle. Progesterone pills are also prescribed to prevent overgrowth of the uterine-lining cells. Also, it is important to take in about 1,500 milligrams of calcium a day as part of your diet. Calcium supplements can also be used, though they are not as well absorbed as dietary calcium. They are best absorbed if taken a few times a day with food. Vitamin D is necessary for absorption of calcium. This vitamin is naturally produced by the body in the fat layer below the skin when a person is exposed to sunlight. Calcium with vitamin D added should be taken only if you live in an area with little sunlight or if you don't often get outside. For most women, calcium alone is sufficient.

What Is the Treatment If Irregular Bleeding Is Due to Missed Ovulation?

For most women, the cause of infrequent but heavy bleeding is a missed ovulation or two that results in a lack of progesterone. Taking progesterone tablets will usually correct the problem. Another alternative is to take birth control pills, which also contain progesterone and will regulate your bleeding. While these treatments will correct your bleeding pattern, they obviously do not correct the original cause of the bleeding. If the stress, exercise, or weight issues continue, the abnormal bleeding may return.

When Is a D&C Necessary for Abnormal Hormonal Bleeding?

If you are younger than thirty-five years old, abnormal bleeding is usually the result of irregular hormones, and hormonal treatment is nearly always effective. However, if the bleeding persists, or if it is very heavy (defined as bleeding through a tampon or pad every hour or two), then a D&C should be considered. The purpose of the D&C is twofold. First, the D&C removes the lining cells so that they can be examined under a microscope, and a precise diagnosis can be made regarding the cause of the bleeding. The pathologist can sometimes tell what the hormonal abnormality appears to be, and then appropriate treatment can be started. Also, any other problem such as polyps or precancerous cells can be detected by the pathologist. Second, the D&C removes all of the lining cells that are bleeding. This often stops the abnormal bleeding and allows the uterus to form a new, healthier lining. The D&C and other diagnostic tests are fully discussed beginning on page 75.

Are There Homeopathic Remedies for Abnormal Bleeding Due to Hormonal Causes?

Remedies prescribed by homeopathic practitioners are based on the type of abnormal bleeding, as well as symptoms of exhaustion, discomfort, or irritability. Before beginning this type of treatment, I urge you to have an examination to eliminate any serious condition as the cause of the bleeding.

What Is Polycystic Ovarian Disease (PCO)?

PCO is a rare hormonal condition associated with infrequent periods, and often with excess hair growth and infertility. This condition has also been called Stein-Leventhal syndrome, but is now more accurately referred to as *persistent anovulation* (lack of ovulation). The ovaries are often filled with many small cysts, the remnants of eggs that failed to ovulate. The normal menstrual cycle depends on the proper balance and interplay of many hormones and other proteins within the body. There are many opportunities for this system to go awry, leading to a failure to ovulate, which in turn leads to hormonal imbalances that further inhibit ovulation, thus starting a continuing abnormal cycle. Persistent anovulation is not dangerous, and most of its symptoms are treatable. About one-third of women with persistent anovulation will have infrequent but heavy periods, and about 50 percent will stop having periods altogether.

Progesterone is not produced if ovulation does not take place, so it must be administered to help bring about bleeding. Birth control pills (which contain progesterone) or pure progesterone pills are prescribed to help regulate the cycles. The lining cells are shed in the bleeding that results, thus preventing cell overgrowth. If no periods, or very few, occur over a number of years, the overgrown lining cells can develop into a precancerous condition called atypical hyperplasia. Progesterone treatment or birth control pills, given on a monthly basis, can prevent the development of these abnormal cells.

Persistent anovulation also leads to an increase in male hormones, small amounts of which are normally secreted by a woman's ovaries. This increase in male hormone can lead to excess hair growth in about 70 percent of women with persistent anovulation. This problem also can usually be controlled by taking birth control pills, which decrease the production of male hormone. Stronger medications are available if this regimen is unsuccessful. Electrolysis is an effective alternative if medical therapy has not solved the problem.

The infrequent and somewhat unpredictable ovulation associated with this condition can lead to problems getting pregnant. Medications can help promote ovulation and fertility with excellent results.

What Is Premature Menopause?

The average age of a woman going through menopause, the time of her last menstrual period, is about fifty-one, but the actual age may range from the early forties to the late fifties. In less than 1 percent of women, menopause occurs before the age of forty. Menopause before the age of forty is called premature menopause.

When you are born, your ovaries contain about 2 million eggs.

However, the natural process of cell death decreases the number of eggs to about 300,000 by the time you have your first period. The number of eggs actually ovulated during your lifetime, about five hundred, is obviously only a small percentage of the original population of eggs. The rest regularly die off over time, even during the times you are pregnant or on birth control pills. In some women, the rate of egg death is very rapid and leads to premature menopause. One cause of this loss of eggs may be an autoimmune disease, a condition in which the body makes antibodies that destroy its own tissue. Some rare genetic diseases and exposure to radiation treatments or chemotherapy lead to early menopause. Premature menopause is very rare, but if you start missing periods or having hot flashes at an early age, you should be evaluated by your doctor.

MENOPAUSAL BLEEDING

What Kind of Bleeding Problems May Develop During Perimenopause and Menopause?

By definition, menopause is the date of your last menstrual period. The onset of menopause signifies that the eggs and the cells surrounding the eggs that produce female hormones are no longer present. Over the months or years preceding menopause, as your ovaries begin to run out of eggs, those that remain may not be quite as responsive to the hormonal signals sent from the pituitary gland. If a normal egg happens to be developing, your level of hormones will be normal. But if a less responsive egg is developing, your level of hormones may be low for that month. This period of time when your hormone levels vary is called perimenopause. Because some or even most of your cycles are normal, it may not be clear that you are entering menopause. Symptoms such as hot flashes or vaginal dryness may be sporadically present, or not present at all. Hormonal tests can fluctuate from month to month and may not reveal what is happening to your body.

The most common pattern of bleeding during perimenopause is lighter periods that are farther apart. If this pattern is accompanied by hot flashes, the approach of menopause may be recognized. However, in some women the diagnosis will not be certain until periods are missed or blood tests clearly show the changes of menopause. Recent studies have shown that osteoporosis may start to develop during perimenopause as estrogen levels begin to decrease. Therefore, consideration should be given to taking hormonal therapy during this time. Taking estrogen and progesterone can prevent both heart disease and osteoporosis, as well as relieve the symptoms of menopause.

What Should Be Done If You Have Abnormal Bleeding During Perimenopause or After Menopause?

As menopause approaches, most women will experience lighter and less frequent periods. However, the likelihood of bleeding from other causes such as hyperplasia (lining overgrowth), polyps, or precancer or cancer of the uterus increases at this time of your life. Bleeding that is irregular, very heavy (requiring a pad change every hour or two), or prolonged (more than seven days) is abnormal and it is important to establish the cause. The best way to accomplish this is to take a sample of the cells from the uterine lining. The diagnostic methods to do this, including hysteroscopy, endometrial biopsy, and D&C, are described beginning on page 75.

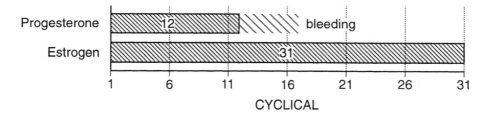

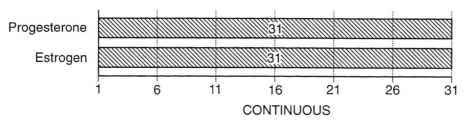

Fig. 3.1. Hormone replacement therapy

What If You Are Bleeding While You Are on Hormone Replacement Therapy for Menopause?

There are two basic regimens for taking hormone replacement therapy (see fig. 3.1). One regimen uses daily doses of estrogen with progesterone taken *cyclically* for about half of each month (twelve days). With this regimen, some monthly bleeding is normal and occurs around the time that the progesterone tablets are finished. Bleeding at any other time of the month is not expected and should be reported to your doctor.

The other commonly used regimen calls for daily doses of both estrogen and progesterone, with no days off. This regimen works well to relieve the symptoms of menopause and is also felt to be effective as protection against heart disease and osteoporosis. During the first six months of this *continuous* therapy, as the uterus adjusts to the hormones, bleeding may be irregular and unpredictable. It is usually not heavy or persistent. After the first six months of therapy, 80 percent of women will have no bleeding at all for as long as they are on the hormones. If you are on continuous therapy, then any bleeding after the first six months should be reported to your doctor. Heavy or persistent bleeding, even in the first six months, should be reported as well. For some women, the lack of any bleeding with the continuous regimen is a plus; other women prefer to have the monthly bleeding with the cyclical regimen. You should discuss the choice of regimens with your doctor. In either case, let your doctor know if bleeding occurs unexpectedly.

POLYPS, FIBROIDS, HYPERPLASIA, AND CANCER

As the uterine lining grows, it normally appears smooth and regular. When menstrual bleeding occurs, the entire lining is shed over the course of a few days, leaving an even surface. Uterine polyps, fibroids, hyperplasia, and cancer can grow within the uterus and disrupt the normal appearance and the bleeding patterns of the lining cells.

What Are Uterine Polyps?

Polyps are fingerlike overgrowths of lining cells that can occur in many areas of the body, including the nasal passages, the intestines, and the lining of the uterus (see fig. 3.2). The cause of polyps is unknown, but in the uterus they are virtually always benign. As the cells of the polyp overgrow, they can become fragile and start to bleed. Polyps are now easy to diagnose in the gynecologist's office. Your doctor uses a very small telescope called a hysteroscope to see into the uterus and detect even small abnormalities that can cause abnormal bleeding (see page 75).

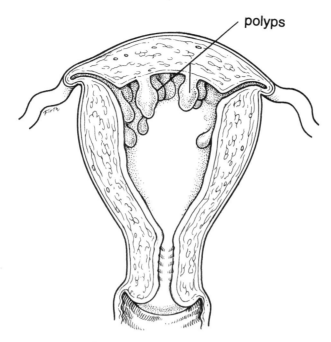

Fig. 3.2.   Uterine polyps

Can Polyps Be Cured?

Polyps are often loosely attached to the lining of the uterus. The hysteroscope is very helpful because it allows the doctor to see exactly where
the polyp is. Then the polyp can be easily removed by performing a
D&C or by grasping it with a small instrument. After removal, the hysteroscope is reinserted to make sure that the polyp has been totally eliminated. In a few cases polyps may be very large or attached to the uterine
lining by thick stalks. A resectoscope may be needed to cut the stalk
of the polyp before it can be removed (see page 51). This procedure is
usually performed in the hospital with anesthesia.

Molly's Persistent Bleeding

Molly is a sixty-six-year-old woman who had been having bleeding after menopause. She had already had three D&Cs and a
variety of hormonal treatments, yet the bleeding persisted. Her
examination was normal, but I suggested that we do a hys-

teroscopy in the office, which had not been done before, to see why the bleeding was not going away. She agreed, and we scheduled it for the next day. After giving Molly local anesthesia, I inserted the hysteroscope. It was immediately apparent that a large polyp was inside the uterine cavity. Loosely attached to the uterine lining by a stalk, it flopped back and forth. Without the benefit of hysteroscopy to pinpoint the exact location of the polyp, the previous D&Cs had missed it entirely. The polyp was easy to remove with a polyp forceps. Another inspection of the uterine cavity with the hysteroscope showed that the polyp was gone. Molly has not had abnormal bleeding again.

What Kind of Bleeding Problems Can Fibroids Cause?

Fibroids, benign overgrowths of the uterine muscle, can interfere with the ability of the uterus to stop the flow of blood once a period begins. As a result, the bleeding associated with fibroids is often heavy and prolonged. Fibroids and their associated problems are discussed in chapter 2.

What Is the Best Treatment If the Cause of Bleeding Is Fibroids?

While fibroids are a common cause of heavy bleeding, they often do not require treatment unless the bleeding is very heavy or persistent; then, removal of the fibroids may be indicated. There are a number of ways to remove fibroids, including the standard treatment of abdominal surgery, as well as some newer developments. Removal of fibroids from within the cavity of the uterus can now be accomplished with a resectoscope, a small instrument passed through the cervix (see page 51). This procedure is very effective for treating heavy bleeding associated with fibroids.

What Is Hyperplasia (Overgrowth) of the Uterine Lining?

The lining of the uterus grows in response to the hormones in your bloodstream. Estrogen causes these cells to grow, and constant high levels of estrogen over a long period of time can cause an overgrowth of the cells called hyperplasia. As this overgrowth occurs, the cells can become fragile and start to bleed unpredictably.

One of the causes of hyperplasia is being overweight. All of the fat cells in your body usually take up the hormones produced by the adrenal glands and change them into estrogen. Therefore, if you are overweight, you have more fat cells to change the adrenal hormones into estrogen.

This results in more estrogen floating around in your bloodstream, which can stimulate overgrowth of the uterine-lining cells. And higher levels of estrogen can affect the brain hormones that regulate the menstrual cycle, leading to less frequent periods, less shedding of the lining, and eventually the accumulation of overgrown cells.

To diagnose hyperplasia, your doctor performs either a D&C or an endometrial biopsy (see pages 75 and 76) to remove some of the lining cells, which are examined under a microscope. Simple hyperplasia is a benign condition. Because the underlying problem is too much estrogen (and not enough progesterone), progesterone tablets are prescribed. Progesterone will thin out the overgrown cells and help avoid further bleeding problems. If being overweight is the cause of the bleeding, then losing weight usually will correct the problem. Another condition called *atypical* hyperplasia also involves the overgrowth of uterine-lining cells. These cells are different, however: They have the potential to develop into cancer. Atypical hyperplasia is discussed on page 242.

Can Abnormal Bleeding Be a Sign of Cancer?

Cancer of the uterus is a rare condition, occurring in about two out of every thousand postmenopausal women and in much fewer younger women. The cause of uterine cancer is unknown but may be related to the presence of high levels of estrogen in the body over a very long period of time. The high levels of estrogen cause continued stimulation and overgrowth of the uterine-lining cells, which may then become cancerous. As cancer cells develop and grow, they burrow into nearby normal cells and cause bleeding. Although bleeding is often the first sign of uterine cancer, there are many causes for abnormal bleeding besides cancer. The good news about uterine cancer is that it is one of the most curable cancers if it is discovered early (see chapter 10). If you have abnormal bleeding, in all likelihood it is not caused by uterine cancer. But report any abnormal bleeding to your doctor, just to be sure.

How Do We Find Out What Is Causing Your Abnormal Bleeding?

The first thing that you should do if you have abnormal bleeding is to let your doctor know. Depending on your age, the type of medications you take, and the amount and timing of the bleeding, your doctor will make some assessment as to what type of evaluation is needed. The first step is usually a pelvic examination. Your doctor will start by placing a speculum in your vagina and examining your cervix. Sometimes infections of the cervix can cause enough irritation to create bleeding, and this can be easily detected by looking at the cervix. Benign cervical polyps, fragile overgrowths of the cells that line the inside of the cervix, can be easily seen. These polyps can also cause bleeding.

Next, your doctor will examine your uterus by placing one hand on your abdomen and pushing the cervix and uterus up from the inside of the vagina. By feeling the uterus, fallopian tubes, and ovaries, abnormal growths like ovarian cysts or fibroids can be detected. If the uterus or ovaries are hard to feel, or if something feels abnormal, a sonogram may be helpful.

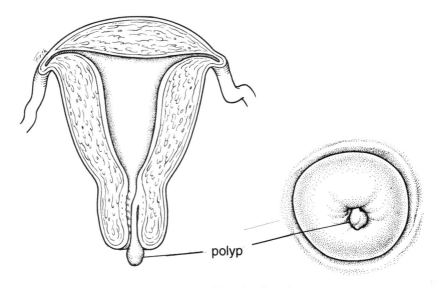

Fig. 3.3.   Cervical polyp

Julie Bleeds After Sex

Julie is a thirty-three-year-old woman who found bright red blood on her sheets right after she had sex. This had been going on for the past three months. Initially she was not alarmed because she just assumed it was a strange but passing thing and that it would go away by itself. Her periods were regular, and she had no pain, nausea, diarrhea, fever, or any other problems. When it didn't "just go away," she and her husband became concerned, and Julie came in for an examination. During her pelvic examination, a small polyp could be seen on her cervix (see fig. 3.3). When touched with a Q-tip, the polyp bled. The rest of the examination was totally normal. Her fallopian tubes, uterus, and ovaries were all the right size, and there was no tenderness or signs of infection. We were able to remove the polyp by grasping it with an instrument and twisting it off its stalk. The procedure required no anesthesia, was painless, and took about two minutes. It put an end to Julie's bleeding.

When Are Further Tests Needed?

If your bleeding is very heavy or prolonged, or if it has not improved after treatment with progesterone as described above, then other tests may be indicated to discover the cause of the bleeding and help determine the appropriate treatment. Tests that may be performed include hysteroscopy, D&C, endometrial biopsy, and sonogram. These tests are described below. As mentioned earlier, if you are approaching menopause or are already postmenopausal and have abnormal bleeding, these tests are virtually always indicated to look for the presence of precancerous or cancerous cells.

What Is Hysteroscopy?

This test allows the doctor to look inside the uterus by placing the hysteroscope, a small telescope, through the vagina and into the opening in the cervix. Once inside the uterus, the lining cells can be inspected. Polyps, fibroids, hyperplasia, and cancer can all be seen with the hysteroscope. Hysteroscopy can be done in the doctor's office in about five minutes and usually does not require any anesthesia. The information the doctor can get from this procedure is invaluable. Because many problems can be clearly seen, diagnosis is often certain. A number of studies have shown that a diagnosis made by hysteroscopy followed by scraping the visualized abnormal area of lining cells is more accurate than when a D&C is performed blindly.

What Happens During an Office D&C?

The cause of abnormal bleeding can often be determined by examining the uterine-lining cells under a microscope. These cells can be removed for examination by D&C, which stands for *d*ilatation (opening the cervix) and *c*urettage (scraping the lining of the uterus). For some women, the procedure may also be used to scrape away the cells causing the bleeding and cure the problem.

In our office, we give the patient mildly sedating medication before the procedure to help her relax. We use small doses of Valium plus a pain reliever, both injected slowly into a vein. Ordinarily, you do not need to be put to sleep, because the entire procedure takes about five minutes, and most women feel only some mild menstrual cramping for a minute or two. Many women have no discomfort at all. Because the medication goes directly into the bloodstream, it works rapidly. It also leaves the body quickly so that you don't feel "drugged" once the procedure is over. In eighteen years of practice, I have had only three patients say they wished they had been asleep during the office D&C. The anticipation is usually much worse than the reality.

After you are relaxed from the medication, a local anesthetic is injected near the cervix to numb it. Then the cervix is held with an instrument and gently dilated so that the hysteroscope can pass easily through it. The uterine cavity can then be viewed and inspected for polyps, fibroids, overgrowth, or cancer. If any abnormalities are seen, the doctor knows exactly where to scrape in order to remove these cells. After the hysteroscope is removed, a small metal instrument called a curette is inserted into the uterine cavity, and the lining cells are scraped out. If any polyps are present, a grasping instrument can be placed into the cavity to remove them.

In order to be sure that all the cells are removed and collected, a tubular plastic instrument is inserted into the uterus, and a suction is attached to vacuum any remaining cells into a container. All of these cells are sent to the laboratory so that a pathologist can examine them. Cancer, precancer, polyps, and hyperplasia can all be detected by the pathologist, who may also be able to see evidence in the cells of any hormonal imbalance that may have caused your abnormal bleeding.

Between the information that the doctor obtains by viewing the uterine cavity with a hysteroscope and the information the pathologist gets from looking at the lining cells with a microscope, the cause of your bleeding can be determined, and the appropriate treatment chosen.

What Is an Endometrial Biopsy?

An office D&C is a far cry from major surgery, but it often requires some form of medication, usually mild sedation and local anesthesia. It also involves a fair amount of expertise and equipment. In an effort to get information about the lining cells of the uterus with a simpler procedure, a smaller biopsy of the lining, called an endometrial biopsy, has been used for years. An endometrial biopsy is performed by placing a small plastic tube about the diameter of spaghetti through the cervix and into the uterus. As the tube is removed it scrapes some cells from the uterine lining. Because this procedure samples only a small area of the lining, it is not quite as accurate as a hysteroscopy and complete D&C. But recently, a number of small suction-type instruments have been developed to improve the accuracy of the procedure. The early results show that in most cases these newer instruments work fairly well. I find an endometrial biopsy most helpful when I am *not* very suspicious that cancer is the cause of the bleeding. But if the results of this test are not 100 percent normal, I think a full office D&C is required to make sure that everything is okay.

However, if the bleeding is persistent or heavy, if you are postmenopausal, or if a sonogram shows increased thickness of the lining cells (see below), which suggests that precancer or cancer is possible, then I always recommend that a hysteroscopy and office D&C be done, since this is the most accurate test we have.

Janet Bleeds on Hormone Replacement Therapy

Janet is a fifty-five-year-old woman who was experiencing irregular bleeding while taking her estrogen and progesterone therapy for menopausal symptoms. One year earlier, Janet had a similar problem while living in another city. Her gynecologist there had performed a D&C and hysteroscopy; lab results showed her to be entirely normal.

Because the D&C had been done within the recent past, another one did not seem warranted. However, some evaluation seemed necessary to be sure that nothing new was developing. Therefore, I recommended that Janet have an endometrial biopsy in the office. No anesthesia or medications were needed, and the test took about two minutes to perform. When the results came back a week later, it showed that the lining cells were not getting enough estrogen, and we just needed to adjust her hormone dose.

Can a Sonogram Be Used to Diagnose the Cause of Abnormal Bleeding?

The equipment and techniques used for sonography have improved enormously. Patterned after ship's sonar, the sonogram machine bounces harmless sound waves off the organs inside your body. The reflected sound waves are picked up and recorded in the form of a black-and-white picture on a screen. Photographs can then be made to record the images. Transvaginal sonography, the newest technique, makes images using a small wand placed within your vagina. The end of the instrument gets very close to the uterus, fallopian tubes, and ovaries; therefore, it is able to sense very small detail, including the thickness and regularity of the lining of your uterus. A thick uterine lining may be associated with hyperplasia, precancer, or cancer. Polyps can show up as irregular structures within the cavity, and fibroids appear as enlarged round areas of tissue growing within the uterine wall. If you have irregular bleeding and the lining appears very thin on the sonogram, you are probably fine. Cancer almost never appears that way. A very recent development called the sonohysterogram uses a small catheter to pass sterile water through the cervix and into the uterus. The water helps to outline any abnormalities present, and the sonohysterogram gives more detail. However, all of this technology is still being developed, and I do not rely solely on sonography to make a diagnosis. Currently, the only way to make a *diagnosis* is by examining the lining cells under the microscope. Perhaps sonography will be accurate enough in the future to use alone to diagnose the cause of bleeding problems.

What Is the Best Treatment If the Bleeding Does Not Go Away?

For some women, the bleeding may persist even after hormonal treatments and the removal of the lining cells by the D&C. The cause of the continued bleeding may be subtle hormonal changes or changes in the uterine lining or muscle wall. After precancerous or cancerous cells have been ruled out by a D&C, one option is to do nothing. As long as the bleeding does not make you anemic, it is not dangerous from a medical perspective. And if the bleeding is not very bothersome, you may choose to live with it. On the other hand, if the bleeding causes severe anemia or is bothersome because it is extremely heavy or continuous, a new treatment called endometrial ablation may interest you. This procedure is appropriate only if you do not want to have children.

What Is an Endometrial Ablation?

Endometrial ablation is an outpatient surgical procedure used to stop or decrease bleeding from the uterus. Using electrical energy passed into the uterus at the end of a hysteroscope, the doctor burns and destroys the lining of the uterus (figs. 3.4a and b). The ovaries continue to make normal amounts of hormone, but without lining cells, bleeding cannot occur.

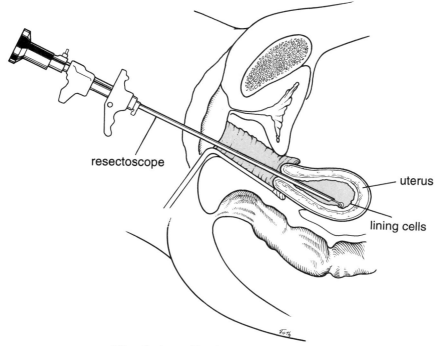

resectoscope

uterus

lining cells

Fig. 3.4a.   Endometrial ablation

All the lining cells are destroyed in 50 percent of the patients, and these women will never have another menstrual period. In 40 percent of women, a few lining cells are left behind, and these women will experience a light flow for a few days each month. No improvement is noted in 10 percent of women. Ninety percent of the women who have this procedure are extremely happy to be rid of the severe and debilitating monthly bleeding they previously had to endure. Women who have had an endometrial ablation are often my most satisfied patients. After surgery, they are able to return to normal activity and life unencumbered by the fatigue and inconvenience associated with heavy bleeding.

Endometrial ablation should be performed only on women who do not want to have children. Once the lining cells of the uterus are destroyed by the procedure, there is no place for a developing fetus to attach within the uterus. Despite this, it is best to use some form of contraception after the procedure. If some cells remain following endometrial ablation, there exists the rare possibility of pregnancy. In the few cases where pregnancy has occurred, termination has been recommended. Doctors are concerned that without adequate cells lining the inside of the uterus, the placenta would grow directly into the muscle wall of the uterus and take hold like the roots of a tree. As a result, the placenta would not be able to separate at the time of delivery, and hemorrhage could occur.

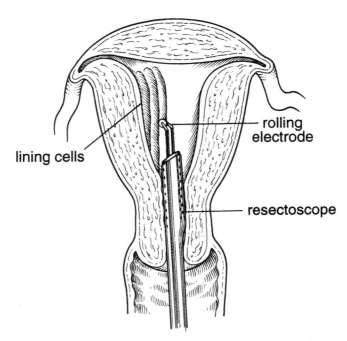

Fig. 3.4b.   Uterine lining cells destroyed

When Is a Hysterectomy Necessary for Abnormal Bleeding?

Hysterectomy should be performed for bleeding only as a last resort. After appropriate evaluation of the problem, hormonal treatment or a D&C will often stop abnormal bleeding. If this fails, you should consider endometrial ablation or, if you have fibroids, resectoscope myomectomy (see page 51). If all of these treatments fail, or if you or your doctor feel they are not appropriate for you, then hysterectomy may be a reasonable option. Recently, the Maine Women's Health Study (see page 281) found that women who had not responded to nonsurgical management of their bleeding were very satisfied with the relief of symptoms and change in quality of life following hysterectomy. Chapter 11 discusses hysterectomy.

What Can Be Done If You Have Uterine Precancer or Cancer?

If uterine precancer is found, treatment with high doses of progesterone may effectively change the cells back to normal. However, often hysterectomy is suggested as a way of removing the abnormal cells in order to prevent the development of cancer (see page 265). If cancer is present, hysterectomy will almost always be the recommended treatment (see page 257). If the cancer appears to be fast growing (the pathologist can see this under a microscope), or has spread deep within the muscle wall of the uterus, or has spread outside your uterus, more extensive surgery and/or radiation therapy will be required. Uterine precancer and cancer are discussed in chapter 10.

BLEEDING PROBLEMS AND PREGNANCY

What If You Are Pregnant and Have Bleeding?

About 20 percent of women with totally normal, healthy pregnancies will have some bleeding in the first three months. As the placenta burrows into the lining of the uterus seeking blood to supply the fetus, blood vessels may be disrupted and bleeding may result. Therefore, most women with light bleeding early in pregnancy should not be concerned. If the bleeding becomes heavy or if it is associated with bad cramping, then the possibility of miscarriage should be considered. At this point, an examination and perhaps a sonogram should be performed by your doctor to help determine whether a miscarriage is occurring. The small fluid-filled sac surrounding the developing fetus should be visible on the sonogram after about five weeks from your last normal menstrual period. If this sac is collapsing, then a miscarriage may be inevitable. Also, if no fetus is seen within the sac by the sixth week of pregnancy, a miscarriage may be likely.

In addition to the sonogram, the blood test measurement of HCG (the main hormone of pregnancy made by the placenta) can help make the diagnosis. If the pregnancy is continuing normally, the level of this hormone continues to rise in early pregnancy. If the pregnancy is destined to end in a miscarriage, then the HCG level starts to drop. Again, most bleeding in early pregnancy is normal and does not indicate a problem with the baby.

What Should Be Done If You Are Miscarrying?

Miscarriage is the body's way of expelling a pregnancy that is not developing properly. This is fairly common, occurring in about 15 percent of all pregnancies. Often miscarriage results from *nonhereditary* chromosomal abnormalities that occur by chance before or during fertilization of the egg. As a miscarriage proceeds, the uterus begins to contract and pushes the pregnancy tissue out through the cervix, causing cramping and bleeding. If you are pregnant and begin to bleed and cramp, then you should be examined by your doctor. The first thing the doctor will do is look at your cervix. If your cervix has dilated, then miscarriage is inevitable. Over the next hours or days the uterus will continue to contract to expel the tissue. On occasion, this process may be uncomfortable or associated with heavy bleeding. Sometimes the uterus may not fully empty, and a D&C may be necessary to completely remove any remaining tissue. Some women may choose to have a D&C as soon as the diagnosis of miscarriage is made in order to avoid prolonging the bleeding and cramping and insure that all the tissue is gone.

If your cervix is not dilated, then the diagnosis may not be certain. A sonogram or a test to measure pregnancy hormone levels in the blood can often establish whether this is a normal pregnancy, a miscarriage, or an ectopic pregnancy (see below). If the diagnosis of miscarriage is established, you may wish to have a D&C in order to avoid the inevitable bleeding and cramping associated with expelling the pregnancy tissue.

While the physical effects of a miscarriage may cause some discomfort, the emotional effects are usually much harder to deal with. The loss of a pregnancy is often accompanied by sadness and even depression. Having your partner, family, and close friends to talk to and cry with is important. Also, it is helpful to remember that having a miscarriage does not make it any less likely that you will be able to go on to have a healthy pregnancy.

Can Bleeding Mean You Have an Ectopic Pregnancy?

In a normal pregnancy, the fertilized egg implants itself inside the uterine cavity. In some women, however, the fertilized egg may not reach the uterus, and it starts to develop within the fallopian tube (see fig. 3.5). Scar tissue from a previous pelvic infection or endometriosis can block the tube. Other factors not yet well understood can slow the movement of the egg down a normal tube. At the time the egg is ready to implant, it is still in the fallopian tube and begins to grow there. The uterus has the remarkable ability to expand enormously with the growing fetus, but the fallopian tube can only grow to about the diameter of your thumb before it begins to tear. As times goes on, this causes pain on the side where the tube is located. The fallopian tube is not able to supply the placenta with adequate amounts of blood, and the placenta fails to develop properly. Without the support of the normal hormones of pregnancy from the placenta, the lining cells of the uterus break down, and bleeding results. If you think you are pregnant and have bleeding and pain, you should see your doctor.

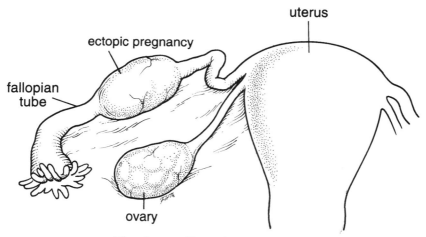

Fig. 3.5. Ectopic pregnancy

How Can the Doctor Tell If You Have an Ectopic Pregnancy?

Enormous advances have been made in the ability to diagnose an ectopic pregnancy early, before it tears the fallopian tube and causes serious bleeding inside the body. Ten years ago the diagnosis of an ectopic pregnancy was usually made only if a woman had a swollen, tender abdomen that had filled with blood as the pregnancy tore open the tube. With good medical care that situation is now a very rare occurrence. We are able to detect an ectopic pregnancy with blood tests and sonograms very early, before it tears the fallopian tube.

As a normal pregnancy develops, the placenta makes increasing amounts of the hormone HCG. If the level of pregnancy hormone does not continue to increase as expected, a miscarriage or ectopic pregnancy is suspected.

Five to six weeks after your last period, the amount of pregnancy hormone should be about 1,500 units or greater (this number may vary from lab to lab). At this point, the pregnancy can be seen as a fluid-filled sac within the uterus. If the level of HCG in the blood is greater than 1,500 units and the pregnancy cannot be seen within the uterus, the possibility of a pregnancy outside the uterus becomes more certain.

Sometimes the growth of the pregnancy in the fallopian tube will cause a tender swelling in the tube that can be felt on examination. However, since the tube and ovary lie so close together, it may be difficult for your doctor to tell whether this tender swelling is a tubal pregnancy or the corpus luteum, the normal ovarian cyst of pregnancy. A sonogram can often help to tell the difference. Using a combination of examination, pregnancy hormone blood tests, and sonogram, the diagnosis can usually be made long before the fallopian tube tears and starts to bleed.

What Are the Possible Treatments for an Ectopic Pregnancy?

Advances in the field of gynecology have totally changed the way we treat ectopic pregnancy. Ten years ago the only way to treat this problem was with major surgery; often the entire fallopian tube was removed along with the pregnancy it contained. A woman who had this type of surgery spent four or five days in the hospital and took six weeks to recover before she went back to normal activity.

One of the first applications of laparoscopic surgery was the removal of a tubal pregnancy. When the laparoscope is placed in the abdominal cavity, the enlarged fallopian tube can be seen. Using a small scissors or a laser, the doctor cuts open the tube and removes the pregnancy tissue. The open tube will heal by itself. The advantage of laparoscopic surgery is that women with ectopic pregnancies can usually go home a few hours after surgery and can return to normal activity within a week or so. Blood tests for HCG are performed following surgery to insure that all of the pregnancy tissue has been removed.

Lee Has an Ectopic Pregnancy

Lee is a twenty-eight-year-old woman who had been trying to get pregnant for about five months. When her period was a week late she went to the pharmacy and bought a home pregnancy test. Much to her dismay, the test came out negative. She felt fine and decided to wait and repeat the test in another week. Within a few days, she noted some light spotting and figured her period was about to start. The bleeding was unusual for her, though, because the spotting went on for a few days and never really turned into her normal flow. At this point she went to see her doctor.

Other than the fact that she was bleeding, Lee's examination was normal. A blood test for pregnancy hormone was performed and it was positive, but at a fairly low level—1,200 units. Lee's doctor explained that she was pregnant, but that the low level of hormone might just mean that the pregnancy was earlier than they thought. She also mentioned the possibility of either a miscarriage or a tubal pregnancy, although there was no evidence for either. Lee was instructed to call her doctor if she developed any heavier bleeding or pain in the pelvic or abdominal areas. She was also scheduled to come back to the doctor's office in two days for a repeat test of the level of pregnancy hormone. Lee was happy about being pregnant but anxious at the same time.

The level of pregnancy hormone just about doubles every forty-eight hours. A smaller rise or any fall in the level signifies either a miscarriage or an ectopic pregnancy. In two days, Lee's blood test came back as 1,700 units. It was higher than before but not as high as it should be, and her doctor ordered a sonogram. Although no pregnancy could be seen in the tube, none was seen in the uterus either. Because at this level of pregnancy hormone a normal pregnancy should have been seen in the uterus, her doctor suspected an ectopic pregnancy. Lee still felt fine and was shocked and upset that anything was wrong.

Because of the likelihood of a tubal pregnancy, Lee was scheduled for a laparoscopy the next day. At the time of surgery, it was clear that she had a tubal pregnancy. Her left fallopian tube was about twice as big as normal, and it was a somewhat darker shade of red than usual. An incision was made in the tube using a laser, and the pregnancy tissue, an unrecognizable clot of bloody tissue the size of a marble, was removed. The rest of the tube looked healthy, as did her other tube and both ovaries. The surgery was completed, and Lee went home that evening. While upset about the loss of her pregnancy, she was relieved that nothing more serious had developed. She was also relieved that the rest of her reproductive organs looked healthy and that future pregnancy was possible.

Bleeding during the first three months of pregnancy is very common and usually does not indicate any problem. However, you should let your doctor know if any bleeding does occur.

What Is the Current Research Regarding Treatment of Ectopic Pregnancy?

In the past few years, an attempt has been made to treat ectopic pregnancies with medication only instead of surgery. A drug called methotrexate had been very successfully used to treat a rare cancer of placental tissue called gestational trophoblastic disease. The drug was so successful that it changed the survival rate for this cancer from about 10 percent in 1965 to almost 100 percent today. Most of the tissue that develops in the tube during an ectopic pregnancy is placental, so researchers felt that perhaps this tissue could be destroyed by methotrexate as well. The drug was tried originally in women who had surgery for an ectopic pregnancy and were later found to have a positive pregnancy test, signaling that not all the pregnancy tissue had been removed. After treatment with methotrexate, the remaining placental tissue was destroyed, and the pregnancy hormone levels went down to zero. Recently, methotrexate has been used to treat early ectopic pregnancies detected by sonogram and blood tests without surgery. The preliminary results are very good, and there are virtually no side effects with the small doses used.

PAINFUL PERIODS

How Common Are Painful Periods (Dysmenorrhea)?

Nearly 50 percent of all women have some degree of pain associated with their periods. About 10 percent of adult women are unable to perform their normal activities because of this pain, and 50 percent of young women miss school for this reason. Painful periods, or dysmenorrhea, can occur at any age. They are uncommon in the first six months after the onset of menstrual periods and relatively uncommon in the years prior to menopause. The most common ages for this problem to occur are in the late teens or early twenties.

What Symptoms Can Occur with Painful Periods?

Dysmenorrhea is cyclical, with pain most often occurring just before or during the first few days of each period. Women with dysmenorrhea often feel sharp, crampy pain below the pubic area, but some may also have pain in the back or down the thighs. A few women have such intense pain that they feel weak and may even feel close to passing out. And some women may also have nausea, vomiting, or diarrhea associated with their painful periods.

What Are the Causes of Painful Periods?

Dysmenorrhea refers only to the pain accompanying a period. While sometimes associated with premenstrual syndrome or PMS (the cyclical change in *mood* associated with a period), the two conditions are not necessarily connected. The symptoms may occur together, but some women have painful periods without mood changes, and other women have mood changes without painful periods.

Most menstruating women have uterine contractions of moderate strength that each last for less than thirty seconds and occur about every three to five minutes. Women who experience severe dysmenorrhea have cramps that last up to ninety seconds with only a few seconds of rest in between. And the strength of the contraction may be up to five times greater than normal.

We now know that dysmenorrhea results from the release of a chemical substance called prostaglandin from the lining cells of the uterus at the time of the menstrual period. The prostaglandin causes contractions of the muscle wall of the uterus that are called menstrual cramps. In fact, if you give prostaglandin to a woman by injection, severe menstrual cramps result. Prostaglandin is used to help start labor contractions in women who, for medical reasons, need to deliver their babies promptly.

Women who have dysmenorrhea produce more prostaglandin in the lining cells of the uterus than woman who do not have cramps. And when the increased amount of prostaglandin is released at the time of the period, stronger uterine contractions are the result. New medications are available that prevent the formation of prostaglandins in the uterus and thus can prevent or decrease menstrual cramps.

How Is the Diagnosis of Dysmenorrhea Made?

Because menstrual cramps are the result of an increased amount of a chemical, there is nothing abnormal for your doctor to feel on your examination. Therefore, the diagnosis of dysmenorrhea can be made by the history of cramping in the presence of a normal pelvic examination. If the pain is severe, it is a good idea to have an examination in order to be sure that other causes of pelvic pain, such as endometriosis (see page 157) or adenomyosis (see page 52), are not present. And unless another condition is suspected, tests such as a sonogram, CT scan (three-dimensional X ray), MRI, or blood work are unnecessary.

What Is the Best Treatment for Painful Periods?

Medications called *n*onsteroidal *a*nti-*i*nflammatory *d*rugs (NSAIDs) work extremely well to control cramps in about 75 percent of women with dysmenorrhea. The medications work by preventing the formation of prostaglandins in the uterine-lining cells. They are more effective if taken before the prostaglandins are formed and *before* the onset of cramps. The pills should be taken *every* six to eight hours (depending on the type of medication) beginning the day before you anticipate the start of the cramps or the day before your period is expected. The pills should be continued until the day after your cramps would normally disappear. If you cannot tell when your period is about to begin, the medication should be started the moment bleeding starts. If you wait until you have cramps, the prostaglandins have already been formed, and the medication may be less helpful.

If you do not get relief from one type of the many NSAIDs available, switching to another may provide relief. Most of these medications are now available over the counter in the form of Advil, Aleve, ibuprofen, etc. Discuss the proper dose and schedule of taking these pills with your doctor.

Birth control pills are another effective way to decrease or even prevent dysmenorrhea. Prostaglandin is produced in the uterine-lining cells and released when the cells begin to disintegrate prior to the menstrual period. The hormone progesterone, present in all birth control pills, makes the uterine-lining cells thinner. As a result, many women on the pill note that their periods are lighter and shorter. But because the cells are thinner, they also produce less prostaglandin. And less prostaglandin means less dysmenorrhea. Accordingly, if you take birth control pills, you may find a dramatic decrease in menstrual cramps. For some women with severe dysmenorrhea, a combination of birth control pills and NSAIDs may be very helpful in controlling the pain of menstrual periods.

Leslie's Painful Periods

Leslie is a twenty-two-year-old woman who had been bothered by painful periods for as long as she could remember. When she was in high school, she had tried over-the-counter remedies for menstrual cramps, but none had been helpful. Over the past few years, she had used increasingly stronger pain medications, and now was fairly dependent on narcotic drugs to get her through those few days every month. She was not happy to be taking these medications but couldn't make it out of her house without them during her periods.

Leslie's pelvic examination was totally normal. I was concerned about her need for narcotics and the potential for addiction and discussed other possible medical treatments for dysmenorrhea with her. Leslie had never taken birth control pills for the cramps, and because she was not sexually active, she was embarrassed and a little reluctant to start taking them now. Therefore, I recommended that Leslie stop using the narcotics and begin to take four Advil (800 milligrams) every six hours, starting the day before her period. I recommended she try this for two months and then call to tell me how she was doing. She agreed.

When she called two months later, she said that she had noted some relief from the Advil, but was still having a lot of discomfort from her periods and still needed to stay in bed for a few days each month. I suggested that she again consider taking birth control pills to help with the pain, and she agreed. After two months of taking the pill, Leslie noted a marked decrease in her pain, but not complete relief. Finally, we had her continue to take the pill along with Advil for the first few days of her period. She now has almost no cramping and has totally tolerable periods for the first time in her life. She is able to work and take part in all of her regular activities every day of the month and has not needed to take narcotics again for pain relief.

Can Homeopathic and Herbal Therapies Be Used for Period Pain?

A number of homeopathic and herbal therapies have been used to treat dysmenorrhea. Tea made from chamomilla may be effective, as may be pulsatilla. Herbs such as cramp bark, rosemary, black haw, kava kava, and lobelia used in combination may bring relief. The type of homeopathic or herbal therapy prescribed depends on the symptoms experienced and your general health. Eight hundred milligrams of calcium, the amount found in three cups of milk or yogurt, and magnesium, found in whole grains, tofu, and vegetables, may also be used to relieve cramps.

Can Acupuncture Be Used to Treat Painful Periods?

Acupuncture has been shown to reduce menstrual pain. Following the use of acupuncture twice a week for six weeks, pain relief may last as long as six months. As always, it is best to find an experienced practitioner. Your doctor may be able to recommend someone.

Can Surgery Help Period Pain?

For women who experience severe menstrual pain that is not relieved by medication, interrupting the nerves that "feel" pain from the uterus can be attempted with a surgical procedure called presacral neurectomy. It is performed by a gynecologist, usually through an abdominal incision, although laparoscopic techniques have recently been developed. Fortunately, cutting these nerves does not interfere with any other function of the uterus, fallopian tubes, or ovaries, including sexual response or the ability to get pregnant, go into labor, and have a normal delivery. In addition, it will not mask the pain from appendicitis or other serious conditions for which pain is a warning signal. Because surgery entails risk, time, and expense, it is appropriate only for those women who have not had relief from other methods of treatment.

What If Your Pain Occurs in the Middle of the Cycle?

Ovulation occurs around the middle of the menstrual cycle, and an egg is released from the ovary into the fallopian tube. The fluid that normally surrounds the egg as it develops is also released at this time. If a large amount of fluid has formed, its release may irritate the inside lining cells of the body, causing pain. This pain has been called *mittelschmerz*, which in German means pain in the middle (of the cycle).

The irritation from the fluid may even lead to a low fever (100°F.) and nausea. The fluid is usually quickly reabsorbed by the body, and the pain and other symptoms should resolve over a few hours or a day. The key to making this diagnosis is the description of sudden onset of pain in the middle of your cycle along with the findings of a slightly tender but otherwise normal pelvic exam. If the diagnosis is uncertain, a sonogram may confirm that fluid is present behind the uterus. Rest and mild analgesics should get you through until the pain goes away. Resting in bed will stop the fluid from moving around inside you and reduce the irritation.

REFERENCES

Cumming, D., C. Cumming, and D. Kieren. 1991. Menstrual mythology and sources of information about menstruation. *American Journal of Obstetrics and Gynecology* 164:472–76.

Duffy, J. 1979. *The Healers—A History of American Medicine.* Chicago: University of Illinois Press.

Ehrenreich, B., and D. English. 1978. *For Her Own Good—150 Years of the Experts' Advice to Women.* Garden City, N.Y.: Anchor Press.

Falk, R. 1994. Ovarian malfunction: when is it exercise induced? *Contemporary Ob/Gyn* October: 187–93.

Kustin, J., and R. Rebar. 1985. Addressing the concerns of amenorrheic athletes. *Contemporary Ob/Gyn.*

Neistein, L. 1985. Menstrual dysfunction in pathophysiologic states. *Western Journal of Medicine* 143:476–84.

Shangold, M. 1985. Factors affecting menstrual flow. *Comtemporary Ob/Gyn* April: 73–81.

Spiroff, L., R. Glass, and N. Kase. 1994. *Clinical Gynecologic Endocrinology and Infertility.* Baltimore: Williams and Wilkins, pp. 183–230.

4

IF YOU HAVE OVARIAN CYSTS

What Are Ovarian Cysts?

An ovarian cyst is simply a collection of fluid within the normally solid ovary. There are many different types of ovarian cysts, and they are an extremely common gynecologic problem. Because of the fear of ovarian cancer, cysts are a common cause of concern among women, but it is important to know that the vast majority of ovarian cysts are *not* cancer. However, some benign cysts will require treatment because they do not go away by themselves, and in quite rare cases some may be cancerous. A cyst may cause discomfort or may be discovered at the time of a routine examination, when you are feeling absolutely fine. The good news is that almost all ovarian cysts are benign and will go away by themselves without any treatment.

What Are the Different Types of Ovarian Cysts?

Ovarian cysts can be divided into two categories: those that go away by themselves versus those that need treatment, and those that are benign versus those that are cancer. Most cysts are benign and will go away by themselves. The distinction that is most important to your health and well-being is whether the cyst is cancerous or benign. Cancerous cysts should be removed as soon as possible. Benign cysts that will not go away by themselves may also need to be removed to prevent further problems. The following chart lists the different types of cysts, and it may be helpful if you refer back to it as you read this chapter. Further explanations of each type of cyst are included later in this chapter.

Cysts That Usually Go Away by Themselves

Benign	*Cancerous*
follicular	none
corpus luteum	
hemorrhagic	

Cysts That Do Not Go Away by Themselves

Benign	*Cancerous*
endometriomas	epithelial cancers
epithelial—serous,	germ cell cancers
mucinous	
dermoid	

What Causes Most Ovarian Cysts?

The most common types of ovarian cysts are *functional cysts*, which result from a collection of fluid forming around a developing egg. Every woman who is ovulating will form a small amount of fluid around the developing egg each month. The combination of the egg, the special fluid-producing cells, and the fluid is called a *follicle* and is normally about the size of a pea. For unknown reasons, the cells that surround the egg occasionally form too much fluid, and this straw-colored fluid expands the ovary from within. If the collection of fluid gets to be larger than a normal follicle, about three-quarters of an inch in diameter, a *follicular cyst* is present (see fig. 4.1). If fluid continues to form, the ovary is stretched like a balloon being filled up with water. The normally white covering of the ovary becomes thin and smooth and appears bluish-gray. Follicular cysts as large as 3 or 4 inches are rare. The majority of these cysts, even the large ones, go away after a month or two as the extra fluid dissolves back into the bloodstream.

At the time of ovulation, the covering of the ovary tears open in order to release the egg. Within hours, this covering heals, and the cells in the ovary form a structure called the corpus luteum. The corpus luteum produces progesterone, the hormone that prepares the uterine-lining cells for the arrival of the fertilized egg. Every menstruating woman forms a corpus luteum every month. However, cells can produce fluid within the corpus luteum and form a cyst. A *corpus luteum cyst* is usually no larger than a small marble, but sometimes so much fluid is produced that a cyst of a few inches results. The good news is that most corpus luteum cysts will go away by themselves in a few weeks. Follicular cysts and corpus luteum cysts are collectively referred to as functional cysts.

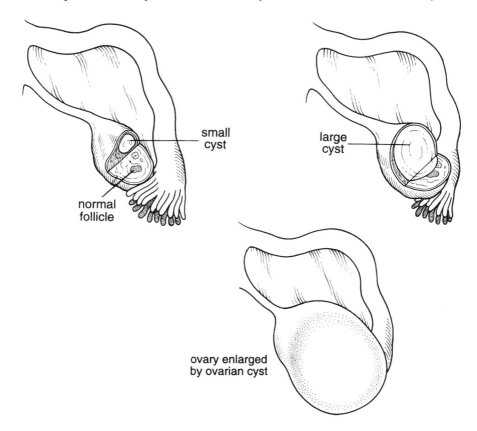

small cyst

normal follicle

large cyst

ovary enlarged by ovarian cyst

Fig. 4.1.   Ovarian cysts

Other types of ovarian cysts can form as a result of the abnormal growth of other cells contained in the ovary. These cysts are less common and are discussed later in this chapter.

If You Are Prone to Developing Functional Ovarian Cysts, Is There Anything You Can Do?

If you have recurrent functional cysts (follicular or corpus luteum), you may want to consider preventing the formation of new cysts, especially if they cause you pain. Since functional ovarian cysts are related to the process of ovulation, anything that stops the development of a new egg will decrease the likelihood of cyst formation. Birth control pills prevent pregnancy by preventing both the development of an egg and ovulation; therefore, they are an excellent way to reduce the risk of forming follicular and corpus luteum cysts, although they will not make an already formed cyst go away. There are many types of birth control pills. A recent study showed that the higher-dose estrogen pills were more effective in preventing the formation of new cysts. However, these pills may cause a few more side effects in some women, such as breast tenderness or weight gain, but may be worth a try because of their greater effectiveness than very-low-dose pills.

Gail's Recurrent Cysts

Gail is a twenty-four-year-old emergency room nurse. She called me late one night to report the sudden onset of pain in her lower abdomen. She had been fine all day but now was having trouble walking because of the pain. I met her at the emergency room. She was visibly uncomfortable, and examining her was difficult because of the pain. A sonogram showed a cyst in her ovary and about a half-cup of fluid floating around near the ovary. This was pretty good evidence that she had ruptured an ovarian cyst. Reassured that nothing more serious was happening, she decided to go home and back to bed. Within two days, the fluid had dissolved back into her bloodstream, and Gail was feeling fine and able to return to work. However, one month later she had exactly the same experience. When she had pain again for the third month in a row, we decided to perform a laparoscopy to make sure we weren't missing anything. The laparoscopy showed a benign ovarian cyst that had ruptured, just as we had expected. After the laparoscopy, Gail and I talked about ways to prevent this from happening again. Since she had endured three painful cysts and a laparoscopy, she was already dreading what would happen next month. We discussed the use of birth control pills, which she agreed to start immediately. She has been taking the pills for a few years and has not had another ovarian cyst.

What Are the Symptoms of Ovarian Cysts?

Many cysts cause no symptoms at all, but pressure or pain in the pelvic area is a common problem that may prompt a woman with an ovarian cyst to see her doctor. As fluid collects in a cyst, making the ovary expand, the covering of the ovary is stretched. This stretching can trigger discomfort or pain. The fluid within the cyst can weigh down the ovary, causing a pulling sensation when a woman moves. In very rare cases, the covering of the ovary tears opens, or ruptures, releasing the cyst fluid into the abdominal cavity. A ruptured ovarian cyst is usually painful.

Jane's Painful Ovarian Cyst

Jane is a twenty-five-year-old woman who felt some pain on the right side of her lower abdomen one morning when she awoke. The pain was mild at first, but then became more bothersome over the next few days. It seemed to be worse when she was walking or being active and was better when she was still. Even though her job as a secretary allowed her to sit much of the day, the pain bothered her when she had to get up from her desk and lift or move things. She made an appointment to come to our office. During the pelvic examination, a small cyst about the size of a walnut was felt on her right ovary. The cyst was slightly tender when touched during the examination. We performed a sonogram, which suggested a simple follicular-type cyst. Jane's discomfort was not too bad overall, and she was reassured that nothing serious was going on. I suggested that she limit her activity at work to avoid aggravating the discomfort. She made an appointment for another examination in two weeks, with instructions to call if the discomfort got worse. Two weeks later she came back to the office feeling fine, and the examination showed that the cyst was already entirely dissolved. Jane was relieved and has not had another cyst.

Can an Ovarian Cyst Cause Severe Pain?

In rare cases, an ovarian cyst can twist the ovary all the way around. This condition is called ovarian torsion. The twisting prevents the flow of blood to the ovary, and the cells in the ovary begin to deteriorate, releasing chemicals that cause severe pain. Often the pain is so bad that you are not able to stand up straight, and in that case emergency surgery may be needed.

Sometimes the diagnosis is not entirely clear, but surgery is recommended in order to discover the cause of the pain and correct it. At the time of surgery, the doctor can see the twisted ovary, which is usually discolored from the lack of blood. If caught early, the ovary can be untwisted, the cyst can be removed, and the remaining healthy portion of the ovary can be saved. If not caught early, the ovarian cells may die, necessitating removal of the entire ovary. If you have a painful cyst, it is unlikely that it is ovarian torsion, which is a very rare occurrence. See your physician if you experience acute of persistent pelvic or abdominal pain.

Sara's Laparoscopy for Her Ovarian Cyst

Sara is a thirty-five-year-old woman who felt a pain on her right side that was strong enough to awaken her from a sound sleep. She noticed that if she turned toward her right, the pain was better, but if she turned to the left, it became more intense and sharper. She called the office, and we asked her to come right in. The examination was difficult because she was so uncomfortable, but it felt like her right ovary was enlarged to the size of a lemon. A sonogram was performed and showed a large ovarian cyst that was filled entirely with fluid and appeared benign. Unfortunately, Sara was in so much pain that she was crying and couldn't move. She and I agreed that immediate surgery should be performed to relieve her discomfort.

We chose to perform a laparoscopy (see page 106) so that we could examine the ovary first and determine what the problem was without making a large abdominal incision. In the hospital, with Sara under general anesthesia, a small telescope was placed through a half-inch incision in her navel in order to look into her abdominal and pelvic areas. During the laparoscopy, we found a large ovarian cyst that was twisted around itself, causing her all the pain. We were able to safely untwist the ovary and then remove the cyst.

Sara felt better immediately after surgery. The sharp pain was gone, and despite being groggy from the anesthesia, she was able to go home that afternoon. Since laparoscopic surgery uses small incisions, the postoperative pain is usually much less than it is with an abdominal incision. At the time of her two-week postoperative visit, Sara was feeling entirely normal and had already returned to work and exercise.

Can an Ovarian Cyst Destroy the Normal Ovary?

The ovary has a remarkable ability to expand without damage to the small eggs contained within its tissue. As an ovarian cyst develops, the normal ovarian tissue containing the eggs spreads out over the cyst. If the cyst goes away by itself, as most of them do, then the ovary shrinks to its normal size over a period of a few weeks without any residual effects. If the cyst needs to be surgically removed, we try to leave as much normal ovarian tissue as possible so that the ovary can heal with healthy eggs remaining. Even with large cysts—those that are more than three inches in diameter—some normal ovarian tissue can usually be saved. The ovaries contain hundreds of thousands of eggs, so the loss of a small number should not make any difference in your fertility or the age at which your menopause will begin.

Can a Cyst Interfere with Your Menstrual Cycle?

The ovaries produce estrogen and progesterone, the hormones that regulate your menstrual cycle. Therefore, when the ovary is disrupted by an ovarian cyst, it may not produce hormones normally, and the result can be abnormal periods. The bleeding may be heavy or light, long or short, or irregular. Abnormal amounts of hormone can cause water retention, breast swelling or tenderness, and even PMS-type symptoms. Once the cyst resolves, your periods and body should return to normal within a cycle or two. As always, if you have abnormal bleeding, you should contact your physician.

Can a Cyst Cause Infertility?

There are two types of cystic conditions that are associated with infertility: the cysts of endometriosis and polycystic ovarian disease. If endometriosis cells get inside the ovary, they will cause blood to collect within the ovary itself, forming an ovarian cyst called an endometrioma. Endometriosis can interfere with a woman's fertility, although the reasons for this are not entirely clear. Current theories suggest that the endometriosis cells produce chemicals that interfere with either the ovary's ability to release the egg or the sperm's ability to fertilize the egg.

In addition, if the endometriosis is severe, bands of scar tissue may form that block the passage of the egg into and down the fallopian tube. Endometriosis is discussed in chapter 6.

Polycystic ovarian disease (PCO), also known as Stein-Leventhal syndrome, is the result of hormonal changes that are associated with infertility. That is to say, the cysts are not the cause of infertility, but rather result from the same problem that causes the infertility. This condition is discussed on page 66. The most common symptom of PCO is infrequent periods. Notable acne, oily skin, and obesity are other symptoms. As the hormonal abnormalities become established, the ovary forms multiple small cysts (about one-quarter inch) that can make the ovaries two or three times larger than normal. These small cysts often can be detected by sonography.

The drug clomiphene is used to treat infertility associated with PCO. This medication fixes the hormonal imbalance long enough for the ovary to produce and release an egg. Clomiphene causes minimal side effects, and it must be taken for a few days every month until you get pregnant. The success rate is fairly good: about 60 percent of women get pregnant. If pregnancy does not occur in the first three months of using clomiphene, other treatments should be tried, such as a new procedure that uses a laser aimed through a laparoscope to puncture the cysts. This technique temporarily brings hormone levels back to normal and often reestablishes ovulation.

How Are Ovarian Cysts Diagnosed?

At the time of a pelvic exam, your doctor will feel next to the sides of the uterus, where the ovaries are located. Normal ovaries are no larger than a small walnut. But if a cyst forms, the ovary can swell a few inches or more. The doctor is often able to feel a cyst as a soft, movable lump. Most cysts feel alike to the physician. Sometimes they are tender, but often they cause no discomfort or pain, and you may be surprised to find out that you have a cyst.

If you are not menopausal and the cyst is not bothersome, nothing needs to be done, because most of these cysts will go away by themselves. A repeat examination can be scheduled in two or three weeks to make sure that the cyst is dissolving. If the cyst is gone by that time, no further treatment or follow-up is needed. If the cyst is still present at the follow-up visit, I usually order a pelvic sonogram. This test can help to determine the type of cyst present in order to plan further treatment.

What Can a Sonogram Show?

The most accurate way to get a picture of the ovary and cyst is with a vaginal sonogram. A small instrument passed comfortably into the vagina bounces harmless sound waves off your uterus, fallopian tubes, and ovaries, forming a picture on a monitor. A sonogram allows the doctor to accurately determine the size of the cyst and to "see" inside it in order to detect whether it is filled with fluid or solid areas. This can help determine the type of cyst. Depending on which cells in the ovary are overgrowing, certain types of ovarian cysts will make fairly reliable patterns on a sonogram (see fig. 4.2).

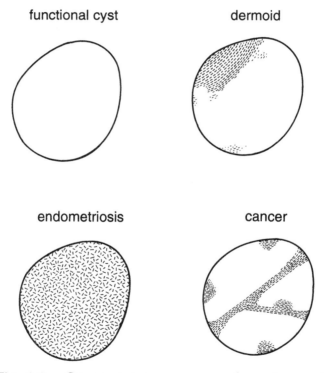

functional cyst

dermoid

endometriosis

cancer

Fig. 4.2.   Sonogram appearance of ovarian cysts

On the sonogram, functional cysts usually appear entirely clear in the middle with smooth walls. The cyst of endometriosis looks like a circle with speckles (blood) floating within. A dermoid cyst (see page 103) may have very white areas, representing the sound waves bouncing off the calcium in teeth or bone. A hemorrhagic cyst (see page 102) often has thick areas of blood clot within the cyst that dissolve in a few weeks. Abnormal cysts often have an overgrowth of cells that stick out from the inside of the cyst wall, making the inside of the cyst appear jagged on the sonogram. Many of these irregularly shaped cysts are benign, but cancer can also appear this way, and, unfortunately, the sonogram cannot be used to make a definite diagnosis. If the sonogram shows solid areas within a cyst, surgery will be needed to remove it, in order to rule out ovarian cancer.

If You Have a Cyst, Should You Have a CT Scan or MRI?

Some doctors may recommend a CT (computer tomography) scan or MRI (magnetic resonance imaging) to get a "better" look at an ovarian cyst. However, neither the CT scan, which is a high-tech X ray, nor the MRI, which uses magnetic forces to form a picture, can give more helpful information than a sonogram. In addition, both of these tests are five or six times as expensive as a sonogram. The CT or MRI may be helpful in diagnosing a dermoid or hemorrhagic cyst if the sonogram result is uncertain. But no test can flawlessly predict benign or cancerous cysts, and surgery will be required to remove any questionable cyst so that a definite diagnosis can be made.

If You Have a Cyst, Should You Get a CA-125 Test?

The CA-125 blood test was developed in an attempt to detect ovarian cancer at a very early stage. Theoretically, cancer cells should produce chemicals that differ from those produced by normal cells. The hope was that these different chemicals could be detected in the blood, and cancer found before it spread. However, these hopes have not been fulfilled. Unfortunately, the CA-125 test received a lot of inaccurate publicity following the sad death of comedienne Gilda Radner from ovarian cancer. Many press reports suggested that *all* women have the CA-125 blood test as a preliminary test for ovarian cancer in order to make an early diagnosis. But the CA-125 is a terrible test for determining who has ovarian cancer in premenopausal women.

In addition, studies showed that in women under the age of fifty who had an ovarian cyst and an abnormal CA-125 result, no cancer was present 65 percent of the time, meaning the test was inaccurate. Conditions commonly found in younger women, such as endometriosis, fibroids, pelvic infections, benign cysts, and pregnancy, can lead to erroneous abnormal results. Perfectly healthy women can have an abnormal CA-125 value as a result of normal variations that occur with the menstrual cycle. Needless to say, getting such a test result would scare you and your doctor. Unfortunately, this fear often leads the patient into unnecessary surgery with all of its attendant risks, expense, and time needed for recovery. Therefore, I feel strongly that the CA-125 test should *not* be done in women younger than fifty who have an ovarian cyst.

The CA-125 test is somewhat more accurate for menopausal women who have an ovarian cyst. For those women, a normal test is reassuring, and an abnormal test still does not mean that ovarian cancer is present. However, the cyst must be removed in order to be sure that there is no cancer. A great deal of research, time, and money are currently being devoted to finding a method of early detection for ovarian cancer; unfortunately, we do not have the answer yet (see chapter 8).

What Is an Epithelial Ovarian Cyst?

The ovary contains many types of cells that are able to form growths within the ovary. At the time of ovulation, the ovary bursts open to release the egg, leaving behind a hollow, raw area inside. Sometimes the epithelial cells that make up the outside coating of the ovary get trapped inside the hollow area as it heals. The trapped cells may form fluid that collects within the ovary and produces an epithelial cyst. There are two types of epithelial cells and thus two types of epithelial cysts. One type, called serous cells, produces a clear, straw-colored fluid within the cyst. The other, called mucinous cells, produces a thick mucous fluid. Because the epithelial cells are trapped within the ovary, they must be removed in order to stop the production of the fluid and prevent further growth of the cyst. Unfortunately, there is no way to treat epithelial cysts other than to remove them surgically.

What Is a Hemorrhagic Cyst of the Ovary?

Sometimes during the growth of a follicular or corpus luteum cyst, the tissue within the ovary tears as it is stretched and begins to bleed. Like the fluid from the cyst itself, this blood becomes trapped within the ovary. This is called a hemorrhagic cyst. Because the bleeding may occur quickly, it can rapidly stretch the covering of the ovary and result in pain. As the blood collects within the ovary, it begins to form clots that can be seen on a sonogram. This type of cyst will almost always go away by itself, but it may take a few weeks. Waiting is fine if you feel well, but in rare cases the cyst causes so much discomfort that it may be desirable to remove it by surgery.

Sandy's Painful Ovarian Cyst

Sandy is a thirty-seven-year-old woman who was awakened from sleep one night with a sharp pain on her left side. The pain persisted during the night, and she came to the office first thing in the morning. Upon examination, I could feel a swelling in her left ovary. This ovary was also fairly tender when I touched it. Because of her discomfort, we performed a sonogram immediately. The sonogram showed a fluid-filled cyst, but there were some other shadows on the picture that looked like clotted blood. It seemed pretty clear that Sandy had a hemorrhagic cyst, which usually would go away by itself. We discussed whether she would be comfortable enough to stay off her feet for a few days until this cyst settled down. The only other alternative was surgery, and Sandy was naturally not too happy about that. We agreed to do nothing for a while and see how she felt in a few days. She spent the next few days in bed and came back to the office feeling slightly better. We repeated the sonogram, which showed a slightly smaller cyst and some shrinking of the blood clots inside the cyst. Within a few more days Sandy was feeling better and was able to go back to work. It took about one month for the cyst to go away entirely. The sonogram had helped Sandy avoid surgery.

What Is a Dermoid Cyst?

The idea of a dermoid cyst is somewhat startling. The ovary contains eggs that, when fertilized, have the ability to form a human being. However, for reasons we don't understand, the cells of the ovary can all by themselves, without the presence of any sperm, start to produce hair, teeth, fluid, and other growing tissues to form a cyst. When removed during surgery, these tissues are clearly seen within the cyst, which is called a dermoid cyst. Dermoid cysts are fairly common, occurring most often before menopause, and are almost never cancerous (less than one in one thousand).

Because of all the unusual types of cells within these cysts, a fairly characteristic appearance can be seen on a sonogram, and often the diagnosis can be made just from this test. Unfortunately, these cysts do not go away by themselves. If dermoid cysts are not removed, they can continue to grow and may crowd out the normal cells to the point where no healthy ovary remains. In rare cases, the cyst can cause the ovary to twist around and stop the flow of blood to the ovary, causing severe pain and the need for emergency surgery. Therefore, these cysts should be surgically removed.

Can Endometriosis Cause an Ovarian Cyst?

At the time of the monthly menstrual flow, the lining cells of the uterus are normally shed through the cervix into the vagina. In some women these cells go out the wrong way, through the fallopian tubes, and end up in the abdominal cavity. If these cells survive, they may attach to the outside of the uterus, tubes, or ovaries and begin to grow. This is called endometriosis (see chapter 6). During subsequent menstrual cycles, these cells are stimulated to grow and bleed just as the lining cells within the uterus continue to do.

If endometrial cells get trapped within the ovary, the blood has nowhere to go, so it collects within the ovary, forming a cyst called an endometrioma. As the blood ages within the cyst, it becomes dark brown and thick, with a strong resemblance to chocolate syrup. For this reason, endometriosis of the ovary has been referred to as a chocolate cyst. The pattern of this old blood looks distinctive on a sonogram, so the diagnosis can often be made by that test. Sometimes endometriosis within the ovary causes pain, but it may also be painless and only discovered at the time of a routine examination. If endometriosis forms in one ovary, it may also be present near the uterus, fallopian tubes, and other ovary. While this condition is not dangerous, endometriosis can lead to pelvic pain and/or infertility and should be appropriately treated. The treatment of endometriosis of the ovary involves removal of the cyst, often by laparoscopic surgery (see chapter 6).

Do Benign Ovarian Cysts Become Cancerous?

We really do not understand ovarian cancer very well, and we certainly do not know what causes it. The evidence seems to indicate benign cysts do *not* turn into cancerous cysts, so if you have an ovarian cyst that seems to be benign upon exam and on a sonogram, waiting for it to go away for two months or so is not risky. There is also no evidence to suggest that women who form benign ovarian cysts are any more likely to develop ovarian cancer than women who have not had cysts.

What Types of Cysts Are Cancerous?

Ovarian cancer is a rare disease. Only one out of every 15,000 women will have the disease at the age of thirty. At forty, only one of every 10,000 women have this disease, and at age sixty, only one of every 1,500 women will have it. Therefore, if a premenopausal woman has a cyst in her ovary, the odds are overwhelming that it is benign. Even in postmenopausal women, an ovarian cyst has more than a 70 percent chance of being benign. Therefore, if a cyst is found on your ovary, it is most likely a *benign* ovarian cyst. However, cancer can develop in the ovary, and its diagnosis and treatment are discussed fully in chapter 8.

TREATMENT FOR OVARIAN CYSTS

The appropriate treatment for an ovarian cyst depends on the type of cyst present, the symptoms you have, and whether you are pre- or post-menopausal. As noted before, if you are premenopausal, if you are not having bothersome symptoms, and if your cyst appears benign on a sonogram, watchful waiting will often allow it to dissolve by itself within four to ten weeks. However, if your symptoms are very bothersome or the cyst appears suspicious for malignancy, then it should be removed.

As discussed earlier, during the normal menstrual cycle small collections of fluid routinely surround developing eggs, and these functional cysts are common. No eggs develop after menopause, and therefore no functional cysts should form. When a cyst forms after menopause, it should be removed to determine what type of cyst it is and to make sure cancer is not present.

Should You Take Birth Control Pills to Make Your Ovarian Cyst Go Away?

The short answer is no. In 1973, a study was published that included 286 premenopausal women with ovarian cysts who were placed on the pill for six weeks and then reexamined. The pill was used because the doctor who performed the study felt it would help to stop ovulation and quiet down the ovary. After treatment with the pill, 90 percent of the cysts disappeared, and the doctor concluded that the pill was the reason why. Unfortunately, the study did not have a control group of women who had cysts but were not treated with the pill. Twenty years later, a study was done that included a group of women not treated with anything. Interestingly, just as many women had their cysts disappear without taking the pill. The conclusion: If the cyst is going to disappear it will do so by itself. Consequently, we no longer use the pill to treat a premenopausal woman who is found to have an ovarian cyst. However, the pill can be used to prevent new ovarian cysts from forming (see page 95).

When Is Surgery Needed for an Ovarian Cyst?

Surgery may be considered necessary if a cyst appears suspicious for cancer on the sonogram, if it causes severe pain, if it continues to grow, or if it does not go away in eight weeks. A number of studies show that cysts that persist longer than eight weeks without decreasing in size have a greater likelihood of being abnormal. This does not mean cancer, but rather an abnormal growth of cells within the ovary that will never go away. If left in place, these cysts may continue to grow and cause discomfort or twist the ovary around and destroy it. In very rare instances (less than 5 percent), these cysts may be cancerous, and early detection and removal are important.

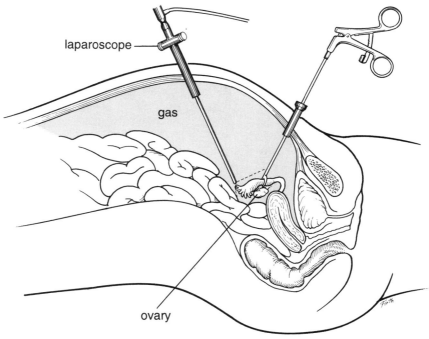

laparoscope

gas

ovary

Fig. 4.3.   Laparoscopy

Can Laparoscopic Surgery Be Used to Treat an Ovarian Cyst?

Instruments are now available that enable the gynecologist to remove a cyst through small incisions in the abdomen. This type of procedure, known as laparoscopic surgery, provides the benefits of outpatient surgery and a quick recovery. Using a telescope placed through the navel and small instruments placed near the pubic bone, the gynecologic surgeon can remove either the cyst alone or the entire ovary.

An ovarian cyst, which looks like a small balloon filled with water, grows from within the ovary and stretches the normal ovarian tissue over it. Removal of the cyst, called a cystectomy, is like taking a clam out of its shell. The thinned-out ovarian tissue is cut open, and the cyst is gently peeled away from inside the ovary (see fig. 4.4). The cyst fluid is then removed with a suction device. The cyst now looks like a deflated balloon and can be easily removed through the small laparoscopy incision. Sometimes the normal part of the ovary that remains needs to be sutured closed, and there are special instruments the surgeon can use to do this. Because recent studies show that the ovary may heal better if it is left alone, we allow the ovary to heal by itself in most situations.

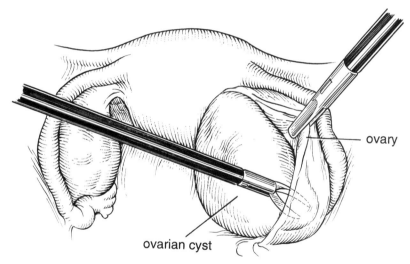

ovary

ovarian cyst

Fig. 4.4. Laparoscopic removal of ovarian cyst

If a cyst has destroyed all the normal ovarian tissue, it may be necessary to remove the entire ovary. A number of ways have been developed to remove the entire ovary with the laparoscope. Using either special sutures or surgical staples, the surgeon can tie blood vessels going to the ovary and then cut away and remove the ovary. In most situations, laparoscopic surgery takes no longer than standard surgery. The benefit of laparoscopic surgery is that you may leave the hospital on the same day and return to normal activity within a week or two.

When Is Major Surgery Needed for an Ovarian Cyst?

The goal of all surgery is to take care of the patient in the safest and most expeditious way possible. Based on the examination and sonogram, if the likelihood of a cyst being benign is very high, then laparoscopic surgery offers the advantage of a quick and easy recovery. If a cyst is cancerous, then more extensive surgery is needed through an abdominal incision, and laparoscopy is not appropriate. If cancer is suspected, there is no reason to subject a woman to the added time, risk, and expense of a laparoscopy only to find that it is necessary for the doctor to switch, while the patient is anesthetized, to the standard abdominal surgery. Therefore, if there is a possibility that a cyst is cancerous based on the examination and sonogram, abdominal surgery should be performed.

Do Large Ovarian Cysts Need to Be Removed?

Most ovarian cysts don't get any larger than two to three inches in diameter. Infrequently, they can grow to five or six inches or larger. When a cyst gets this large, it almost never goes away by itself, and surgery is needed, because it may crowd out and destroy most of the normal ovary. In that case, the entire ovary must be removed. We always try to save some of the ovary, if possible, in all premenopausal women. Some doctors may make more of an effort to do this than others, so it is a good idea to discuss the possibility of saving the ovary with your doctor *before* surgery.

If You Are Premenopausal, Do You Need to Have Your Entire Ovary Removed If You Have an Ovarian Cyst?

In most cases, the answer is no. If you are premenopausal, the ovary contains eggs that make the female hormones estrogen and progesterone and also allow you to get pregnant. As long as there is healthy ovarian tissue remaining, it is a good idea to leave the ovary in place and remove just the benign cyst. The procedure to remove only the cyst is called a cystectomy (see page 107) and usually can be performed for all types of benign cysts. In rare instances, the cyst destroys all the normal ovarian tissue, and there is nothing left to save. Removing the entire ovary is then necessary.

Laurie's Large Ovarian Cyst

Laurie is a nineteen-year-old woman who began to feel a vague discomfort near her right groin about two weeks before she came to our office for an examination. Since the pain had not gone away, she thought she should be examined. At the time of her pelvic examination, it was immediately apparent that her right ovary had enlarged to the size of a cantaloupe. The ovary was mildly tender to touch, but otherwise Laurie was reasonably comfortable. Despite the large cyst, she had not noted any other symptoms or changes in the way she felt or looked. A sonogram showed that the ovary was filled with a six-inch (twelve-centimeter) cyst. There were a few shadows inside the cyst, and although it did not appear to be malignant, these shadows and the large size of the cyst raised the possibility that it could be cancerous. Of course, Laurie was upset and shocked that something this size could have grown without her even knowing, and she was concerned about the possibility that this was cancer. I reassured her that the chance of cancer at her age was extremely small, but I felt that surgery should be performed within the next week so that the cyst could be removed to make a certain diagnosis. Because laparoscopic surgery is usually appropriate only for benign cysts, and since this cyst did not clearly appear to be benign on a sonogram, we chose to make a standard abdominal incision.

During surgery, the outside of the cyst looked smooth and clear, so there was no obvious evidence of cancer. However, the normal cells of the ovary had been stretched so thinly over the large cyst that the ovary could not be repaired and had to be entirely removed. After the ovary was removed, the pathologist performed a "frozen section." A portion of the cyst was quickly frozen, cut into thin sections, and examined under a microscope to determine if the cyst was benign or malignant. The pathologist came back into the operating room about ten minutes later with a smile on her face to tell us that it was a benign growth.

Can an Ovarian Cyst Form After Menopause?

The ovary no longer produces eggs after menopause and, therefore, it is not possible for a follicular or corpus luteum cyst to form. But other types of benign ovarian cysts do occur after menopause. In fact, the most likely types of ovarian cysts after menopause are still benign cysts. However, because the incidence of ovarian cancer increases with age, any cyst or growth in the ovary after menopause should be evaluated with a sonogram. Once again, the sonogram can be helpful in predicting whether the cyst is benign, or if it is suspicious for cancer. In addition, if you have a cyst *after* menopause, the blood test CA-125 should be done. As previously noted, this test is inaccurate in premenopausal women, but it is more accurate in postmenopausal women. After menopause, women do not usually have endometriosis, fibroids, or other conditions associated with menstruation that yield a false positive result. If the sonogram shows a benign pattern and the CA-125 test is normal, then the ovarian cyst is probably benign. However, the ovary containing the cyst should be removed in any case so that it can be entirely examined under a microscope to be sure that cancer is not present. If a benign cyst is suspected, laparoscopic surgery may be performed to remove the ovary. We recommend that both ovaries be removed in order to completely evaluate the tissue for the presence of cancer and also to prevent the future development of either benign or malignant ovarian cysts.

If the sonogram looks suspicious or if the CA-125 test is abnormal, then the cyst may still be benign. However, major abdominal surgery should be performed because of the possibility of cancer. A larger incision allows the doctor to remove all the cancer, especially if it is present in other organs. In any case, any cyst found after menopause must be removed to make sure it is not cancer.

Molly's Ovarian Cyst

Molly is a seventy-five-year-old woman who went to see her internist because of a vague sense of discomfort and pain on the left side of her abdomen. She had no other symptoms, no nausea or vomiting, no fever, no problems urinating or moving her bowels. In fact, at first she chose to ignore the discomfort, but after a while she decided to see her family doctor. At the time of her pelvic examination, the doctor felt a swelling near her left ovary and ordered a sonogram, which showed a large ovarian cyst about five inches across. Molly was pretty nervous by the time she got to my office the next day. When I examined her, I could feel the cyst as a soft, smooth swelling where her left ovary was. It wasn't at all uncomfortable for Molly to have the cyst touched. Because of Molly's age, it was clear that surgery would be necessary to remove the cyst in order to make sure it wasn't malignant. This was recommended even though this cyst didn't feel the way cancer often feels. Cancer usually grows irregularly, not in the smooth way that this cyst felt. Cancer also often feels hard, and this cyst felt soft. Lastly, cancer sometimes gives off a clear fluid into the patient's abdominal cavity, which causes swelling and bloating. Molly had none of this, and I thought she probably had a benign cyst. I looked at her sonogram, and it did not show any of the features of a cancer. Two days later the CA-125 test came back totally normal. All of the signs now pointed to a benign cyst, but unfortunately none of these tests are 100 percent accurate. Surgery would still be needed to remove the cyst and make a diagnosis.

Since we felt the cyst was probably benign, I talked to Molly about the possibility of removing her ovary with laparoscopic surgery rather than through a larger abdominal incision. She was thrilled about the low risk of cancer and eager to try laparoscopic surgery so that she could get out of the hospital quickly and back to her normal routine. At the time of her surgery, we removed her left ovary and sent it immediately to the pathologist, who viewed it under the microscope. Within ten minutes the pathologist confirmed that the cyst was benign. We removed her right ovary as well, to prevent the future occurrence of either benign or cancerous ovarian cysts. The surgery had taken less than an hour, and that afternoon a relieved and elated Molly went home.

If You Are Postmenopausal, Should Your Entire Ovary Be Removed If You Have a Cyst?

If you have gone through menopause, two things need to be considered when making a decision about removal of the entire ovary if you have a cyst. First, as you get older the risk of ovarian cancer, while still not great, increases. If the entire ovary is removed, the pathologist can examine it completely to make sure no cancer is present. And if the ovary is removed, then the possibility of it developing cancer in the future is eliminated. Along these lines, we have also been recommending that the other (normal) ovary be removed during the same surgery. This takes very little additional time and prevents growths, both benign and malignant, from forming in the future.

The other issue relates to hormone therapy. After menopause the main function of the ovary, the production of estrogen, ceases. If you already take hormone replacement therapy, then the removal of your ovaries will not change the way you feel because your body is already getting estrogen from the medication. If you do not take hormones, no change will be noted either, since your ovaries are not producing estrogen anyway. However, after menopause the ovary does continue to produce some testosterone, a male hormone that helps libido or sex drive. Some women who have their ovaries removed notice a decrease in sexual feelings after surgery. If this happens, testosterone pills can be prescribed along with estrogen to enhance sexual feelings. Women always cringe when I mention this, imagining that their voice will deepen, and they will soon grow a beard. The amount of testosterone needed to enhance sexual feelings is *very small*, and side effects are extremely rare. In addition, some women note that testosterone has a positive effect on their mood; they feel better and more energetic than if they take just estrogen.

Is a Hysterectomy Needed If You Have an Ovarian Cyst?

In the past, if a woman had completed her family and had a benign cyst that needed to be removed surgically, a hysterectomy was routinely performed at the same time. Doctors felt that performing a hysterectomy made sense because the woman's abdomen was already cut open, and the healing would be the same no matter what additional surgery was performed. Also, if the uterus was removed, then it could not go on to develop a cancer at a later time. This practice has recently been questioned by a scientific study that showed the risks of surgery were greater if, in addition to removing the ovary, a hysterectomy was also performed to remove a normal uterus. This makes sense—more surgery leads to more risk of blood loss, more risk to injury to other organs, and more time under anesthesia. Also, the risk of developing uterine cancer is fairly low. About 3 percent of American women will get this disease in their lifetime, and it is often diagnosed at an early stage. I hope the idea of limiting surgery to just the problem area will be adopted by more gynecologists. If you have an ovarian cyst and your doctor is recommending hysterectomy, ask her why she thinks it is necessary. If you are not satisfied with the answer, you should consider getting a second opinion. The issues concerning hysterectomy are discussed in chapter 11.

REFERENCES

Canis, M., G. Mage, J. Pouly, A. Wattiez, H. Manhes, and M. Bruhat. 1994. Laparoscopic diagnosis of adnexal cystic masses: a twelve year experience with long-term follow-up. *Obstetrics and Gynecology* 83:707–12.

Finkler, N., B. Benacerrat, F. Lavin, C. Wojciechowski, and R. Knapp. 1988. Comparison of serum CA-125, clinical impression, and ultrasound in the preoperative evaluation of ovarian masses. *Obstetrics and Gynecology* 72:659–64.

Gambone, J., R. Reiter, and J. Lench. 1992. Short term outcome of incidental hysterectomy at the time of adnexectomy for benign disease. *Journal of Women's Health* 1:197–200.

Jacobs, I., and R. Bast. 1989. The CA-125 tumour associated antigen: a review of the literature. *Human Reproduction* 4:1–17.

Maiman, M., V. Seltzer, and J. Boyce. 1991. Laparoscopic excision of ovarian neoplasms subsequently found to be malignant. *Obstetrics and Gynecology* 77:563–65.

Parker, W., and J. Berek. 1990. Management of selected cystic adnexal masses in postmenopausal women by operative laparoscopy: a pilot study. *American Journal of Obstetrics and Gynecology* 163:1574–77.

Parker, W., and J. Berek. 1993. Management of the adnexal mass by operative laparoscopy. *Clinical Obstetrics and Gynecology* 36:413–22.

Parker, W., R. Levine, F. Howard, B. Sansone, and J. Berek. 1994. Laparoscopic management of selected cystic adnexal masses in postmenopausal women: a multicentered study. *Journal of the American College of Surgeons* 179:733–37.

5

IF YOU HAVE BLADDER PROBLEMS OR PROLAPSE

by Amy E. Rosenman, M.D.

Approximately 10 million American adults, the majority of whom are women, have problems controlling their bladders. Over $10 billion a year are spent on medical care and absorbent products to manage these problems. Those facts should go a long way toward pointing out that if you have a problem with the loss of urine, you are very far from alone. We hope that knowing that you are not alone will encourage you to seek help. New techniques in the fields of urology and gynecology are enabling us to help more and more women with bladder problems. Sadly, despite the enormous number of women suffering from bladder problems and despite a variety of new treatments available, many women are still reluctant to seek treatment and relief.

The problems of incontinence and prolapse of the pelvic organs are not new. Dame Trotula, a medical teacher in the eleventh century, fully described the same problems we deal with today. However, the thinking at that time placed the blame for prolapse on cold air entering the uterus as a result of a woman sitting on a cold stone or bathing in cold water. By the nineteenth century, medical thinkers were sure that abnormal positions of the uterus were at the root of all female ills. Treatments have included the use of aromatic herbs, sea water douches, and the application of leeches directly onto the cervix. Hanging a woman upside down in an effort to encourage the uterus to go to its proper position was another common treatment. Pessaries, devices that hold the uterus in place, were somewhat less refined than those used today. Then, they were made from pomegranates cut in half. We have come a long way since those times, and our current understanding of these problems and their treatments is the subject of this chapter.

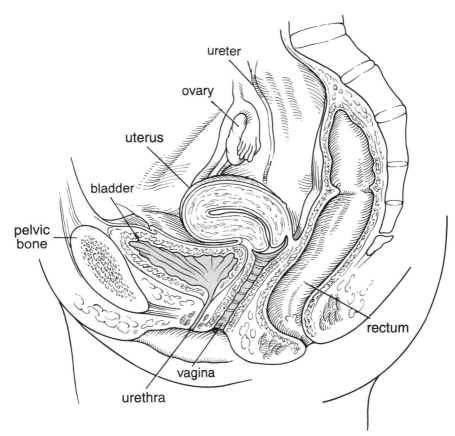

Fig. 5.1.   Normal position of pelvic organs

How Does the Bladder Normally Work?

The bladder has two jobs: storing and emptying urine. It functions in two phases. First, we expect the bladder to store our urine as it is produced by our kidneys. The bladder must give us quiet messages as it fills, and then it must loudly inform us that it is almost full, while still giving us plenty of time to find a bathroom. All this is accomplished while the bladder expands and collects urine painlessly. We then sit on a toilet and tell our pelvic muscles to relax, while our bladder muscle contracts and pushes the urine out the urethra and into the toilet . . . MISSION ACCOMPLISHED. When all works well, it becomes second nature to us. This is a complicated system that, for most of us, functions every day with little conscious effort or consideration. The normal position of the bladder, uterus, and rectum is illustrated in fig. 5.1.

What Is Incontinence?

Incontinence is the inability to control when and where your bladder empties. We all learned to control our bladders as young children, and it then became second nature to us as adults. We come to depend on this control for confidence in social situations. We are not prepared to have to reconsider our bladder control again later in our lives. The good news is that with understanding and treatment you can once again make normal bladder function second nature.

What Is Prolapse?

Prolapse is the dropping of the uterus or the bulging of the bladder or rectum into the vagina. These changes may or may not be accompanied by incontinence. The problems and treatment of prolapse are described on page 141.

Why Do So Many Women Endure Incontinence in Silence?

There are many reasons. Many women feel that incontinence is embarrassing because they think they should be able to solve it themselves. Lack of control over anything to do with one's body is hard to accept. Some women mistakenly and silently decide that they should be able to fix this problem on their own. Embarrassment is clearly the biggest obstacle to seeking appropriate care for incontinence. Many women won't even bring up the problem with their own doctor or close friends. If you are reading this chapter, we assume that you have some interest in the problem of bladder control. Please know that this is a condition that deserves the same attention you would give to other medical conditions such as abdominal pain or a broken arm. This is a medical problem. It is not a case of poor manners, bad behavior, or faulty upbringing. Fixing the problem will help get rid of the embarrassment.

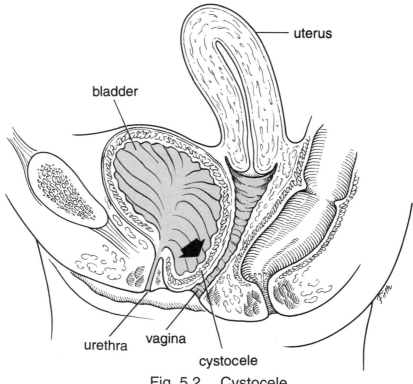

uterus

bladder

urethra   vagina

cystocele

Fig. 5.2.   Cystocele

Does Incontinence Always Occur Following Childbirth?

Some women think urine loss is an inevitable consequence of child-birth. Pregnancy and delivery cause stretching and strain of the bladder and the tissues that hold the uterus in the proper place. This sometimes results in the widening of the vagina and a dropping of the womb lower into the vagina. The muscles that are on top of the vagina and that hold the bladder up may be weakened over time, allowing the bladder to drop down. This bulging of the bladder into the vagina is called a cysto-cele (see fig. 5.2). The urethra, the tube that you urinate out of, also then drops down. A second type of problem that could occur as a result of childbirth is that the pressure of the baby's head in the birth canal may damage the nerves in this area. Therefore, the messages meant for the muscles around the bladder, vagina, and rectum may not be transmit-ted properly. This nerve damage can be permanent if it repeatedly hap-pens in two or more deliveries. The combination of the changes in the normal position of the bladder and urethra and the abnormal nerve signals may interfere with the bladder enough so that urine leaks out. Likewise, the muscle below the vagina that holds the rectum down may be weakened so that the rectum bulges up into the vagina. Bulging of the rectum into the vagina is called a rectocele (see fig. 5.3). These are common but often nonbothersome problems resulting from pregnancy and childbirth.

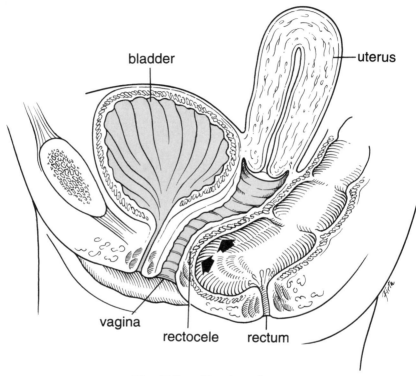

Fig. 5.3.   Rectocele

But remember, the majority of women, despite age and childbearing, are dry. If you have delivered children and now leak urine, you can be helped. The truth is that most causes of incontinence are treatable. If you do suffer from bladder problems, I hope you now are feeling a bit hopeful. Keep reading—the picture gets rosier.

Is Incontinence a Normal Part of Aging?

Many people erroneously believe that loss of urine, called incontinence, is a normal part of aging. It is not. Although it is more common in women over age sixty, the majority of women, regardless of their age, are not incontinent. And, regardless of your age, we are able to evaluate and treat most of the causes of incontinence. You are never too old or too young to seek care for this troubling problem.

Will Incontinence Affect Your Sexuality?

Until recently, women who had incontinence or pelvic prolapse—the dropping of the uterus into the vagina—were thought to have more discomfort with intercourse and were thought to be less sexually active than women without these problems. However, a new study found no difference in sexual activity, pain with intercourse, frequency of sexual desire, or satisfaction with relationships among women with and without incontinence or prolapse. Although some women found that severe prolapse impeded intercourse or was psychologically distressing, overall sexual activity was not different from the group of women without this problem. Therefore, you should not assume that incontinence or prolapse will lead to sexual problems.

Is All Incontinence the Same?

Incontinence is a symptom of an underlying problem, and there are a number of causes of incontinence. The most common types of incontinence are called *stress* incontinence, *urge* incontinence, and *overflow* incontinence. Sometimes more than one type may be present at one time, and this is called *mixed* incontinence. Because the particular types of incontinence have different causes, the treatments are also different.

TYPES OF INCONTINENCE

Stress incontinence: Small amount of urine loss with cough, sneeze, activity, laughter

Urge incontinence: Variable quantity of urine loss associated with a sense of needing to urinate before reaching the bathroom (due to spasms of the bladder)

Mixed incontinence: Urine loss with aspects of both stress and urge. That is, it includes leakage with cough or sneeze as well as episodes of bladder spasms causing leakage before reaching the bathroom.

Overflow incontinence: Urine loss occurring when the bladder fills to capacity and does not empty properly (due to neurologic problems or blockage). Excess urine then dribbles out.

Urgency and frequency: The constant sensation of needing to urinate associated with a sensitive bladder or bladder spasms. This does not necessarily cause leakage.

Total incontinence: A constant loss of urine resulting from an inability of the muscle that controls urination to close properly. This is very rare and requires continual use of protective pads.

How Can the Doctor Tell Which Type of Incontinence You Have?

Stress, urge, or mixed stress and urge incontinence affects the vast majority of people who leak. Most women cannot determine the type of incontinence that they have on their own. So do not be concerned if you feel somewhere in between these categories. These determinations can be made in collaboration with your doctor after a thorough evaluation.

If you are being evaluated for bladder problems, you can expect to be asked a lot of questions. Your doctor should listen carefully to your answers because your medical history is essential to your evaluation. Here are some of the questions I ask:

What activities or circumstances cause the episodes of leakage?

Is the amount of urine lost small, or do you flood?

Is urine loss preceded by an urge to urinate?

Are you experiencing frequent urination?

Does your bladder feel empty after you urinate?

Is there pain or burning when you pass urine?

Do you have any difficulty initiating a stream of urine?

Do you feel any dropping of your bladder or uterus?

Do you feel any bulging from the vagina?

Do you experience a pulling or pressure in the pelvis, especially when you are on your feet for any length of time?

Do you have any neurological problems, especially of the lower back or legs?

Do you have diabetes?

The answers to these questions begin to give us an idea of what type of incontinence you have. The specific types of incontinence are described in more detail below.

What Is Stress Incontinence?

Sometimes incontinence occurs when a cough, sneeze, exercise, or change of positions leads to the loss of small quantities of urine. Because the loss of urine occurs as a result of the pressure or stress from a cough, for example, this type of incontinence is called *stress* incontinence. When you cough, the muscles of your abdomen tighten and increase the pressure inside your abdomen and against your bladder. If the pelvic muscles, which normally support the urethra and keep it closed, are weakened, the urethra may be forced open by the cough, and urine will leak out. Many activities cause increased pressure in the abdomen and the bladder. A cough, a strain to lift a heavy piece of luggage, aerobic exercises, or even a hiccup can be a challenge to a woman with this problem.

What Causes Stress Incontinence?

As we already discussed, pregnancy and childbirth can damage pelvic ligaments that connect the uterus and bladder to the bones of the pelvis. The nerves sending messages to the muscles supporting the uterus and bladder may also be altered due to childbirth. They may not work as efficiently as before. This all leads to weakness of the pelvic muscles and sagging of the uterus and bladder into the vagina. This sagging is known as *prolapse* of the uterus and bladder.

In addition, the hormonal changes that occur with menopause can cause thinning of the tissues of the urethra. Try to visualize the urethra as a tube—if you cut across it, it will appear like a doughnut. As we have less and less estrogen in our bodies, the material making up this doughnut shrinks, which results in a larger hole. This larger opening in the urethra allows urine to leak out.

Obesity may add pressure to an already weakened system. When a woman carries extra weight in her abdomen, it often presses on the bladder, which can aggravate the problem of leakage. The combination of one or more of these factors may lead to stress incontinence.

What Is Urge Incontinence?

Urge incontinence is urine leakage that results from an involuntary, uncontrollable desire to urinate. Because this urge to urinate cannot be suppressed, this type of incontinence is called *urge* incontinence. With a healthy bladder, we are in control, and we can decide when to wait and when the urge to go is strong enough that we need to interrupt our activities. We then walk to the bathroom and voluntarily empty our bladder. You probably have not put too much thought into the act of emptying your bladder before. However, some women have a spasm of the bladder muscle that causes it to contract and push out urine without the conscious control that we are used to. The loss of urine often begins before reaching the toilet and may lead to soaked clothes or puddles in embarrassing places. Urge incontinence is the leakage that can occur when one returns home, parks the car, rushes up the path to the front door, and puts the key in the door. Since this happens quite commonly, it's actually called the key-in-door symptom and helps alert the doctor to the possibility of urge incontinence.

What Causes Urge Incontinence?

The most common cause of having frequent, strong urges to urinate or involuntary loss of urine is a bladder infection. The infection causes inflammation of the bladder that leads to spasms of the bladder muscle. The spasms cause the bladder to contract and push out some or all of the urine from the bladder. However, bladder infections cause only *temporary* incontinence and usually have no permanent effect on your bladder if they are treated. So, if you have had occasional bladder infections, you do not need to worry that this might lead to future incontinence.

For most women with urge incontinence, no specific cause is discovered. Perhaps the cause is a mild change in the nerves of the bladder, but at this point we just do not know. Other rare conditions such as interstitial cystitis, polyps in the bladder, and stone formation in the bladder can also cause bladder spasms. These are uncommon problems that are easily evaluated by a physician who looks into the bladder with a small telescope called a cystoscope. This is a painless office procedure that usually requires only the use of a topical gel anesthesia. It is necessary only in the case of multiple bladder infections, perhaps more than three in one year, or an infection that is not cured with one or two courses of antibiotics. Cystoscopy may also be performed when symptoms of infection are present, but urine samples show no evidence of infection.

What Causes Urgency and Frequency?

Women who have a constant urge to empty their bladder and need to make frequent trips to the toilet find these symptoms disabling. These women do not necessarily leak urine, but their lives are governed by their bladder problems. The causes of this problem are similar to those of urge incontinence. The bladder is basically misbehaving. Instead of quietly collecting urine, it is constantly whining and making a nuisance of itself. This is perceived as constant bladder pressure. The bladder feels as if it was always full, but, in fact, most trips to the toilet are a waste of time, producing no more than a few ounces of urine. Urgency and frequency is a frustrating problem that does have solutions. The treatment for this condition enlists many techniques that are described on page 128. These include the use of medication to reduce the spasms as well as exercises that can also reduce spasms. These can be used with techniques that increase the time a woman can wait between trips to the bathroom. This behavioral technique is known as *timed voiding* or *bladder drills* and is discussed in detail on page 130.

What Is Overflow Incontinence?

Overflow incontinence is the leakage of small amounts of urine when your bladder is full. It usually occurs because you are unable to fully empty your bladder when you urinate. The urine continues to collect in the bladder until it overflows.

What Causes Overflow Incontinence?

Overflow incontinence can be caused by an obstruction to the urethra, the bladder opening. Sometimes a contraceptive diaphragm can press on the urethra, and emptying the bladder with the diaphragm in place becomes difficult. Or, the bladder may drop as you get older and kink the urethra, which prevent you from fully emptying your bladder. You may feel that your bladder is quite full, but as you attempt to urinate only a small amount of urine is passed and you do not feel empty. After the bladder fills to capacity, any additional urine leaks out, resulting in overflow incontinence.

Overflow incontinence is sometimes caused by an injury to the nerves that go to the bladder. This could be a temporary injury to your back, which puts pressure on your spinal cord, or it could be permanent, the result of paralysis due to a serious accident. If the proper messages cannot get from the brain to the bladder, loss of urine may result.

What Is Total Incontinence?

Total incontinence, which is uncommon, is the complete loss of control of the bladder so that there is a constant loss of small amounts of urine. With total incontinence, you need to wear a pad at all times and have no control at all of when and where you urinate.

What Causes Total Incontinence?

Total incontinence occurs when the urethral muscle, called the sphincter, just won't stay closed completely. This is a very rare problem, sometimes related to an injury to the sphincter at the time of childbirth or previous surgery near the bladder. Another very rare cause of total incontinence is a fistula, a hole in the bladder that drains into the vagina. This problem can result from a difficult childbirth during which the vagina and bladder may be torn, or it may result from an operation near the bladder, vagina, or uterus.

What Can the Doctor Tell from an Examination?

The first part of an examination for incontinence and prolapse is performed in the same way a routine exam is done in a gynecologist's office, lying on your back with your feet in the stirrups. The pelvic organs are examined to confirm that the vagina, uterus, fallopian tubes, and ovaries feel normal. In addition, the position of the uterus and any weakness in the muscles supporting the bladder or rectum can be evaluated by observing how much movement occurs with coughing or straining.

The second part of the exam is performed while you are standing. Although this may sound odd, the problems of a dropped bladder or uterus may only be apparent when you are sitting or standing. As awkward as it may sound, it is in no way painful. With one of your feet elevated on a stool, the doctor can observe any bulge at the vaginal opening from the dropping of the uterus, bladder, or rectum.

Gravity, menopause with weakening of pelvic ligaments, aging, and heredity may also contribute to the problem of sagging or dropping of these organs. Luckily, there are solutions to these problems.

What Are the Q-tip and Stress Tests?

Other tests may be used after the examination in order to help determine which type of incontinence you have. Two simple tests are the Q-tip test and the cough stress test. The Q-tip test is performed with you lying on the exam table with your feet in stirrups. A cotton-tipped applicator covered with some anesthetic gel is inserted painlessly into the urethra, the bladder opening. You are then asked to cough and strain, and the movement of the Q-tip is measured. The cough stress test is performed in the same position. You are again asked to cough with a full bladder to see if that causes leakage of urine. Excessive movement of the Q-tip or loss of urine with coughing indicates *stress* incontinence.

Next, you will be asked to empty your bladder. A small tube, called a catheter, is then painlessly passed through the urethra into the bladder, and any remaining urine is collected and measured. The amount of urine left in the bladder after normal urination is called the postvoid residual. It is normal to have up to two ounces left in the bladder after urinating. If more is found, this indicates a problem with incomplete emptying and suggests that overflow incontinence is present. The sample of urine from the catheter is then cultured to see if any infection is present in the bladder. If an infection is present, treatment with antibiotics is started.

What Is a Voiding Diary?

A voiding diary is like any diary you might keep. It is intended to be an ongoing record of your normal urination and any leaking you have during a few days or a week. Because a written record is better than relying on memory, the voiding diary is a very accurate method of telling just how significant the incontinence problem is and how different treatments work for you. In addition to documenting when you urinate during the day and night and when any accidents occur, you may also be asked to include the volume of urine passed as well as the time, type, and amount of fluid you drink. The urine volume can be measured with a special basin that fits under the seat of any normal toilet. This basin has ounces written on it and you simply read off the amount and record it in your voiding diary. The urine is then discarded in the toilet and flushed away.

Claire Develops a Problem

Claire is a seventy-three-year-old woman who is a very active photographer. She is so active that she routinely works into the wee hours of the night in her darkroom, developing film and printing photographs. She also drinks lots of tea throughout those wee hours.

When Claire came into the office, she complained of flooding her bed in the morning. She is sometimes unpleasantly awakened, surrounded by puddles. We learned from her voiding diary that this happened on the average of two or three times a week, between eight and nine a.m., and only on the nights she stayed up late working. We talked about changing her schedule and avoiding the late nights, but Claire really enjoyed those quiet times to work on her art, undisturbed by telephones or visitors. From looking at the diary, I found that Claire's problem was a bladder spasm that emptied her bladder only when it was very full (from the tea), and when she was very tired (from the late work). I suggested a loud alarm clock at seven and a quick trip to the toilet before the critical volume was reached. The puddles are gone, and Claire is dry. The problem was simply solved, and Claire is delighted.

What Is Urodynamics Testing?

In order to find out how well the bladder is functioning, we must see if the muscle that makes up the wall of the bladder is doing what it is supposed to do. The test for this is known as *urodynamics*, or UDS for short. And, despite the name, this has nothing to do with jet planes or aerodynamics. UDS is done in the office and is painless. The muscular sac we call the bladder is supposed to relax and comfortably stretch out while it collects and stores urine made by the kidneys. Then, when you are ready to urinate, it is supposed to contract and force the stored urine out into the toilet. The urodynamic study allows us to measure the pressures in the bladder with a small tube painlessly placed in the bladder. In order to calculate the appropriate pressures, we must also know the pressure in your abdomen as measured by another catheter painlessly placed in either the vagina or the rectum. In addition, a specialized tampon is inserted into the vagina that can measure the strength of the pelvic muscles.

Although you may feel "wired for sound" during this exam, this test does not hurt at all, and we can get a wealth of information that can lead to a specific diagnosis for the cause of incontinence. Is this a big bladder contraction or a spasm pushing out the urine? Or, is this stress incontinence, leakage due to increased abdominal pressure from a cough or a sneeze? Many neurological conditions affecting the bladder, such as back injuries, strokes, diabetes, and multiple sclerosis, may also be apparent on UDS. Once we know the underlying cause, we can choose the best remedy.

Sarah Gets Some Well-Deserved Support (at Her Bladder Neck)

Sarah, a thirty-seven-year-old mother of four, came to see me complaining of urinary loss whenever she coughed, sneezed, or exercised. Due to the distress caused by this condition, Sarah had greatly scaled back her activity. She no longer attended her aerobics class because she was too uncomfortable with bulky pads under her leotard. She also had stopped running and jumping with her children. During the allergy season, she could barely leave her house.

Sarah first noted urine leakage immediately after the birth of her fourth child. With pelvic floor exercise, she was able to manage for a few years. These are the exercises women are often taught after childbirth to strengthen the muscles around the vagina. Then the situation deteriorated, and she needed to wear protection. First she only wore pads to aerobics or when she had a cough or a cold. Soon she wore them daily, and then she started cutting back on her activity. This whole process was slow and insidious, but one day she woke up and realized that her life had become narrow and restricted, all because of her bladder.

Massively frustrated, Sarah decided to take action. She came in for an exam and consultation. We discussed her medical history in detail, and then I examined her. The uterus, fallopian tubes, and ovaries felt normal, but the bladder and urethra were bulging into the vagina. Further inspection of the vagina showed that the rectum was also bulging into the vagina (see figs. 5.2 and 5.3).

To evaluate the bladder opening, a Q-tip with anesthetic gel was painlessly placed into the urethra. Sarah was asked to strain, and the movement of the Q-tip was assessed. In fact, this demonstrated movement and dropping of the bladder opening, an indication of stress incontinence. The swab was removed, and she was asked to cough. I could see the leakage of a few drops of urine during the cough. My examining fingers then gently elevated the bladder back to a normal position, and Sarah was asked to cough again. This time there was no leakage. Sarah was also examined while standing to assess the dropping of her pelvic organs. Although her bladder was dropping, her uterus was in the normal position. The entire exam was no more uncomfortable than a routine pelvic exam with a Pap smear.

A tiny tube was then passed into Sarah's bladder to see if

she had emptied it completely. The tube is usually passed only one or two inches into the urethra and does not hurt at all. She had very little urine left in the bladder, which indicated that she had emptied normally. A urine culture performed on this sample of urine showed that she did not have a bladder infection.

We then went together to the UDS lab. This exam room in the office has an automated chair that moves into several positions while keeping the patient comfortable, as well as computerized equipment for recording and interpreting the bladder pressures correctly. We have a specially trained nurse who, under my supervision, assists with the testing. While the bladder is filling and emptying, we are constantly observing the computer readouts and can see from the measurements just what is going on in the bladder when leakage occurs. Sarah's test showed that coughing caused urinary loss without any bladder contraction or spasm. This is what we see with stress incontinence.

Surgery to repair the muscles in the vagina and suspend the bladder (see page 134) was recommended to Sarah, and she decided to proceed. Two months after successful surgery, Sarah was once again running and playing with her children.

TREATMENT FOR INCONTINENCE

The good news is that there are many options for the treatment of incontinence that include exercising, using a pessary, taking medication, and surgery.

Can Exercise Treat Incontinence?

Just as doing sit-ups helps keep your stomach flat and provides extra support to those aching backs, exercise of the pelvic floor muscles helps you keep control of your urine. These exercises were first described by Dr. Arnold Kegel in the late 1940s. The Kegel exercises aren't difficult to do, but they must be done regularly.

Here's how it works. The correct muscles are identified by sitting on the toilet with your legs apart. You should try to stop the stream of urine without moving your legs. If the urine stream stops, you have identified the correct muscle. If not, keep trying. One-on-one instruction with an incontinence expert (either a doctor or a nurse) may be helpful. Once the correct muscle is identified, you can exercise the muscle by tightening it for a slow count of five and then relaxing the muscle. These isometric exercises should be done in sets of ten in the standing, sitting, and reclining positions at least three times per day. This exercise routine requires no special equipment and can be easily incorporated into a daily routine. You can combine these exercises with other activities for maximum efficiency, such as while brushing your teeth or driving to work. Improvement should be noticeable in weeks to months. Once the desired improvement is attained, continued exercise is necessary to maintain the good results.

Consciously contracting these muscles can stop a bladder spasm and, therefore, can help you control urge incontinence. Also, if you build up adequate muscle strength, these muscles can be contracted prior to a cough or sneeze and prevent stress incontinence. It has been shown that reinforcement and education are imperative to the success of pelvic floor exercise. If needed, there are many ways to get this education and reinforcement, as discussed below.

Can Biofeedback Help Me Learn These Exercises?

Biofeedback is one successful method to learn the proper way to strengthen the pelvic muscles. By using a special sensor placed in the vagina and rectum, the contractions of these muscles can be displayed on a screen. You can then exercise different muscles while watching the screen and learn how to contract the appropriate muscles. If the exercise is improperly performed, the monitor will display this as well. By using your visual sense to reinforce correct exercising, we are using a biofeedback technique. These techniques are easily and painlessly learned one-on-one with a trained nurse or physical therapist. In a large study involving several thousand patients who were incontinent for many reasons, women were taught pelvic floor exercise in small classes with a physical therapist over six months. At the conclusion of the study, 70 percent of the women were dry, significantly more than if no instruction was given. Most of my patients get the hang of this relatively quickly and are very proficient after one forty-five-minute session with the nurse. I suggest a review session two weeks later and another one a month later. With this training, most women are able to master these techniques. As with any part of your body, you may lose the benefits if you stop exercising. Therefore, the exercises should be done daily.

What Are Vaginal Cones?

Another method to help you become aware of exactly which muscles need strengthening uses small weighted cone-shaped objects that you place in the vagina. These look like smooth white vaginal suppositories and vary in weight from less than an ounce to a few ounces. They are inserted one at a time like a tampon, and their slippery nature causes the user to have to grip the pelvic muscles in a tight contraction so the cone won't fall out. The cones are only used for exercise sessions lasting about ten minutes, sometimes several times a day, and are removed at the end of each session with a string attached to the weight. The weights are graduated, and you can increase the weight until you regain bladder control. All pelvic floor exercises are associated with a good chance for improving bladder function as well as sexual function and satisfaction.

What Are Bladder Drills?

The bladder drill, also known as timed voiding, is based on the accepted premise that bladder control is a *learned* behavior. We all began as babies in diapers with absolutely no bladder control—our bladders had a life of their own. As we grew to the ripe old age of two or three, we noticed what it felt like to have a full bladder and a wet diaper. We learned to listen to the signals telling us that we had to urinate and learned how to hold our urine until we reached the toilet.

The bladder drill is a form of behavior modification that reteaches us how to control when and where we urinate. The goal is to increase the time between urinations according to a timed schedule. For example, if you now feel the need to urinate every hour, you would not allow yourself to urinate before an hour and fifteen minutes by the clock. After a few days this time can be increased to an hour and a half, and eventually to two or three hours. Pelvic floor contractions are used to suppress bladder spasms and the urge to urinate, while you try to space trips to the toilet. Medication to control spasms can be added if needed. Put all these techniques together, and when you feel you need to urinate, you will be able to control the urge. Ultimately, a normal voiding pattern can be reestablished.

The average, healthy woman makes about eight trips to the toilet in a twenty-four-hour period, assuming a normal fluid intake of about a quart and a half of liquid per day. Women with urinary urgency are uncomfortable and always have the sense that they need to void. This is distracting and distressing, and in many situations socially limiting. Many women avoid overnight visits, car trips, the theater, public transportation—anything that limits immediate access to a toilet. The bladder drill's goals are to increase the capacity of the bladder and increase the interval between trips to the toilet. This is important to women with urinary frequency and urgency.

Carol Gets a Grip

Carol is a sixty-year-old psychotherapist who was facing a difficult dilemma. Her patients were seen in blocks of two to three hours, but unfortunately her bladder was on a different schedule. She had to run to the toilet down the corridor and back in the one minute between her patients. She was quick, but this was ridiculous. Her bladder was running her ragged. If she did not heed the call of her bladder, she was punished with a wet episode. What a predicament. Carol came into the office and had a complete history and physical examination, Q-tip test, urine culture, and postvoid residual test. She then kept a voiding diary for three days and nights. Next, we went to the laboratory and performed UDS.

Carol's diagnosis was mixed stress and urge incontinence. She was started on a program of biofeedback to learn proper pelvic floor exercise and weighted vaginal cones to increase muscle strength and decrease bladder spasms. After she became skilled with these tools, she was instructed in timed voiding to increase the interval of time between trips to the bathroom. Carol is now listening to her patients again, instead of her bladder, and remaining dry.

What Is Electrical Stimulation?

This is a technique to help identify the pelvic muscles for a woman with very weak pelvic muscles or someone who has had trouble figuring out the right muscles to contract. I always fantasize about how great it would be to be able to exercise with only a minimum of effort on my part. Electrical stimulation works very much in this way. A small instrument is inserted into the vagina or the rectum to deliver a tiny electrical pulse that actually contracts the muscle for the individual. It feels like a hum in the muscle and is not at all uncomfortable. This technique can be used to initiate a program of pelvic floor exercise when the muscles are weak, with some gain in muscle strength resulting.

Electrical stimulation has also been shown to reduce bladder spasms in women with urge incontinence. The treatment involves use of the device for one to two hours, three times a day, on a schedule outlined by a professional. Once you get the hang of this program, it is easy and produces noticeable improvement in muscle tone and bladder control.

Can Medications Be Used to Treat Incontinence?

Stress, urge, mixed, and overflow incontinence may all be treated with medications that can improve symptoms. Different drugs affect the bladder in varying ways. Some medications relax the bladder muscle and reduce spasms that can cause accidents. Other medications increase the strength of the urethral muscle and keep the bladder closed during coughing or sneezing. Medication can be used alone or in conjunction with exercises and bladder drills.

Can Estrogen Improve Incontinence in Postmenopausal Women?

Estrogen is often helpful for women with incontinence who are either entering menopause or who are postmenopausal. Both the bladder and the urethra need estrogen in order to stay healthy. Therefore, menopausal women who are not taking estrogen replacement may notice a worsening of their symptoms over time. There may be more bladder spasms that can cause accidents. Remember that image of the urethra as a doughnut? As the urethral tissues atrophy and thin, the hole of the doughnut gets larger, and there is more leakage. Estrogen prevents this thinning so that the urethra stays closed and stops leaks. If you have already gone through menopause and have not taken estrogen, starting it now can often reverse the bladder and urethral changes and improve your symptoms.

Estrogen can be used in several forms: as a vaginal cream inserted two to three times a week at bedtime, as an oral tablet taken daily, or as a skin patch applied daily. If you have your uterus, progesterone should be prescribed as well to prevent overgrowth, or even cancer, of the uterine lining (see page 243). Estrogen can be taken safely by most women with minimal side effects. Discuss the form and dose of the estrogen with your doctor.

Can Medication Be Used for Urge Incontinence?

Urge incontinence can often be treated with medications that reduce bladder spasms and sometimes just a small dose of one of these medications is all that is necessary to live a normal life. And when a comfortable and effective medication is found, it may be used indefinitely. Some medications that have been used for urge incontinence are Ditropan, Tofranil, and Levsin. These drugs can be used alone or in combination and have been found to help over half of the people who try them. As all these medications require a prescription and medical supervision, you may want to discuss them with your doctor. There may be some side effects such as a dry mouth or constipation. Rarely, women may experience slight confusion or dizziness. If taken in small doses, side effects are minimized and benefits are maximized. Also, side effects may differ from one medication to another; therefore, changing the medication may eliminate any problems.

Can Medication Be Used to Treat Stress Incontinence?

Stress incontinence occurs when the urethral muscle (sphincter) does not stay sufficiently closed, especially when you cough or sneeze. Therefore, drugs that help close the sphincter can prevent urinary loss. Interestingly, these drugs are found in some common cold decongestants such as Sudafed. Many women do try Sudafed for occasional bad days, but most cannot tolerate it daily because of the side effects of dry mouth or headache. Rarely, it may also cause increased blood pressure or rapid heartbeat; therefore, it should not be used if you have high blood pressure. Other frequently used drugs for stress incontinence are Ornade and Tofranil, which are prescription drugs and must be supervised by your doctor. As mentioned before, in postmenopausal women, estrogen should be used in combination with these medications.

What Medications Can Be Used for Mixed Incontinence?

Mixed incontinence is a combination of problems that requires a dual solution. The bladder wall has spasms, and the pelvic muscles are weak and cannot prevent leaking. Therefore, a drug that relaxes the bladder wall muscle is used in conjunction with a drug that keeps the bladder closed. Estrogen is also added for postmenopausal women.

Can Medication Be Used to Treat Overflow Incontinence?

Remember that overflow incontinence results when you are not able to empty your bladder, and the urine continues to fill the bladder until it overflows and spills out. This problem can be treated with drugs that relax the urethral sphincter and allow the urine to pass more freely. Other medications may be used to encourage the bladder to contract and force the urine out. These medications can assist in better emptying of the bladder so that overflow does not occur.

What Can Be Done If You Can't Empty Your Bladder at All?

Very rarely, a woman will not be able to empty her bladder at all. There is another simple technique that is easily taught to solve this problem. While sitting on the toilet, a small tube is painlessly inserted into the urethra to empty the urine into the toilet. This technique is known as self-catheterization and may be safely performed several times a day as required.

Can Surgery Be Used to Treat Incontinence?

Yes. One of the goals of surgery for the treatment of incontinence is the restoration of the normal position of the bladder and urethra. There are many techniques available that can accomplish this. Most women who have given birth vaginally have some degree of prolapse. This begins unnoticed and asymptomatically in most women and *remains* that way for the majority. There are no health risks to this condition, so surgery is only necessary when you have discomfort or incontinence that cannot be corrected by the simple techniques described earlier.

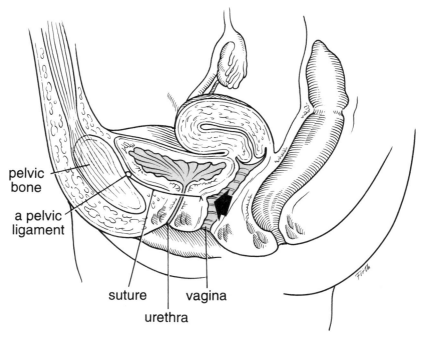

pelvic bone

a pelvic ligament

suture | vagina

urethra

Fig. 5.4.   Burch procedure (abdominal bladder suspension)

What Kind of Surgery Can Treat Stress Incontinence?

If the stress incontinence results from the dropping of the bladder that occurs with a cough, sneeze, or exercise, the goal of the surgery is to suture the bladder back in the correct place so that it cannot drop. The standard way to do this is with an operation known as an abdominal bladder suspension. This surgery is done through an abdominal, bikini-type incision, and the tissue near the bladder opening is stitched to the ligaments of the pelvis (see fig. 5.4). The operation described above is also called a Burch procedure or a Marshall-Marchetti-Krantz procedure (named after the doctors who developed them) and is successful over 80 percent of the time.

Another operation for the treatment of stress incontinence is called the vaginal needle suspension. This operation is done primarily through an incision in the vagina, rather than with an abdominal incision as described above. Through this vaginal incision, stitches are placed near the bladder and urethra, then passed behind the pubic bone with a long needle and tied above the pubic bone (see fig. 5.5). By avoiding a large abdominal incision, the recovery is quicker and less painful than with the abdominal suspension. However, this operation is slightly less effective, with cure rates in the 70 percent range.

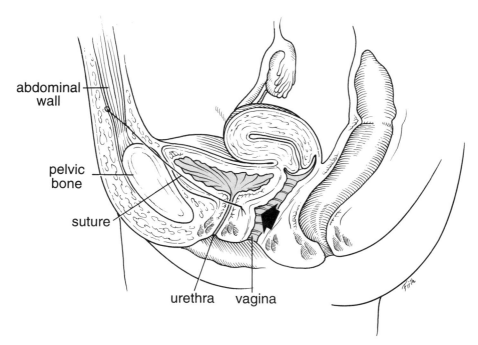

Fig. 5.5.   Vaginal needle suspension

What Is a Laparoscopic Bladder Suspension?

A bladder suspension technique may now be performed through the laparoscope. This is an appealing idea because it gets around the necessity of an abdominal incision and allows most patients to go home the day of surgery. It also results in a decrease in the pain and time needed for recovery.

However, this operation is new and is still being evaluated from the point of view of long-term success rates. Studies are now being performed to compare the effectiveness over time of this new approach with the more traditional operations. It must also be noted that the laparoscopic procedure is technically difficult and requires specialized skills. I suggest that you discuss your doctor's personal preference regarding these operations and his or her experience in performing these surgeries.

What Is an Anterior Repair?

An anterior repair is an operation performed through a vaginal incision in order to strengthen the tissue beneath the bladder and push it back up to its original position. It is a very good procedure for treating a dropped bladder, but not too effective if used alone for the treatment of incontinence. There are simply too many failures and recurrences of urine leakage after this operation. If leakage is the reason for the surgery, the anterior repair must be accompanied by a bladder suspension for good results.

Can Surgery Be Used to Treat Mixed Incontinence?

In the event that the diagnosis is mixed incontinence, there are several issues to understand before agreeing to surgery. As the name implies, there is more than one abnormality in this case. Surgery can put things back where they belong, but this may only cure the *stress* component of the incontinence. However, the bladder's errant spasms may continue to cause urge incontinence and wetness. To provide complete dryness, in many cases surgery can be combined with any of the treatments for urge incontinence.

In cases of severe prolapse and mixed incontinence, it has been shown that appropriate surgery to fix the prolapse and suspend the bladder can, in about two-thirds of women, successfully treat the bladder spasms as well. About one-third of women with mixed incontinence will continue to experience abnormal bladder spasms after surgery, but this may be associated with less leakage. Women who are somewhat improved by the operation usually consider it a major success even if they still continue to have an occasional spasm.

How Successful Are These Operations?

There is an excellent study that has followed women for five years after they have had surgery to correct incontinence. The women with abdominal bladder suspensions have the best five-year success rate, about 80 percent. The women with needle bladder suspensions had success rates in the 70 percent range, and the women with anterior bladder repairs had the lowest success rate, in the 60 percent range. While the women with the abdominal incisions had the longest success, they also had the more painful surgery with a longer recovery. The women with vaginal needle bladder suspensions were up and around sooner with less pain, but slightly less long-term success. These trade-offs must be considered when contemplating surgery and when deciding what's best for you. The anterior repair is not designed to correct leaking, and the long-term success was only a little better than fifty-fifty. However, this operation is good for a dropped bladder, and if incontinence is a problem, the anterior repair can be performed in conjunction with one of the bladder suspensions to treat the incontinence.

Katherine's Difficult Decision

Katherine came into my office seeking a third opinion. She is a forty-six-year-old attorney, employed full time, and spends a good part of her day lugging heavy legal briefs all over town. She is also busy with her two children, playing competitive tennis, and exercising three times a week. She was suffering from stress incontinence and was not satisfied with the results of the nonsurgical interventions she had tried. She was advised by one doctor to have a needle suspension because that's what he did on all his patients, and they all did well. Another doctor recommended an anterior repair because she'd been doing them for thirty years, and she liked the procedure.

Since Katherine is young, healthy, and active, long-term results were important to her, and she was willing to tolerate the longer recovery time and increased discomfort following an abdominal operation. She decided to have an abdominal bladder suspension, where the bladder neck would be stitched to the firm ligaments under the pubic bone. Katherine was admitted to the hospital and had surgery the same day. The next morning, self-catheterization was reviewed, and her catheter was removed. She was started on food and was walking by the afternoon. She did so well that she was able to go home the following day. Katherine was driving in two weeks and back to work in six weeks. She has continued to do well during the several years since her surgery—a long dry stretch, you might say!

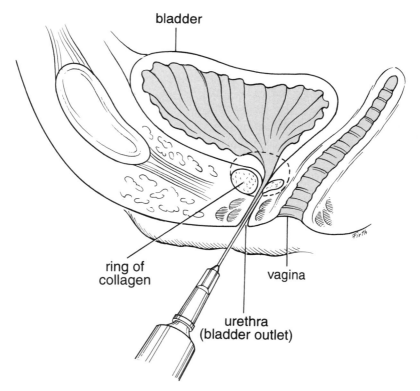

Fig. 5.6.   Collagen injections

Can Collagen Injections Be Used to Treat Incontinence?

If the bladder sphincter works properly, the bladder suspension operations can often correct stress incontinence caused by dropping of the bladder and urethra. However, in about 10 percent of women the urethral sphincter does not work properly, often because of scarring from prior surgery for incontinence. The scarring interferes with the natural ability of the bladder to close and keep urine in the bladder. With the bladder partially open all the time, it is easy to understand why these women complain of constant wetness. This condition cannot easily be corrected by a suspension operation, and until recently, these have been some of our most unhappy patients.

However, there is a new and effective treatment for this problem that has changed the lives of many women who have leaked for years. With minimal risk or discomfort, collagen is injected near the opening of the bladder to narrow the urethra and keep the urine in the bladder (see fig. 5.6). This procedure is performed in the hospital with local or general anesthesia, and the patient may go home the same day and resume normal activity the next day. And you will know immediately if the injections are successful. If only partial success is noted, an additional injection can be scheduled one month later. Often the treatments last for up to two years. If leakage recurs at a later date, reinjection can be performed. Although collagen is appropriate for only a small number of women, it is enormously important because these women often had prior surgical failures and were the most difficult to cure. These women are very grateful for this new technique.

Nancy's Bladder Problem

Nancy is a sixty-three-year-old with her own business that requires some travel. Nancy packs a suitcase for her clothes and a separate tote just for her incontinence pads. She has been doing this for fifteen years and not because she hasn't sought solutions. Fifteen years ago she had a vaginal hysterectomy and anterior repair for mild stress incontinence. She had been dry for two years when her stress incontinence returned. Three years later, she had a needle procedure that kept her dry for five years, but her stress incontinence returned with a vengeance.

She was evaluated again and told there was excessive scarring near her bladder that had to be removed through an abdominal incision in addition to needing an abdominal bladder suspension. These surgeries had been performed, and although they were properly performed, the leakage returned six months later. In our office, a complete evaluation showed that the bladder was in the right position, but the urethra was open all the time. This is why Nancy leaked.

Collagen injections had just become available and I suggested she try this new technique. A few hours after the injections she was urinating normally and she returned to work the next day. She wore her usual large incontinence pad to work (old habits are hard to break), but after three days of staying dry she gave them up. The following week, she went on a business trip and packed only her clothes!

What Is the Recovery Like Following Bladder Operations?

Surgery near the delicate area around the bladder leads to some swelling, and the pressure of this swelling on the urethra temporarily prevents the normal emptying of the bladder. Therefore, immediately after surgery the bladder needs to be emptied with a small tube called a suprapubic catheter that is placed in the bladder. The tube, inserted at the time of surgery while you are under anesthesia, exits through a small hole above the pubic bone, where it is taped in place. Hospitalization is usually required for two to three days, and many women are discharged with the suprapubic catheter in place. The catheter is easy to care for and is well tolerated by women of all ages. It can be easily and painlessly removed in the office soon after surgery, when urine is once again passing normally through your urethra. This may take a few days to a few weeks, although rarely it can take a couple of months. Another way to empty the bladder is self-catheterization: You are taught how to insert a small tube through the urethra to drain the bladder until this can occur naturally.

The discomfort of surgery may last a few weeks. Walking and stairs are safe to tackle immediately post-op. Driving can usually be resumed two weeks after surgery. Light activities are perfectly safe, but lifting anything heavier than five pounds is not recommended for the first two months. Physical exercise should also wait until the two-month period of healing is over. This is true for all bladder surgeries, including laparoscopic surgery. Lifting anything heavier than twenty pounds should generally be avoided for life, in order to prevent weakening of the repaired tissue. Luggage should be carried by someone else or wheeled. Furniture moving should be left to the experts! The results of the surgery can only be judged a couple of months after the operation when all the swelling has gone away and healing is complete.

How Do You Decide Which Operation Is Best for You?

This is a decision that takes into account many factors and is made in collaboration with your surgeon. Age and general physical condition are considered. Is surgery planned for prolapse *and* incontinence? What type of incontinence do you have? What is the severity of the incontinence? What level of activity is anticipated in your lifestyle?

If incontinence is a major problem, an abdominal bladder suspension is best. If prolapse is the primary problem, a repair of the weakened tissues will need to be performed through the vagina, and a needle suspension of the bladder through the vagina may be the most appropriate operation. If the sphincter is scarred open, collagen injections may be the best answer. A careful history and physical examination, proper testing, and an understanding of your problems and wishes are all important parts of this decision.

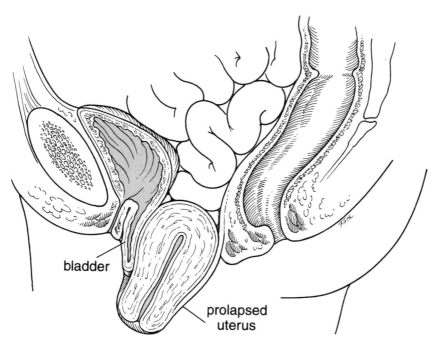

bladder

prolapsed
uterus

Fig. 5.7.   Severe uterine prolapse

PROLAPSE

What Can Be Used to Treat Prolapse?

Prolapse is defined as the dropping of the uterus, or the bulging of the bladder or rectum into the vagina (see fig. 5.7). If your symptoms are mild, either no treatment or the use of a pessary may be considered. If your symptoms are very bothersome, surgery can be used to put things back where they belong. If the uterus is falling down and you have completed your family, hysterectomy may be warranted. At the same time, repair of the bladder and rectum can be performed through vaginal incisions.

What Is a Pessary?

A pessary is made of rubber and is placed in the vagina in order to elevate and support the uterus, bladder, and/or rectum when these organs are dropping (see fig. 5.8). Women who only experience symptoms of prolapse or incontinence in limited settings may benefit greatly from the use of a pessary. Pessaries are also very useful for women who wish to defer surgery for a while or who cannot have surgery for medical reasons. Pessaries are not particularly helpful for incontinence, but with better support, some women experience less urinary incontinence. However, in rare cases, a pessary can *increase* leaking.

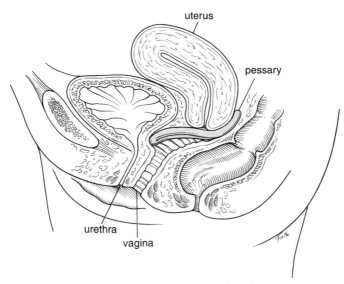

Fig. 5.8.   Pessary in place

Pessaries come in many shapes, sizes, and materials. Some look like contraceptive diaphragms, others like rubber doughnuts. Usually we can find one that will help. The pessary should be fitted by a professional, either a doctor or a nurse practitioner or physician's assistant with special training. The process has been compared to fitting shoes. We try several pessaries and choose one that reduces the prolapse, is comfortable, easy to insert, stays put, and is easy for the patient to remove and reinsert. If the pessary is the proper size, it should be small enough so that you are not able to feel it at all, but large enough so that it does not fall out, even with straining. And it should not cause the incontinence to get worse.

But just like with shoes, we sometimes find that in a few days the fit is not right. If the first size does not work, do not be discouraged. In general, most women can be properly fit with a pessary. A follow-up visit is usually planned within a week of the initial fitting to see if any changes are needed. This is also an opportune time for the patient to learn how to remove and reinsert the pessary herself, a fairly simple task. If you feel comfortable removing your own pessary, you may do this as often as you like. It also needs to be removed before intercourse. Wash the pessary with mild soap and water and reinsert it. If you wish, the doctor or nurse can do this on a regular basis every month or so.

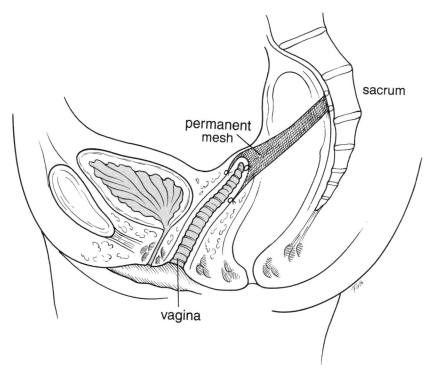

Fig. 5.9.   Vaginal suspension

The possible side effects of wearing a pessary are irritation of the vagina that can cause vaginal discharge or, rarely, vaginal bleeding. If you have these symptoms, you should be seen by your doctor or nurse practitioner. Use of estrogen, either in vaginal cream or pill form, will make the vaginal tissues healthier and eliminate or greatly reduce vaginal irritation and discharge. It also softens the vaginal tissue and adds to the comfort of pessary use.

Can Prolapse Occur After Hysterectomy?

Sometimes the vagina can actually begin to protrude even years after hysterectomy as the supporting ligaments weaken over time. When there is permanent protrusion, something should be done to protect the tissues, allow normal urination, and give a woman relief from what is a debilitating and demoralizing situation. Surgery to correct this problem involves stitching the top of the vagina back to the proper place (see fig. 5.9). This type of surgery may be performed at any age, as long as a woman is reasonably healthy and active.

Miriam Proves You Are Never Too Old

Miriam is an eighty-five-year-old widow who lives alone. She still works part-time in a family business and is quite active and vital. Over the past year, she noted increasing prolapse—first occasionally, then daily. Finally, the bulge just wouldn't go back inside the vagina. She was fitted with a pessary, which initially helped. However, as the prolapse got worse, the pessary would not stay in, and a better-fitting pessary could not be found. Miriam wanted to have surgery because she did not want to give up her job and her independence, but she was concerned that she was too old for an operation. After reassurance that she could handle the surgery just fine, she underwent a vaginal hysterectomy, repair of the vagina near the bladder and rectum, a needle suspension of the bladder, and a suspension of the top of the vagina to a strong ligament in the pelvis. The day after surgery she was sore but out of bed and walking. The next day she was discharged to her home. A visiting nurse checked in on her daily for one week until she was urinating normally, and her catheter could be removed in the office. One month later, she was back to her part-time job with no regrets. She has done extremely well and has offered to speak to other older women contemplating surgery to offer reassurance.

Are There Any Minor Surgical Procedures for Prolapse?

In certain unique situations where a pessary has failed and the patient is not healthy enough or active physically or sexually, a minor operation may be used to correct prolapse. This procedure, called the Le Fort procedure, can tuck back the prolapsed organs inside the vaginal canal. The top and bottom of the vaginal walls are then sewn together in order to hold things up where they belong. The advantages to this operation are that it is relatively simple, has few surgical risks, and can be done as an outpatient with either local, light general, or spinal anesthesia. Recovery is easy. The disadvantages are that closing the vagina may have an effect on self-image and sense of femininity and should be explored with each woman before surgery. Also, if the uterus is present and there is any abnormal bleeding, an evaluation with a D&C is more difficult. As always, there are risks and benefits to any medical procedure.

How Do You Choose a Doctor for Your Bladder or Prolapse Problems?

Experience counts. Ask questions. Make sure you are evaluated fully and properly. Inquire as to whether your doctor does urodynamics or works with someone who does. Make sure your treatment is tailored to your particular needs and that your doctor has a large repertoire of treatments and is choosing what is best for you. If surgery is necessary, make sure she or he performs these procedures successfully several times per month. Either a gynecologist, a urogynecologist, or both a gynecologist and urologist working together may be appropriate if they have the right experience. A urogynecologist is a doctor who completes the full training in gynecology and then gets further training in the evaluation and treatment of incontinence and pelvic prolapse. This is a developing field, and you want your care to be the best that is available.

There are many types and causes of incontinence and pelvic prolapse. Fortunately, there are also many solutions. Incontinence is not a normal part of aging, nor is it inevitable after childbirth. It is a medical condition with many possible treatments and cures. So throw away those diapers and pads and take an active part in your evaluation and treatment. Solving this problem will improve your life and get you out and active again. Don't be afraid or embarrassed. It can only get better.

REFERENCES

Weber, A., M. Walters, L. Schover, and A. Mitchinson. 1995. Sexual function in women with uterovaginal prolapse and urinary incontinence. *Obstetrics and Gynecology* 85:483–87.

6

ENDOMETRIOSIS
by Ingrid A. Rodi, M.D.

Endometriosis is one of the most common gynecological conditions in the United States. We don't know exactly how many American women suffer from this disease, but best estimates set the number at about 5 million. Women of all ages, races, and backgrounds have been found to have endometriosis.

Recent information suggests that the disease is becoming more prevalent. Some 2 million women had hysterectomies for pelvic pain related to endometriosis between 1965 and 1984. Over that time period, the number of hysterectomies performed per year for this condition doubled. In addition, the proportion of all hysterectomies performed because of endometriosis rose from approximately 10 percent to 20 percent.

Endometriosis can also affect fertility, and about 30 percent of infertile women are found to have endometriosis. The symptoms and problems related to endometriosis lead to the hospitalization of a substantial number of women every year.

What Is Endometriosis?

The tissue that lines the uterus and is shed during the menstrual period is called the endometrium. In some women, this same tissue can be found growing outside of the uterus, where it does not belong. When this occurs, endometriosis is said to be present. The tissue that normally lines the uterus may be found in or on the ovaries, the fallopian tubes, the outer surface of the uterus, or other areas of the peritoneum (the membrane that lines the abdominal cavity and surrounds the internal organs). Occasionally, endometriosis may be found on the bowel or bladder. And very rarely, it has been found in locations far from the pelvis, such as in an old abdominal scar or even the lungs.

The lining cells of the uterus normally go through cyclic changes in response to the varying levels of the female hormones estrogen and progesterone produced by the ovary throughout the month. During the menstrual cycle, as estrogen levels rise, the tissue first grows and builds up, and then, as the levels of both estrogen and progesterone fall at the end of the cycle, the tissue breaks down and is shed as menstrual blood (see page 56). When a woman has endometriosis, the lining cells are present in locations where they are not intended to be, yet they respond to hormonal changes in much the same way as if they were still within the uterus.

So if endometrial cells are sitting on the outside of the lower intestine, for example, those cells will grow lush and full as if they were in the uterus preparing for a fertilized egg. During the menstrual period, as normal uterine-lining cells begin to bleed, the endometrial cells present outside the intestine—endometriosis—also begin to bleed. The blood from these endometrial cells, however, is contained inside the body and accumulates. This accumulation of blood and other substances given off by the endometriosis often causes irritation, and even damage, to the surrounding areas. If these cells are present near the uterus, bladder, or bowel, the irritation may lead to pain in those locations. The body's natural response to irritation and injury often ends with the formation of scar tissue, which also increases the likelihood that discomfort will be experienced (see chapter 7). The scar tissue can also interfere with the passage of the egg into the fallopian tube and lead to infertility. Thus, the abnormal location of uterine-lining cells leads to the symptoms and problems that we associate with the condition called endometriosis.

What Does Endometriosis Look Like?

The appearance of endometriosis is variable and changes over time. Areas of endometriosis may be small, only a millimeter, or larger than a few centimeters. We think that new endometriosis appears as small, almost clear, raised areas on the surface of the uterus, fallopian tubes, ovaries, or inside lining of the abdomen. Over time, these areas, called implants, continue to collect the pigment contained in the blood they secrete. As this occurs the areas become pink, then dark red, and finally a dark brown color. The darker areas have often been called "powder burns" because of their color and shape. In order to evaluate a woman for the presence of endometriosis, a careful inspection of the entire pelvis and abdomen must be performed, looking for all the possible appearances of endometriosis, some of which are fairly subtle (see fig. 6.1).

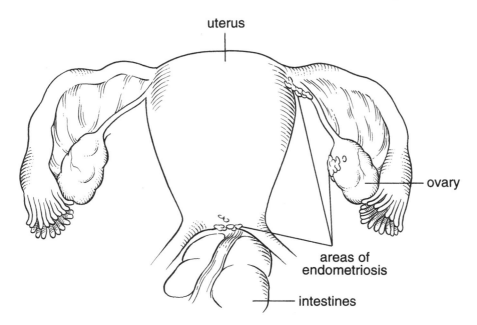

uterus

ovary

areas of
endometriosis

intestines

Fig. 6.1. Mild endometriosis

What Is an Endometrioma?

The cells of endometriosis can get trapped inside the ovary. During the menstrual period, when there is bleeding from this endometriosis, the blood accumulates inside the ovary, forming a cyst. These blood-filled cysts are called endometriomas (see fig. 6.2). As the blood ages and becomes more concentrated, it assumes a dark brown, chocolate color. When these cysts are opened at the time of surgery, they are usually easy to recognize because the dark brown fluid appears quite different than the normal clear fluid of common ovarian cysts. For this reason, the cysts are sometimes called "chocolate cysts." The size of these cysts can range from very small to the size of a grapefruit, and there can be more than one present at a time (see chapter 4).

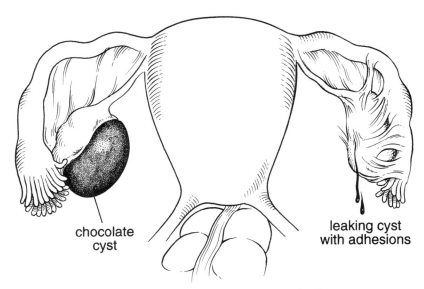

Fig. 6.2.   Severe endometriosis

What Causes Endometriosis?

A great deal of research and effort has gone into trying to clarify the cause of endometriosis. Several theories have been proposed suggesting more than one possible cause, and there is evidence to suggest that any, or all, of these theories may be possible. It may be that endometriosis has different causes in different women. At present, the most probable explanations are the passage of menstrual blood out the fallopian tubes and into the abdomen, or the spread of uterine-lining cells through the bloodstream or lymph system. In addition, it is likely that the immune system plays some role in allowing the development of this condition. All of these concepts are discussed in detail below. The hope is that clarification of the causes of endometriosis will lead to better treatment, or perhaps even prevention, of this common condition.

What Is Retrograde Menstruation?

At the time of the menstrual period, most of the blood and endometrial tissue flows out of the cervix and into the vagina. However, some of the blood and endometrial lining cells can also go out the wrong way, through the ends of the fallopian tubes. This is known as retrograde menstruation and occurs commonly. In fact, if surgery happens to be performed on a woman coincidentally during her menstrual period, menstrual blood and tissue are frequently found at sites outside the uterus, in areas where endometriosis most commonly occurs.

However, even though we know that this "backward" menstruation occurs in most women, the cells usually do not take hold and grow. But, when the cells do take hold and grow, endometriosis is the result. Women who have periods closer together, or that last longer, or are heavier, have an increased amount of blood that flows out of the tubes, and they have a greater chance of developing endometriosis. But still, only in the occasional woman is the tissue able to take hold, grow, and develop into endometriosis. Why the tissue grows outside the uterus in only some women and not in others is not known, although the immune system may be a factor (see page 152).

Can Endometriosis Be Caused by Abnormalities of the Uterus?

Some women have an abnormality of their uterus that may lead to a greater likelihood of developing endometriosis. Very rarely, a woman may be born with a narrowed, or even closed, cervix that prevents the lining cells from leaving the uterus during menstruation. Then, the only way these cells are able to get out of the uterus is through the tubes, where they fall into the abdominal cavity. A large number of lining cells exiting through the tubes probably increases the likelihood that the cells will take hold, grow, and develop into endometriosis.

In the rare case where a woman is born with a closed cervix, she may experience all the symptoms of a period, including menstrual cramping, without any visible bleeding. These women often see a doctor at a young age because the cells start to accumulate after menstrual periods first begin, and pain follows shortly thereafter. A laparoscopy is often performed to determine the cause of the pain, and the diagnosis of endometriosis is made. Surgery can also be performed to open up the cervix and prevent further problems. For reasons that are not clear, it appears that these women have a less aggressive type of endometriosis, with less formation of scar tissue.

Connie's Fibroid Caused Her Endometriosis

Connie came to see me with a history of severe pelvic pain and abnormal bleeding. She was in her midtwenties and had normal periods until two years prior to her visit when she noted bleeding between her periods. She also was experiencing increasingly heavy menstrual bleeding, and she suffered from severe cramping. An evaluation by her doctor found nothing abnormal, and she was given some pain medication.

This did not help very much, and she came to see me for a second opinion. When I examined Connie, her uterus was larger than normal, suggesting that a fibroid might be present. On ultrasound examination, a fibroid was seen in the lower part of the uterus, enlarging her uterus and partially blocking her cervix. Most likely, the fibroid was preventing menstrual blood from leaving the uterus through the cervix, and the blood from her period was accumulating in her uterus. When enough blood collected, the uterus would try to squeeze the blood out, and a severe cramp would result.

The pain with her periods was so bad that Connie requested that something be done to end her discomfort. Unfortunately, no medication is available to treat this type of fibroid problem, and surgery was the only answer (see chapter 2). Unexpectedly, at the time of her surgery, we found a lot of endometriosis around her uterus, fallopian tubes, and ovaries. We suspected that the fibroid had blocked the flow of menstrual blood out of the uterus and forced it out of the tubes, leading to the development of the endometriosis. We were able to remove all the visible endometriosis by using a laser. The fibroid was then surgically removed to prevent further obstruction of the cervix.

Connie did very well for a number of years after surgery. However, a few years later Connie was found to have a new, even larger fibroid that had grown in the wall of her uterus. This fibroid was pressing on her bladder and causing her a great deal of discomfort, and she again requested surgery. At the time of this second surgery, we noted that this new fibroid was not blocking her cervix, and no new endometriosis had formed. We were able to remove the fibroid, and Connie has done extremely well for the past few years. Stories like Connie's give some credence to the theory that obstructions to the flow of the menstrual blood can lead to endometriosis, and relief of the obstruction can prevent endometriosis from forming.

What Does Your Immune System Have to Do with Endometriosis?

Some researchers feel that a woman's immune system plays a part in the development of endometriosis. Components of the immune system include antibodies and white blood cells that attack foreign invaders. It is possible that, in most women, when endometrial cells exit through the fallopian tubes, the body is able to recognize that these cells are in the wrong place, and the antibodies and white blood cells destroy them. However, if the immune system does not recognize and destroy the misplaced tissue, it can take hold, and endometriosis develops. Many research studies have examined the immune system in women who have endometriosis, but none has found any clear evidence of cause and effect. It should also be stated that women with endometriosis are not more likely to get other conditions or illnesses, suggesting that the immune system otherwise works normally.

Is Endometriosis an Inheritable Disease?

It is probable that some women are more prone to develop endometriosis because of a genetic predisposition. A woman who has a mother or sister with endometriosis has an approximately 7 percent risk of developing the disease compared to a 1 percent risk in the general population. The reasons for this are not clear but may be related to an inherited inability of the immune system to recognize endometriosis and destroy it.

Can Endometriosis Spread Through the Bloodstream or Lymph System?

The body has a vast network of veins and arteries that distribute blood to the body. It also has a separate, but similar, network that carries lymph, a fluid involved in the body's defense system, throughout the body. Some researchers think that endometrial tissue can be carried through either the bloodstream or lymph system to distant locations. This mechanism has been proposed in order to explain how endometriosis gets to areas remote from the uterus. In fact, endometriosis has been discovered in areas such as the navel or the lung at the time of surgery. However, it is extremely uncommon to find endometriosis in these distant locations.

What Are the Symptoms of Endometriosis?

If you have painful periods, chronic pelvic pain, pain during or after sex, premenstrual backache, painful bowel movements, the sudden onset of pelvic pain, or a problem with fertility, your doctor will consider endometriosis as one of the possible causes for your problem. On the other hand, many women with endometriosis have no symptoms at all, and the condition may be discovered inadvertently during surgery for another reason.

Katie's Abdominal Pain

Katie is a thirty-nine-year-old woman who had noted pain under her rib cage on her right side for about two months. The pain came and went, but seemed to be present mostly after she ate. Then it became increasingly severe, and she saw her internist for the problem. A series of tests were done, and stones were discovered in her gallbladder. Although the problem was not serious, the pain was very bothersome, and Katie decided to have surgery.

Katie's general surgeon removed her gallbladder using laparoscopic techniques that have recently been developed. However, after the gallbladder was removed, the surgeon examined the pelvic area and saw multiple areas of adhesions and endometriosis. The surgeon called me at my office and asked if I could come right over to have a look. Within ten minutes I was in the operating room, looking at Katie's uterus, fallopian tubes, and ovaries on the video monitor. Katie had three children and felt well, so the endometriosis did not appear to be a significant problem despite the fact that it was present near her ovaries and behind the uterus. Thinking that if the condition continued unabated it might cause problems with pain in the future, we elected to gently remove the scar tissue and areas of endometriosis. This took only about twenty minutes, and then the general surgeon finished closing the small incisions. After surgery, Katie was surprised to learn about the unexpected findings of scar tissue and endometriosis, but she was glad they had been treated.

Can Endometriosis Cause Pain with Your Period?

Painful menstrual periods are very common in women who have endometriosis. We often find that women with endometriosis have pain just before their periods begin. When the ovarian hormone estrogen is produced during the menstrual cycle, it acts on both the normal lining of the uterus and the endometriosis to make all these cells grow. Toward the end of the menstrual cycle, the ovary stops the production of estrogen, and both the lining cells of the uterus and the endometriosis start to break down and bleed. As the endometriosis breaks down, it releases substances such as prostaglandin that can irritate the surrounding tissues of the uterus, bladder, and bowel and cause pain. However, endometriosis can lead to other patterns of pain as well.

Can Endometriosis Lead to Adhesions (Scar Tissue)?

Endometriosis causes the release of blood and chemical substances onto the tissue inside the abdominal cavity. This tissue is delicate and easily damaged by blood and chemical substances. Normally, the body heals itself from such an injury by increasing the growth of cells in the damaged area to replace those that have been damaged. This is the process that forms scar tissue to mend a wound. Unfortunately, scar tissue inside the body, called adhesions, may form between areas that are not normally connected.

Sometimes adhesions can make the uterus, fallopian tubes, or ovaries stick to each other or to nearby organs such as the intestines (see fig. 6.2). Because scar tissue is not elastic like normal tissue, it doesn't stretch easily, and the pulling and tugging of scar tissue on normal tissue that occurs with activity or sex may lead to pain (see chapter 7).

Teresa Was Missing Work

An unhappy Teresa, thirty-two years old, came to see me one morning in the office. She told me her period had gotten so bad that she was missing work, and she didn't know what to do. She had been placed on birth control pills by her previous physician, in an attempt to decrease her menstrual cramping (see chapter 3). In addition, she had been given a prescription for a strong pain pill, but the pain continued. At one point in our conversation, she started crying, and she confided that she was afraid she would become addicted to the pain pills.

On examination, I didn't find anything unusual, so I recommended a sonogram so that I could "see" the uterus. The only unusual finding was a small cyst in her ovary, about one inch in diameter. Usually a cyst that size would be of no concern. However, this particular cyst had an unusual pattern on the sonogram, the kind of pattern we often see when endometriosis of the ovary, called an endometrioma, is present. It appeared that the sonogram might have found the cause of Teresa's pain—endometriosis.

I was concerned because endometriosis of the ovary cannot be cured with medication, and surgery would therefore be needed. I suggested that we take a look with the laparoscope in order to determine if an endometrioma was, in fact, present. If so, we would then be able to remove the endometriosis with the laparoscope and perhaps treat her pain. She was panicked: "How long will I be out of work? I don't have many more sick days left." I was glad to be able to reassure her that we could do her surgery on a Friday, and she would be back to work on Monday.

During the laparoscopy, I could see that she did, in fact, have a one-inch-wide cyst of endometriosis deep in her left ovary. There was also some scarring from additional endometriosis around the tube and ovary. I was able to remove both the cyst and the scar tissue with a laser aimed through the laparoscope. By thoroughly burning away the abnormal cells and scar tissue, pain from endometriosis may often be relieved. During her visit following surgery, I recommended a three-month course of GnRH agonist (see page 162) in order to shrink any remaining endometriosis that had not been visible during the surgery. Teresa did have some hot flashes and vaginal dryness from the medication, but was able to tolerate these side effects knowing they would go away when the medication was soon stopped. Six months after her surgery, the medication was stopped. When she came for her checkup, she was smiling when I walked into the room. "I haven't missed a day of work, and my periods are so easy I don't even have to take an aspirin!"

Can Endometriosis Cause Pain with Sex?

When the endometrial cells come out of the fallopian tubes, they often fall down directly into the pelvis. The pelvis is the most common location for endometriosis, and the cells often land on the supporting ligaments that attach the uterus to the back of the pelvis, close to the top of the vagina. The endometriosis may lead to scar tissue in this area. The stretching of the scar tissue during intercourse can therefore cause pain (dyspareunia).

Can Endometriosis Cause Backache?

If endometriosis is present near the muscles in the back of the pelvis, the cells can secrete chemicals that can irritate these muscles and cause them to go into spasm. This leads to back pain. In addition, the ligaments that support the uterus are attached inside the pelvis near the back. These ligaments are commonly affected by endometriosis, with pain felt near the back as well. Also, a very large endometrioma can lay against the pelvic muscles and nerves and can lead to back pain.

Can Endometriosis Cause Painful Bowel Movements?

Very rarely, endometriosis can grow into the part of the bowel that surrounds the uterus, fallopian tubes, and ovaries. If this occurs, the scar tissue that results may lead to pain at the time of bowel movements, when stool stretches the intestines as it moves down. If the endometriosis grows all the way through the wall of the bowel, bleeding that occurs from these cells during menstruation can show up in the bowel movement. This is an extremely rare situation.

Can Endometriosis Cause Painful Urination?

It is not uncommon for small areas of endometriosis to grow on the outside surface of the bladder. As long as the endometriosis stays outside the bladder, it causes very few symptoms. In very rare cases, the endometriosis grows into the wall of the bladder, irritating the bladder and causing a frequent urge to urinate. More rarely still, the endometriosis grows through the wall, to the inside of the bladder. If this occurs, at the time of the menstrual period, the blood produced by these cells can be found in the urine.

Can Endometriosis Cause Chronic Pelvic Pain?

Chronic pelvic pain is one of the most common symptoms of endometriosis. The pain often comes on gradually, and may be sharp or dull, constant or intermittent. Interestingly, there is no correlation between the amount of endometriosis present and the severity of the pain experienced. Significant pain may result from small, as well as large, areas of the disease. In contrast, women with large areas may have no symptoms at all, adding to our confusion about this medical condition. Medications may be used to treat pelvic pain from endometriosis over the short term, but often surgical removal of the endometriosis is the most effective way to achieve pain relief. These treatments are explained below.

Can Endometriosis Cause Sudden Pelvic Pain?

Very rarely, sudden, severe pain can result from the rupture or twisting of a large ovarian cyst associated with endometriosis. These cysts, called endometriomas (see fig. 6.2), are filled with endometriosis and the blood that these cells have produced. Very often, surgery is required when endometriomas are suspected, to both make the diagnosis and treat the condition.

Robin Missed the Show

I remember first meeting Robin, a twenty-seven-year-old woman, in the emergency room. She was all dressed up, and I asked her where she had planned to go that evening. "I was on my way to the Music Center when I experienced this horrible pain in my side. I told my husband to get me to the nearest hospital, and he brought me here."

On examination, her abdomen was very tender, and a sonogram was performed, which showed a cyst in her right ovary. The sonogram showed that the cyst was about the size of a tennis ball but appeared to be partially collapsed and was surrounded by a lot of fluid. These findings suggested that a ruptured ovarian cyst might be present. Robin was having severe pain; she could not even stand up, and it seemed clear that she would need surgery to remove the ruptured cyst and end the pain.

Once I explained the need for surgery to Robin, she understood and agreed immediately. We performed a laparoscopy, and during the operation, I found that her ovary contained an endometrioma, a cyst that contains a collection of blood and endometriosis. This cyst had burst open, causing Robin the sudden onset of severe pain. We examined all of her pelvic organs and other areas inside her abdomen and could not find any other endometriosis. Using laparoscopic surgery, we were able to remove the cyst and all the fluid that had come out of it. We were also able to repair the remaining healthy portion of her ovary, and the results of the surgery appeared excellent.

The next morning when I told Robin what I had found, she was surprised. "I thought women with endometriosis have pain with their periods, and mine are very easy," she said. I explained that many women do have pain with their periods when they have endometriosis, but that rarely women have no pain until the endometriosis forms a cyst that then ruptures. Robin has done very well since that time and has not had any recurrence of the endometrioma.

Can Endometriosis Cause Irregular Menstrual Periods?

As described in chapter 3, the menstrual cycle is the result of a finely tuned interplay of a number of female hormones. One of the important parts of this system is the production of progesterone following ovulation (the release of the egg from the ovary). Ovulation may be disrupted by the presence of endometriosis, leading to abnormal amounts of progesterone and a disrupted menstrual cycle. For reasons that are not clear, it appears that even if ovulation occurs, it may not be normal, and irregular cycles may result.

Can Endometriosis Cause Infertility?

Infertility has long been felt to be associated with endometriosis, but the reason endometriosis might cause difficulty in getting pregnant has not been established. In fact, it may be that the cause of the endometriosis may also independently cause infertility. We know that about 5 percent of women who have had children and request tubal sterilization will be noted to have areas of old endometriosis at the time of their surgery. Therefore, the presence of endometriosis does not, per se, imply that a woman cannot get pregnant.

However, it does appear that the chance of getting pregnant is decreased somewhat if you have endometriosis, and the more endometriosis you have, the less likely you are to get pregnant. Endometriosis appears to start as small areas of abnormally situated endometrial lining cells. As the tissue grows and bleeds, scar tissue forms around it, increasing the amount of damaged tissue. The scar tissue may even grow around the fallopian tubes and ovaries in a way that blocks the passage of the egg down the tube.

The probability of a healthy woman getting pregnant is about 25 percent per month. For women with mild endometriosis, where the endometriosis is present in small amounts and has not caused any scarring, the pregnancy rate is about 7 percent per month. For women who have severe endometriosis, where extensive scarring, blockage of the fallopian tubes, and large cysts in the ovaries are present, it is not hard to understand why pregnancy rates are extremely low, without treatment.

Can Endometriosis Cause a Miscarriage?

Some studies in the medical literature have suggested that women with endometriosis have a higher risk of having repeated miscarriages. However, recent and better-designed studies do not confirm these findings. Our best information today suggests that women with endometriosis do not have rates of miscarriage any higher than those of other women.

Can Endometriosis Lead to Mood Changes or Depression?

Some women may have pain with endometriosis despite medical or surgical treatment. Under those circumstances, living with endometriosis can be difficult. If the symptoms come back after treatment or you are having trouble getting pregnant, the frustration and pain might lead you to become depressed. If you are in this predicament, don't suffer in silence. Discuss your feelings with your family and doctor in order to get the support and the relief you need. Several options are available, including counseling, support groups (see page 168), and occasionally medication.

How Can Endometriosis Be Diagnosed?

Endometriosis may be suspected if tender, thickened areas are felt near the uterus on a pelvic examination. If an ovarian cyst is present, sometimes a sonogram may exhibit the patterns suggestive of an endometrioma (see page 100), and the diagnosis may then be suspected. Unfortunately, we do not have any test presently available that can reliably predict whether or not endometriosis is present. Neither sonography, MRI, CT scan, nor blood tests are accurate in this regard.

The diagnosis of endometriosis can only be confirmed by looking at the pelvic organs at the time of surgery. Areas with the characteristic appearance of endometriosis (see page 164) can then be seen. Usually a minor surgical procedure called laparoscopy is performed under general anesthesia for this purpose. A small lighted instrument is inserted through the navel, and the surgeon looks through the instrument directly or, with the aid of a camera attached to the laparoscope, the pelvis can be projected on a TV screen.

At times, the diagnosis of endometriosis is made during a laparotomy, abdominal surgery that is performed under either general or regional (such as epidural) anesthesia. The incision in the abdomen ranges from approximately two to five inches in length. This abdominal surgery may be needed when a large endometrioma has been identified by the sonogram or if a pelvic mass of uncertain cause is found on examination. In addition, endometriosis may be incidentally found during an abdominal surgery performed for another reason, such as fibroids, an ovarian cyst, or even surgery for appendicitis.

What Is the Endometriosis Classification System?

A classification system has been developed based on the amount and location of endometriosis present and the amount and location of any scar tissue associated with the endometriosis. The system was devised in order to help to evaluate the success of different treatments in helping women achieve pregnancy. In this system, endometriosis is graded as minimal, mild, moderate, or severe, according to established criteria. Unfortunately, it appears that the present classification system does not accurately predict a woman's chance of getting pregnant, and new systems are being developed to fulfill this objective.

TREATMENT FOR ENDOMETRIOSIS

Treatment is aimed at reducing the symptoms of endometriosis, usually either pain or infertility. Treatment is divided into three paths: observation, medication, or surgery.

Observation: Is Any Treatment Needed for Endometriosis?

Women who have minimal or mild endometriosis and do not have pain may not require any treatment other than careful follow-up. In practice, however, if the diagnosis of endometriosis is made during laparoscopy, most gynecologists will burn or cut away these cells. However, a few studies have demonstrated that this treatment of mild endometriosis does not enhance fertility. For women with mild endometriosis, fertility rates are good even if no treatment is performed.

Can Medication Be Used to Treat Endometriosis?

It is known that estrogen causes endometriosis to grow. Endometriosis is extremely rare before a young woman begins to produce estrogen and starts to have periods and the disease usually disappears after menopause, when estrogen production stops. Therefore, one goal of treatment with medication is to lower, or stop, the production of estrogen. Reducing the levels of estrogen "starves" the endometriosis and causes it to shrink and sometimes even disappear. Two classes of drugs have been developed that lower the amount of estrogen in a woman's body: Danocrine and GnRH agonist. Progesterone can also be used to treat endometriosis.

What Is Danocrine?

Danazol (trade name Danocrine) is a man-made steroid similar to the male hormone testosterone. It lowers the body's production of estrogen, increases the amount of male hormone in a woman's body, and stops the growth of endometrial tissue. Pain relief is improved in up to 90 percent of women taking the medication, but after Danocrine is discontinued, pain often returns within six months. Pregnancy rates, unfortunately, seem to be unaffected following treatment with Danocrine.

One of the advantages of Danocrine is that it can be taken orally. However, the medication can cause a number of unpleasant male hormone–related side effects that include weight gain, decreased breast size, acne, growth of facial hair, or deepening of the voice. One of these symptoms occurs in 80 percent of women who take the drug, but only 10 percent of women have side effects to the degree that leads them to stop the medication. Nevertheless, these unpleasant side effects do limit the use of this medication, and today doctors rarely prescribe it.

What Are GnRH Agonist Medications?

Gonadotropin-releasing hormone (GnRH) agonists stop estrogen production in the ovary. The medications all work by preventing the pituitary gland from sending the signals to the ovary that cause the production of estrogen. Three preparations are available in the United States. Leuprolide (trade name Lupron) and goserelin (trade name Zoladex) are usually administered by a monthly injection given in the arm, and nafarelin (trade name Synarel) is given by nasal spray twice a day.

The medications all cause similar side effects, which are a direct result of the reduced levels of estrogen. This effect is sometimes referred to as "medical menopause" because the symptoms are similar to the ones many women experience during natural menopause. However, the symptoms go away entirely after the treatment has been completed and the medication wears off. To some degree, women experience side effects that may include hot flashes, night sweats, insomnia, vaginal dryness, headaches, mood changes such as irritability and sadness, and loss of interest in sex. However, these medications do not produce any male hormone–related side effects such as weight gain, acne, or hair growth. Because decreased estrogen levels may also lead to osteoporosis, some women may have a small reduction in bone mineral density if the treatment is given for long periods of time. If needed, estrogen, in doses low enough to prevent regrowth of the endometriosis, may sometimes be given to reduce the loss of bone. This is called add-back therapy.

What Is "Add-Back Therapy"?

The side effects of GnRH-agonist therapy often limit the use of these medications. In order to relieve side effects but maintain the beneficial suppression of the endometriosis, we can "add back" small amounts of estrogen and progesterone after the GnRH has stopped the ovary from producing normal amounts of hormone. It appears that it may take different amounts of estrogen to affect different parts of a woman's body. For example, a small dose of estrogen may be sufficient to prevent hot flashes, insomnia, and bone loss, and at the same time not be enough estrogen to allow endometriosis to grow. To date, studies have shown this regimen to be effective. The estrogen can be given orally or by a skin patch. If vaginal dryness is a problem, vaginal estrogen creams are often helpful. Progestins, man-made progesterones, are also used in "add-back" treatment plans to further shrink the endometriosis and help alleviate the hot flashes.

Can Progesterone Be Used to Treat Endometriosis?

Progesterone was the first medication used in an attempt to treat endometriosis and is still used today. Given by injection or pills, it causes endometriosis to wither, thus achieving pain relief over a period of time. Fertility rates do not seem to be improved following the use of progesterone. Side effects of progesterone include bloating, water retention, and weight gain, which are usually tolerable. More bothersome side effects are irregular bleeding and depression. Decreasing the dose of progesterone may help alleviate these problems, and adding small doses of estrogen may also be tried once pain relief has been provided.

Can Birth Control Pills Be Used to Treat Endometriosis?

All oral contraceptive pills contain progesterone and have been used for many years as a treatment for endometriosis. While they are not quite as effective as danazol or GnRH agonists, they work fairly well, have very few bothersome side effects, and are much less expensive. It also appears that women who are on birth control pills seem to have a lower chance of developing endometriosis in the first place. However, it is still unclear whether a woman who has had endometriosis can prevent the disease from returning by taking oral contraceptives. Although the FDA has not approved oral contraceptives solely for the treatment of endometriosis, they are commonly used for this reason.

Can Pregnancy Cure Endometriosis?

The role of pregnancy in curing endometriosis is still uncertain. During pregnancy, the placenta produces large amounts of both major female hormones, but more progesterone than estrogen. Progesterone is known to suppress the growth of endometriosis, and therefore it makes some sense that pregnancy would relieve the pain associated with endometriosis. This beneficial effect may sometimes last for many months, or even years, after delivery.

Can Surgery Be Used to Treat Endometriosis?

Since endometriosis was first described almost a century ago, surgery has been the mainstay of both diagnosis and treatment. Until the middle of the twentieth century, the usual treatment for symptomatic endometriosis consisted of removing the uterus, fallopian tubes, and both ovaries. This is defined as *radical* surgery. In contrast, removal of just areas of endometriosis without the removal of the ovaries or uterus is called *conservative* surgery.

What Is Conservative Surgery?

Conservative surgical treatment is considered when a woman needs surgery for pain or infertility associated with endometriosis, and she desires to preserve her pelvic organs. The goal of this approach is to remove as much endometriosis and scar tissue as possible and restore the uterus, fallopian tubes, and ovaries to their normal positions. Conservative surgery can be performed using laparoscopic surgery or an abdominal incision. Newer modalities involving laparoscopic surgical techniques and use of instruments such as lasers have allowed for surgery to be performed through very small incisions with the benefit of a shorter hospital stay and quicker recovery time. However, laparoscopic surgery requires special training, expertise, and experience on the part of the surgeon. Conservative surgery may provide a cure, but it may also provide only temporary relief of symptoms. A woman may elect to have conservative surgery in order to complete her family, and then, at a later time, she may elect to undergo radical surgery. And some women may require more than one conservative surgical procedure before they need to have, or are willing to consider, a more extensive operation. Yet, for some women, multiple conservative operations may provide relief of symptoms.

If a patient undergoes a conservative surgical procedure for infertility, her chance of getting pregnant is related to the amount of endometriosis found at surgery. Women who have mild endometriosis have about an 80 to 90 percent chance of becoming pregnant within five years whether they have the endometriosis removed surgically or not. Women who had moderate endometriosis treated surgically have about a 60 percent chance, and women with severe disease have about a 35 percent chance of getting pregnant.

What Is Radical Surgery?

Radical surgery is the term used to define the complete removal of all the pelvic organs as treatment for severe pain sometimes associated with endometriosis. In addition to total hysterectomy and removal of the tubes and ovaries, all obvious areas of endometriosis are removed in an attempt to provide a cure. This surgery is usually effective, even if estrogen replacement therapy is given following the operation. However, in rare instances, the pain from endometriosis can return with the estrogen, and the medication may need to be discontinued for relief.

Can Endometriosis Come Back After Treatment?

Unfortunately, endometriosis recurs quite frequently, with some evidence of the disease visible in 30 percent of women within eighteen months of surgery. A woman who has not completed her family may require multiple surgical procedures and courses of medical treatments to be able to have the desired number of children. Some women will need radical surgery—hysterectomy and removal of the ovaries—in order to prevent recurrence of endometriosis. At the time of menopause, the decreasing amounts of estrogen cause endometriosis to become inactive, and symptoms usually resolve. Most postmenopausal women can take estrogen replacement without recurrence of the endometriosis, because the doses of estrogen given are less than the level needed for endometriosis to survive.

Jessica's Story

Jessica came to see me for the first time when she was twenty-six years old. Her main complaint was severe pelvic pain. Two years before, she had had abdominal surgery for a large endometrioma in her right ovary. The endometriosis had destroyed her entire ovary, and it was removed during the surgery. Following the operation, she was treated with danazol for about six months, but decided to stop the treatment because of the weight gain and mood changes she experienced.

One year later she developed severe pain on her left side

and underwent a laparoscopy to diagnose the cause. The endometriosis had come back and was now found on the left ovary, the bowel, and the bladder. Again, we were able to remove the visible endometriosis using laparoscopic surgery. I discussed the options with Jessica and her husband. Her options included getting pregnant as soon as possible now that the endometriosis had been surgically removed, a trial of birth control pills, and a new drug called Lupron. She did not want to get pregnant at this time and opted to take Lupron. She was on that medication for six months. Her pain improved, but the hot flashes were a problem, and she had insomnia and depression.

Jessica started attempting pregnancy, but the pain came back and was so severe she opted to have another laparoscopy, which was successfully performed. Not long after that, Jessica became pregnant, and we were all delighted. Unfortunately, she had a miscarriage (unrelated to the endometriosis). Jessica and her husband knew that the pain would be too severe to attempt pregnancy on their own again. They decided to undergo IVF (in vitro fertilization). The procedure was successful, and she was pregnant.

At first she had a lot of pain, but as the progesterone from the placenta started to cause the endometriosis to wither, the pain disappeared. She delivered a beautiful little boy and had no pain while she was breast-feeding him. However, after her body returned to normal hormone levels, the endometriosis started to grow again, and the pain returned. Again, it became intolerable. We restarted the Lupron for another six months, which controlled her symptoms. Jessica knew that she would have to postpone having a hysterectomy if she wanted to try for another baby.

She underwent another laparoscopy. Luckily, there was no evidence of endometriosis, and we were able to remove some areas of scar tissue around her fallopian tubes and ovaries. Two months later she was pregnant. The pregnancy went extremely well, and she was again pain free. This time she had a beautiful little girl. But a year later the pain was back. Jessica and her husband had already decided that they had completed their family. She realized that this disease had controlled her life for the past several years, and she now requested radical surgery, a hysterectomy. At the age of thirty-four, ten years after her first abdominal surgery, she underwent a laparoscopically assisted vaginal hysterectomy and removal of her remaining ovary and fallopian tube. Shortly after her surgery, she was placed on hormone replacement therapy and has done extremely well. She is not entirely pain free, but she is able to enjoy her life and her family.

What Happens to Endometriosis After Menopause?

After menopause, the ovaries stop secreting estrogen, the endometriosis begins to shrink, and the symptoms of endometriosis go away. Menopausal women who have had endometriosis can usually take estrogen replacement therapy, because the dose of estrogen needed to relieve hot flashes, insomnia, and vaginal dryness and to protect the heart and bones is usually less than the dose that would cause the endometriosis to grow back.

Can Holistic Treatments Be Used to Treat Endometriosis?

Some women have found relief from symptoms of endometriosis with alternative approaches, including acupuncture, traditional Chinese medicine, and homeopathic remedies. No formal comparisons have been undertaken to compare the effectiveness of these alternatives with standard Western treatments, so we are unable to say how successful these approaches are.

What Kind of Research Is Being Done on Endometriosis?

There are still large gaps in our knowledge of endometriosis. Ongoing studies are attempting to better define the causes of endometriosis down to the level of the gene. Easier, less expensive ways of making the diagnosis are being sought. Special chemicals that are attracted to areas of endometriosis have been attached to molecules that can be detected by imaging techniques. It remains to be seen whether this can result in a nonsurgical diagnosis of endometriosis. In addition, adapting these chemicals to provide treatment as well as diagnosis might eliminate the need for surgery entirely. Other studies are looking at novel approaches to treatment, and still others are investigating which women need not be treated at all.

Are There Any Places Where You Can Get Help If You Have Endometriosis?

If you want more information or help, consider contacting the following resources:

Endometriosis Association
8585 North 76th Place
Milwaukee, WI 53223
(800) 992-3636

The Endometriosis Association is a self-help group with chapters around the country. It offers meetings, crisis counseling, medical resources, a newsletter, and literature on endometriosis.

The American Society for Reproductive Medicine
2140 11th Avenue South, Suite 200
Birmingham, AL 35205-2800
(205) 978-5000

Resolve
1310 Broadway
Somerville, MA 02144-1731
(617) 623-0744

Resolve is a national organization with chapters across the country. It is dedicated to supporting people who are having difficulty becoming parents. It offers meetings, lectures, publications, referrals to specialists, and counseling services. In addition, Resolve is involved in lobbying on behalf of its members.

REFERENCES

Schenken, Robert, M.D., ed. 1989. *Endometriosis: Contemporary Concepts in Clinical Management.* Philadelphia: J. B. Lippincott.

7

IF YOU HAVE PELVIC PAIN

What Is Pain?

We all know what pain means. You are injured, and you feel pain. Yet what seems so simple, something that hurts, is actually quite complex. Pelvic pain in particular often bewilders both those who suffer from it and those who attempt to treat it.

It may be helpful to know the general medical thinking on pain in order to get the full picture. The classic view of pain is defined as the sensation of discomfort that results when a part of your body has been damaged. We also expect that the amount of pain is related to the degree of damage: A major injury should result in severe pain, while a minor injury should be less painful. And yet, this classic view may not always be accurate. With chronic pain in particular, the degree and duration of the pain may no longer be related to the amount of injury present.

The sensation of acute pain begins with the stimulation of a nerve, either from extreme heat, severe pressure, or the inflammation of tissue. These nerves then send pain signals to the brain, and both the number and types of nerves that carry these signals influence what message the brain receives. However, in order to "feel" pain, your brain must also interpret the signals it receives. Brain chemicals called neurotransmitters influence the way your brain interprets the signals. Two main neurotransmitters, endorphins and serotonin, are involved in the perception of pain. Some people are said to have a high or low "threshold" of pain, and some studies have found that people who feel more pain actually have less endorphins.

These same neurotransmitters are also involved with the regulation of mood. Therefore, your perception of pain and your mood are interrelated. We all know that there are times when we are able to ignore or withstand more pain. For example, when you are fatigued, you are likely to feel pain more intensely. If you have spent time with a cranky, tired child you know that the smallest injuries can cause huge howls simply because the child is tired. This process is at work in adults as well. As you can see, the perception of pain involves the interplay of different elements, which can sometimes become quite complicated.

There are two basic types of pain, acute and chronic. This chapter will discuss acute and chronic pelvic pain as the result of both gynecologic and nongynecologic causes. Medical science is starting to pay much more attention to the causes of pain, the way people perceive pain, and treatment for people who have pain.

What Is Acute Pain?

You feel acute pain after your body has been injured, and an immediate release of chemicals in the skin, or deeper muscles, excites the nerves in that area. The nerves carry the pain signals directly to the brain. With acute pain, the amount and duration of the pain usually will be related to the severity of the damage. The greater the injury, the more pain you feel, because more chemicals are released in the skin and muscle. As long as the chemicals are stimulating the nerves, you feel pain. As you start to heal, the amount of these chemicals is reduced, and the sensation of pain decreases. As noted above, your psychological state and mood can alter your perception of pain because your brain is responsible for interpreting these signals. When you are tired or upset, you generally feel acute pain more intensely.

What Can Cause Acute Pelvic Pain?

The relatively sudden onset of pain in the pelvis, the lower part of your abdomen, is called acute pelvic pain. The most common gynecologic causes of acute pelvic pain are twisting or rupture of ovarian cysts; infection of the uterus, fallopian tubes, and ovaries; degeneration of fibroids; and tubal pregnancy. Women often describe acute pain as sharp or stabbing, and it may be so intense that normal activity is impossible. Often, causes of acute pain are associated with other symptoms such as nausea, vomiting, fever, or diarrhea. Many of the causes of acute pelvic pain are fully described elsewhere in this book. Acute pain resulting from ovarian cysts is discussed in chapter 4, pain from ectopic pregnancy is discussed in chapter 3, and pain from fibroids is discussed here and in chapter 2.

Can Fibroids Cause Pelvic Pain?

Most fibroids in and of themselves do not cause pain. However, if fibroids grow to be large, they may press on nearby organs, such as the intestines and the bladder, which can result in discomfort, though it would be unusual for this to be severe enough to cause pain. Very rarely, fibroids undergo a process of degeneration, or cell decomposition, that causes the release of chemical substances that produce pain. This type of pain usually starts suddenly and may be severe, but goes away by itself over a few days. Fibroids that form on a stalk (pedunculated fibroids) can twist around on the stalk and cause sudden and severe pain. These very rare cases need to be treated by surgical removal of the fibroid. These problems can cause acute pain, but not chronic pain. Fibroids and their symptoms and treatments are discussed in detail in chapter 2.

What Can Cause Pain with Intercourse?

There are a number of causes of pain during or following intercourse. A vaginal infection that irritates the lining of the vagina can cause pain, often right at the beginning of intercourse. Signs of infection, such as discharge or odor, are usually present. Infections may be either yeast or bacterial, and the diagnosis can be made by examining the discharge under a microscope to see which organisms are present. Infections are usually easily treated with specific antibiotic or antifungal creams or oral medication.

The tissue of the vagina needs estrogen in order to stay healthy and elastic. Many months, or even years, after menopause, vaginal lubrication decreases, and this tissue becomes thinner and less elastic. As a result, the vagina is unable to stretch during intercourse, and pain results. If taken when menopause begins, estrogen in either vaginal cream or pill form is very effective in preventing these changes. If you have gone through menopause and the tissue is already thin, reversing the process with estrogen can be successfully accomplished, but it may take six to twelve months. Homeopathic remedies such as calendula cream, vitamin E oil, or progesterone cream can also be helpful for women who cannot or do not want to take estrogen. Frequent intercourse or manual stretching of the vaginal tissue also helps to maintain its elasticity.

Vaginal dryness can also lead to pain with intercourse. Normally, if a woman is sexually aroused, a lubricating fluid is produced that coats the vaginal walls and protects the tissue from irritation. Sometimes infection or other irritation can cause the vagina to make less fluid, and discomfort during intercourse results. The hormonal changes that result from breast-feeding, taking birth control pills, or menopause may have the same effect. As a consequence of this discomfort, some women may anticipate pain with intercourse. This feeling of anxious, fearful anticipation of pain is thought to bring on a further reduction in the amount of lubrication and further adds to the discomfort.

Liberal use of a nonpetroleum lubricant for every sexual encounter over the course of a few weeks often provides comfort and allows a woman to relax and experience sexual intercourse as pleasurable again. After a while, the lubricant can be discontinued, or used when you think it will help you enjoy your sex life more fully.

Another cause of painful intercourse is vaginismus, involuntary spasm of the vaginal muscles. For some women, this may occur to such a degree that intercourse is not possible. Vaginal infection, irritation, or dryness that causes pain with intercourse may lead to vaginal muscle spasms in response to the pain. Another source of vaginal muscle spasms may be prior sexual or physical abuse. Fear of intercourse, regardless of the reason, may also lead to the same problem. For women who have this condition, exercises that contract and relax the vaginal muscles called Kegel's exercises can teach improved muscular control and may result in comfort during intercourse. Emotional questions and issues that result from abuse are best resolved under the care of a therapist trained to deal with sexual problems.

Scar tissue near the uterus, fallopian tubes, or ovaries from previous infection, surgery, or endometriosis may also cause pain during intercourse. Pain from these causes is usually felt deep in the pelvis rather than in the vagina. Scar tissue is discussed on page 175 and endometriosis on page 177.

What Is Chronic Pain?

Acute pain and chronic pain are very different. Unlike acute pain, chronic pain persists after your body has had a reasonable time to heal from injury. It appears that chronic pain results from changes in your nervous system that cause the brain to feel pain even after the original injury has healed. Common examples of chronic pain include low back pain, frequent headaches, and chronic pelvic pain. Chronic pain can cause a change in your ability to do physical activity and/or cause a change in your mood. It also can lead to fatigue, sluggishness, insomnia, and depression. Anyone who is forced to endure long-term pain will be worn down by it and will likely find that his or her life has been changed by the pain. Fortunately, increased understanding of chronic pain in general has given us a better grasp of chronic pelvic pain.

By the time pain becomes chronic, there are usually both physical and psychological factors contributing to it. Let me make it clear that this does *not* mean that people with chronic pain are "crazy," or that the pain is "all in their minds." The pain is real and is conveyed by neurotransmitters, chemicals made by the brain that regulate both pain perception and mood.

Although pain is not all in the mind, the way you feel pain depends on psychological factors. For example, if you are afraid that pain is the result of a serious problem or is likely to be long-lasting, that fear about your condition may heighten the way your brain perceives the pain. Therefore, in addition to medical therapy, the best approach to chronic pain may be a multidisciplinary approach that often includes medical and psychological methods, as well as modification of diet and physical activity.

What Is Chronic Pelvic Pain?

Pelvic pain that lasts six or more months and is not associated with the menstrual period is called chronic pelvic pain. (Menstrual pain is discussed in chapter 3.) Chronic pelvic pain is a fairly common problem. It is estimated that about 20 percent of the visits to gynecologists are for pelvic pain, and one out of every seven hysterectomies is performed for this reason. Chronic pelvic pain can lead to significant distress and even disability. In recent years, a great deal of effort and research has been focused on helping women with chronic pelvic pain and people suffering from all types of chronic pain. Because of this, we are able to help people diminish the effects of pain.

What Can Cause Chronic Pelvic Pain?

Interestingly, when you were developing as a fetus, the same type of cells that went on to form the uterus, fallopian tubes, and ovaries also developed into the bladder. Furthermore, the bladder, the intestines, and the pelvic organs share similar nerves, and your brain may not be able to differentiate pain in one area from that in another area. Lastly, the bladder, the intestines, and the pelvic organs are close together in the abdominal area (see fig. 1.1), and it may be difficult for you to tell exactly where a pain originates. Therefore gynecologic problems, as well as bladder problems, intestinal problems, and neuromuscular problems can all be felt as "pelvic" pain. In this chapter we will discuss all these causes in detail.

What Can Be Done to Evaluate the Cause of Chronic Pelvic Pain?

Finding the cause of pelvic pain sometimes can be thought of as a puzzle that requires careful and methodical examination until the correct solution comes to light. There are many different causes of pelvic pain, and many of them are nongynecological.

The best way to start to solve the puzzle and get to the source of your pain is to provide your doctor with a detailed description of the pain. Keeping a daily pain diary that you fill out in the morning, afternoon, and evening can help you track the pain: Where is it? When does it occur? What makes it better or worse? Does eating affect it? Is it accompanied by nausea, vomiting, or diarrhea? Do you have any bladder symptoms? The location of the pain, its severity, and any relationship to physical activity or eating will help determine what organs could possibly be involved. The presence of other symptoms may also help focus on particular areas of the body that may need further testing.

A thorough physical examination is the next order of business and should include evaluation of the bladder, intestines, abdominal wall muscles, and pelvic organs. Often, a "multidisciplinary approach" will be the most helpful way to approach the pain. This method uses a team of medical professionals, combining their experience and problem-solving skills in order to solve the puzzle, find the source of the pain, and treat it. The team often consists of a gynecologist, a specialized pain-management physician, and a psychologist. While "pain clinics" have been developed for this purpose, these professionals can also be assembled by your primary care physician or gynecologist. The gynecologist is responsible for evaluating possible gynecologic causes of pain, and the pain-management physician should be skilled in the diagnosis and treatment of other causes of pain. In addition, consultants such as a urologist (urinary system), gastroenterologist (stomach and intestine), or orthopedist (muscles, joints, and bones) may be needed. The therapist is trained to evaluate stress, family, or marital problems, or feelings of helplessness or depression, which all can affect pain. The therapist can also help design an effective plan for stress reduction and pain relief. This may sound like a lot of work, but a pain-free life is a goal worth working toward.

Can Pelvic Infection Cause Chronic Pain?

Infection of the uterus, fallopian tubes, or ovaries is usually associated with fever, nausea, and sometimes vomiting. While infection can certainly cause acute pelvic pain, it is probably an infrequent cause of chronic pain.

However, many women who have chronic or recurrent pelvic pain are often assumed by their doctors to have chronic pelvic infections and are treated with repeated courses of antibiotics. Many of these women are later found to have endometriosis or other causes for their pain. Consequently, they were inappropriately treated, sometimes for years, while their real problem went undetected. Often, viewing the pelvis by means of laparoscopy can make the correct diagnosis for women who are suspected of having chronic pelvic infection.

Can Pelvic Scar Tissue (Adhesions) Cause Chronic Pelvic Pain?

An injury to the pelvic organs can result from infection, endometriosis, or wounds from surgery. Following an injury, the body forms scar tissue as part of the healing process. Unfortunately, this scar tissue, called *adhesions*, may form between areas of the body that are not normally connected. For example, the fallopian tube may stick to the ovary (see fig. 7.1), or the intestine may stick to the top of the uterus.

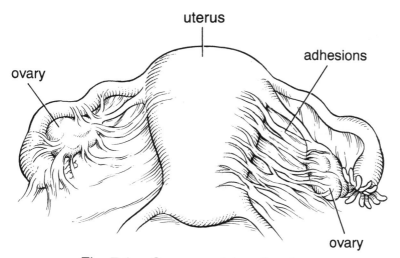

Fig. 7.1.   Severe pelvic adhesions

Although the uterus is anchored inside your body near the cervix, the top of the uterus, the fallopian tubes and the ovaries are only loosely connected by thin, weak ligaments. These ligaments normally allow some movement of the pelvic organs during activity or intercourse. But scar tissue is not elastic like normal tissue; it doesn't stretch easily. If inflexible adhesions form around the pelvic organs, their normal motion may be impaired. The pulling and tugging of scar tissue on normal tissue, which is filled with nerve endings, may lead to pain. Consequently, scar tissue may lead to pain during activity or intercourse.

Adhesions form within a few weeks following an infection or surgery, and once they form they do not get any better or worse over time. It is common to have adhesions without having any pain, especially if the scar tissue forms in areas that do not normally move during activity. Some areas are just less sensitive. However, if the adhesions are the cause of chronic pelvic pain, removal of the adhesions can be performed surgically. Traditionally, this has been done by abdominal surgery, but now laparoscopic techniques (see page 178) are effective and have the benefit of a shorter recovery period. Nonsurgical techniques such as biofeedback and relaxation techniques should also be considered. These techniques are often helpful for the relief of pain from adhesions.

Dianne's Pelvic Pain

Dianne is a thirty-three-year-old woman who had felt lower abdominal and pelvic pain for the past six or seven months. The pain was crampy and came and went from time to time. She seemed to have the most discomfort a few hours after eating, although she did not have any other symptoms of bowel problems such as nausea or diarrhea. She had seen her family physician, who had treated her with a medication to help relax any spasm in the intestines, but this had not helped. Because the symptoms seemed most likely to be intestinal, her family physician referred her to a gastroenterologist.

The gastroenterologist agreed that the problem seemed to be intestinal and performed a series of X-ray tests of the small and large intestines. These tests were also normal. I was asked to see Dianne at this point to determine if any gynecological problem could be found to explain her pain. The only significant part of her gynecologic history was a vague and mild pelvic infection that she had a year ago. The infection had been quickly diagnosed and treated with antibiotics and she was able to return to work in about two days.

Dianne's pelvic examination was normal, but to be sure that I wasn't missing anything, I ordered a pelvic sonogram. The sonogram was also normal. The only thing left to offer Dianne in order to try to determine the cause of her pain was a diagnostic laparoscopy. Even though her pain was not severe, Dianne was frustrated and worried, so she decided to have the laparoscopy performed. During surgery, the cause of her pain became immediately apparent. Probably as a result of her prior pelvic infection, numerous thick bands of scar tissue had formed from her uterus and fallopian tubes to her intestines. The intestines were kinked in such a way that as digested food passed through the intestines, the movement cause the scar tissue to pull on the uterus, thus causing the pain. This explained why her pain seemed to be worse following meals. Using laparoscopic scissors, we were able to carefully cut away the scar tissue from the intestines and the uterus and fallopian tubes. The surgery was difficult and required patience. The end result looked good. She appeared to be free from all the scar tissue. In addition, the ends of Dianne's fallopian tubes appeared to be fairly healthy, and we were hopeful that she would be able to get pregnant in the future. Surgical removal of scar tissue relieves pain about two-thirds of the time. In this case, the surgery relieved Dianne's pain, and it has never returned.

Can Endometriosis Cause Pelvic Pain?

As described in chapter 6, endometriosis results from the growth of uterine-lining cells outside the uterus. These cells remain under the influence of hormones made by the ovary and, to some degree, go through the changes of the menstrual cycle.

However, at the end of the menstrual cycle, when bleeding occurs with your period, the misplaced cells cause a small amount of bleeding inside your body. The blood and other chemicals released from these cells, which do not belong in this area, irritate the pelvic organs. Over time, this irritation leads to injury of the cells covering the pelvic organs, and scar tissue can result, causing pain.

How Can the Pain from Endometriosis Be Treated?

One form of effective treatment for the relief of pain from endometriosis involves the surgical removal of the areas where the endometriosis has begun to grow. Once the source of the misplaced bleeding is removed, pain often improves. Removal of areas of endometriosis can now be accomplished by laparoscopic surgery, using either a laser, electrosurgical instruments, or laparoscopic scissors. All of these techniques are equally effective. Thorough removal of the diseased tissue seems to give the best results, but surgery for extensive endometriosis is difficult to perform. Therefore, it is probably best to choose a gynecologist who has experience treating women with this condition.

Should You Have a Laparoscopy Performed?

Laparoscopy is a surgical procedure that involves placement of a thin telescope through an incision in the navel in order to see inside the abdomen and pelvis. It is often utilized to help establish the cause of pelvic pain and, in many cases, can be used to treat the cause of the pain as well. The procedure is performed in a hospital or outpatient surgery center under general anesthesia. With the laparoscope, the doctor is able to see the uterus, fallopian tubes, ovaries, intestines, appendix, gall bladder, and liver. With a careful inspection, gynecologic problems such as endometriosis, pelvic infection, adhesions, ovarian cysts, and tubal pregnancy can be diagnosed. Inflammation or infection of the appendix, intestines, or gall bladder may also be detected so that appropriate treatment may be started. In addition, by using specialized instruments during the laparoscopy, many of these problems may be treated at the same time. Adhesions and endometriosis may be cut away, and ovarian cysts or a tubal pregnancy removed.

Although new adhesions can sometimes form as part of the healing process after any surgery, many women found to have significant adhesions at the time of the laparoscopy will feel better after the adhesions are surgically removed. Laparoscopic surgery for moderate or severe endometriosis has been shown to provide pain relief about 70 percent of the time. However, the presence of thin adhesions or a small quantity of endometriosis does not often cause pelvic pain; therefore, surgery for these problems should be approached cautiously.

In as many as 30 percent of women who have laparoscopy for chronic pelvic pain, a normal uterus, fallopian tubes, and ovaries are found. A normal pelvis may suggest the need for other tests to determine if the problem is elsewhere. But if the findings during the laparoscopy are normal, it is extremely unlikely that any serious problem exists with the pelvic organs, and this information can be very reassuring.

While not major abdominal surgery, laparoscopic surgery does have risks and should be considered only when other nongynecologic causes of the pain have been excluded. Be sure that any surgery is warranted and will provide the relief you are seeking. However, the information acquired at the time of laparoscopy can be valuable. Nothing else—not ultrasound, nor CT scan, nor MRI, nor blood tests—can diagnose problems such as endometriosis or adhesions at an early stage. Therefore, the procedure can be helpful when used appropriately.

Is There a Relationship Between Sexual or Physical Abuse and Pelvic Pain?

Women who have been physically or sexually abused are more likely to suffer from chronic pelvic pain than women who have not been abused. It has been estimated that 30 percent of all women in the United States have been sexually abused by the time they reach their midteens. The understanding of the relationship between sexual or physical abuse and physical symptoms or emotional problems that may be experienced at some point later in a woman's life is a relatively new concept. Abuse is probably evidence of only one of a family's many failures to provide the quality of emotional comfort and support needed for emotional development and growth. Women who have been abused are more likely to have frequent doctor visits, unexplained medical symptoms, and a higher incidence of surgery.

You should consider discussing any history of abuse with your physician or with a therapist. Appropriate counseling can provide the support and guidance that you need to help with your chronic pain, your emotional state, and your recovery. Counseling will allow you to actively participate in the management of your pain and have some control over it, rather than having it control you. This support is essential to emotional healing and helps to pave the way toward relief of your pain.

Sandra's Confusing Pelvic Pain

Sandra is a thirty-year-old woman who was first referred to me for evaluation of chronic pelvic pain that had been present for about a year. At first the pain had been infrequent, but now it was occurring almost daily. There was no apparent relationship between the pain and her physical activity, eating, or menstrual cycle. Pain medications had failed to help, and Sandra was understandably frustrated. She had alternated between trying to be philosophical and stoical about the pain, to being depressed and angry that her life had become so entrapped by discomfort. She was hoping that I would find something that her other doctors had missed.

Her pelvic examination and the rest of her physical examination were entirely normal, and a sonogram, performed just to make sure we were not missing anything, was also normal. Since she had a long history of pelvic pain that was increasing in intensity and frequency, Sandra and I discussed performing a laparoscopy to enable me to truly "see" if there was something wrong. She and I both agreed that laparoscopy was a reasonable thing to do at this point. Sandra was becoming increasingly worn down by her pain and frustrated that no cause had been found. Being only thirty years old, she had begun to wonder what the rest of her life was going to be like with this amount of daily discomfort. Her usual optimism was diminishing, and she had been unable to make any plans in terms of her career or her personal life. It was time to try something else.

During the laparoscopy, we looked at her uterus, fallopian tubes, and ovaries, as well as her appendix, liver, gall bladder, and intestines. Everything appeared normal and healthy. When I discussed this with Sandra after surgery, she was both relieved and disappointed. It was good to know that all her organs were healthy, yet what could be causing this pain? I reassured Sandra that everything appeared to be perfectly normal and suggested that we allow some time to see if the pain would resolve by itself.

For the next year or so, Sandra was cared for by her family doctor. At times her pain was better and at times worse, but it never went away. Tests of her intestines were performed but were also normal. Then one day she developed the sudden onset of sharp and severe pelvic pain. She came back to see me. On examination, she was extremely tender. Because of the severity of the pain, we felt that another laparoscopy was indicated to diagnose this problem. We performed the surgery that day and found a twisted and dying appendix, which we were able to remove with laparoscopic instruments. This seemed to be the cause of this episode of pain but did not explain her more chronic pain. In fact, shortly after the surgery, her chronic pain reappeared. Now we were all depressed. My heart went out to her, but unfortunately my medical expertise and experience were not enough to provide her with the pain relief she so badly needed.

Sandra continued to see her family doctor for her regular medical care. But at her next gynecologic visit with me, she appeared to be more relaxed and told me that her pain was gone. She then went on to tell me that she had been having a problem in her relationship with her boyfriend and had begun therapy. During the therapy, she discussed the fact that, as a child, she had been sexually abused on multiple occasions by a close relative. Working through this problem with her therapist culminated in a confrontation with the abusive relative. This had gone a long way toward helping her deal with the pain and fear she felt. Her pelvic pain also began to go away during this time. By the time I saw her, she was entirely pain free. She and her therapist felt that the pain was a manifestation of the abuse that had occurred years before. I have seen Sandra every year since, about ten years in a row, and she has never had the pain again and is now happily married.

I learned a great deal from Sandra's experience. I had been unfamiliar with the association of abuse and pelvic pain before seeing Sandra's recovery. Now I am very aware of the issues of sexual and physical abuse and discuss the subject with women who have chronic pelvic pain. For most women, abuse has not been part of their lives, and the discussion ends there. If, however, someone has experienced abuse and is interested in getting help, I refer them to a therapist who is specially trained to deal with these issues. Many women benefit from this therapy.

What Types of Bladder Problems Can Cause Pelvic Pain?

Bladder infections can cause pain that is commonly felt just below the pubic bone. However, the pain usually develops quickly and is associated with other symptoms such as frequency of urination, the feeling of urgency to urinate, pain with urination, or, rarely, blood in the urine. These symptoms differentiate a bladder infection from pain that originates in the pelvic organs or intestines. The diagnosis can be made by examining a urine sample under a microscope for the presence of bacteria and white blood cells.

Chronic mild infections of the urethra (the tube that you urinate out of) may also cause pelvic pain. These urethral infections are also often associated with urgency, frequency, and pain with urination. But sometimes irritation of the urethra occurs in the absence of infection. This condition, called chronic urethral syndrome, may result from eating spicy foods or drinking caffeinated or alcoholic beverages that end up in the urine and cause irritation as they pass through the urethra. This diagnosis is often made when, despite treatment with antibiotics, the urethra remains tender and the feeling of urgency persists. Your doctor will discuss dietary changes with you that restrict irritants like spicy foods, alcohol, or caffeine. Often, these changes will relieve the symptoms without any medication. Some women find that Kegel's exercises (see page 128), which tighten and then relax the vaginal muscles, help them to relax the muscles around the urethra, reducing spasm and pain.

What Is Interstitial Cystitis, and Can It Cause Pelvic Pain?

Interstitial cystitis is a condition that causes chronic inflammation of the bladder lining, without any evidence of infection. Women with interstitial cystitis have almost constant bladder pain or pressure and feel the urge to urinate when there are even small quantities of urine in their bladders. This frequent urination often leads to sleepless nights.

The cause of this condition is unknown. Researchers suspect that the coating layer inside the bladder, which normally protects the bladder from irritation, may be absent in women with this problem. A urologist can diagnose interstitial cystitis by looking inside the bladder with a small telescope called a cystoscope. The procedure is performed while you are under anesthesia. After examination with the cystoscope, the bladder is filled to capacity with water. If interstitial cystitis is present, small areas of bleeding will appear in the bladder wall. A biopsy of the bladder wall examined under a microscope can confirm the diagnosis.

What Is the Treatment for Interstitial Cystitis?

Treatment for interstitial cystitis is difficult, because no available therapy can restore the missing inner protective layer of the bladder. However, for reasons that are not understood, filling the bladder during the cystoscopy with large amounts of water while you are under anesthesia often will relieve discomfort and urgency for months. This treatment can be repeated, if needed.

Other types of therapy may also be helpful. Learning to relax the pelvic floor muscles may relieve symptoms for many women; others may require medication to relieve spasm and pain. Treating the bladder with chemical solutions such as the common solvent called DMSO provides relief for some women with this problem, but pain may recur. For women with interstitial cystitis, a therapy that replaces the missing protective layer of the bladder will, hopefully, be developed soon.

What Types of Intestinal Problems Can Cause Pelvic Pain?

We all know that even simple constipation can cause a fullness or sense of pressure in the pelvis. Intestinal conditions such as irritable bowel syndrome and inflammation or infection of the intestines can also cause lower abdominal and pelvic pain. Oftentimes, we can clearly point to the intestines as the cause of pelvic pain because of the presence of intestinal symptoms. Usual clues that the pain may be intestinal are nausea, vomiting, diarrhea, or constipation. Likewise, a decrease in appetite, a sensation of bloating, or a visible swelling of your abdomen is often the result of intestinal problems. Any blood or mucus in the stool is virtually always the result of intestinal rather than gynecologic disease. Specific intestinal problems are discussed below. If you suspect any of these problems, you should be evaluated by a primary care doctor or gastroenterologist (a specialist in conditions of the stomach, intestines, and liver).

What Is Irritable Bowel Syndrome?

Irritable bowel syndrome is one of the most common causes of lower abdominal and pelvic pain. Some studies have shown that up to 66 percent of women with chronic *pelvic* pain actually have irritable bowel syndrome. The cause of irritable bowel is uncertain. However, as food and gas move through the intestines, people with irritable bowel seem to be overly sensitive to the stretching of the intestines that normally occurs. This leads to crampy pain about an hour or so after eating and seems to be worse at times of stress. The pain may be accompanied by bloating and may last for hours, days, or even weeks. Constipation or, rarely, diarrhea may also be present.

What Is the Treatment for Irritable Bowel Syndrome?

The most effective treatment for irritable bowel syndrome combines medication, dietary changes, and stress reduction. Diets high in fiber (fruits and vegetables), in addition to medications that increase fiber and water in the stool, will help promote normal movement of stool through the colon and lessen the discomfort. Therapy designed to reduce stress, such as relaxation techniques or biofeedback, has also been found to be very effective in decreasing the frequency of attacks. In some women, medications to reduce stress may also be helpful.

Kathy's Pelvic Pain

Kathy is a twenty-eight-year-old woman who first saw me for lower abdominal and pelvic pain and bloating that had been getting worse over the past few months. The pain was crampy and came and went without much warning or apparent reason. Kathy assumed the pain was from her ovaries because it seemed to be in that general area. As we talked, it became apparent that the pain was not related to her menstrual periods, her activities, or intercourse. In fact, the one thing that seemed to make the pain more likely to occur was stress. Kathy had been under an increasing amount of stress on her job, as continuing layoffs of other workers had increased her workload and made her worry that she might be next. She had also noted some diarrhea recently but felt this was due to her increased nervousness about her job and her health.

The examination of her uterus, fallopian tubes, ovaries, and abdomen was normal. Kathy was relieved that she didn't have anything wrong with her ovaries, because she now admitted that she was worried that she had ovarian cancer. She thought that if she had mentioned that possibility, she would have somehow increased the likelihood of having the disease simply by uttering its name. But despite that enormous relief, she was still physically uncomfortable, and we discussed having her get further evaluation. Because of the diarrhea, I recommended that she see a gastroenterologist. When this consultation was completed, the gastroenterologist agreed that her examination was totally normal. Based on Kathy's symptoms, he concluded that she probably had irritable bowel syndrome. Before beginning a series of X-ray tests, the doctor recommended that she try a medication to increase fiber and water in her intestines, as well as some stress-reduction exercises. Kathy's symptoms got better over the next few weeks. The diet changes and medication made her move her bowels more regularly, and the crampy pain gradually seemed to disappear. In addition to the relief of knowing that nothing serious was wrong with her, the relaxation exercises really helped to decrease her stress level. What had appeared to be a gynecologic problem, and in Kathy's mind was ovarian cancer until proven otherwise, turned out to be a common and fairly easy to treat intestinal condition.

What Is Inflammatory Bowel Disease?

Two uncommon conditions, Crohn's disease and ulcerative colitis, produce inflammation of the inside lining of the intestines and cause abdominal pain. Crohn's disease often begins between the ages of fifteen and thirty, but occurs in less than two out of ten thousand people. It is usually associated with diarrhea and sometimes rectal bleeding, and fever is common. Episodes of pain and diarrhea may last for days, or even weeks. Ulcerative colitis is also a rare disease, occurring in about four out of every ten thousand people, most often near the age of thirty or forty. It is usually associated with acute abdominal pain that is often relieved by a bowel movement. Diarrhea and rectal bleeding are common.

Because both of these conditions cause predominantly intestinal symptoms, we commonly suspect the cause to be intestinal disease rather than pelvic problems. Evaluation by a primary care doctor or gastroenterologist should lead to the diagnosis. Then appropriate treatment can be started.

What Is Diverticulitis?

Diverticulosis is a condition common in men and women as they get older. Forty percent of people over the age of sixty have this condition, which by itself causes no symptoms. Diverticulosis develops as a consequence of weakening in the wall of the large intestines. With progressive weakening, small folds and pockets appear in the intestinal wall. These pockets can trap stool, and when stool and the swarm of bacteria contained in it get trapped, an infection may result.

The resulting infection is called diverticulitis and leads to abdominal pain and fever. But this infection is rare, and diverticulitis occurs in fewer than 20 percent of people with diverticulosis. Sometimes a smoldering type of infection may develop and cause a more long-lasting form of pain. The diagnosis of diverticulitis can be made with a specialized X-ray test called a CT scan. Antibiotics are successfully used to treat this illness.

Can Intestinal Cancer Cause Pelvic Pain?

The most common symptom of colon cancer is a change in bowel habits, either diarrhea, constipation, or a narrowing of the stool. Abdominal pain and rectal bleeding occur in about half of the people with colon cancer. Colon cancer becomes more common with age; it is uncommon before age forty. A history of a close family member with intestinal polyps or colon cancer can increase your risk of developing this disease. A yearly test of blood in the stool should be performed after age forty. If it is positive, or if you have bowel symptoms that persist, an inspection of the lower colon and rectum with a small flexible telescope (flexible sigmoidoscopy) should be performed to make the diagnosis. Inspection of the upper colon with colonoscopy may also be recommended.

Can Muscle Problems Cause Pelvic Pain?

The abdominal muscles are situated over the pelvis and attach to the pubic bone. Muscular spasms that result from a previous injury to the muscle or from muscular tension may be confused by both the patient and physician with pain of gynecologic origin.

The nerves that "talk" to the brain are shared in the pelvic area by the uterus, ovaries, muscles, and joints, and you may not be able to tell exactly what part of your body is feeling pain. Therefore, it is not uncommon for muscle or joint pain to be confused with true pelvic pain. For that reason, the right diagnosis is often hard to establish. It might be helpful to keep a pain diary for a few days to see if there are any patterns as to when and where you feel the pain. Pain from muscles or joints is often dull and aching and is usually worse when you are active. What you learn about your body will help your doctor determine the cause of the pain.

What Can Cause Musculoskeletal Pain?

Your parents probably told you to stand up straight, and they were right. Poor standing posture, slumping while you sit, or other poor sitting habits can overstress both muscles and joints and lead to back pain or pelvic pain.

Any previous back or pelvic injuries from work, falling off a horse, playing with the kids, making home repairs, tennis, aerobics, etc., may cause pelvic pain. Arthritis resulting from an old injury or simply the aging process may lead to spasm in the muscles around the joint and cause pain. Sometimes trigger points, very small areas of muscle spasm, are found near previous incisions or areas of prior injury. Women may also have areas of muscle spasm due to poor posture. The doctor can detect these trigger points by pressing into the abdominal and back muscles. Tenderness in the muscle, rather than in the underlying pelvic organs, will confirm this diagnosis.

TREATMENT FOR PELVIC PAIN

What Can Be Done to Treat Musculoskeletal Pain?

Physical therapists and chiropractors are well trained to treat the musculoskeletal causes of pelvic pain. Treatment usually involves teaching you how to stand and sit properly, as well as the use of heat, cold packs, and massage. Stretching and exercise can also be used to relieve muscle spasm, as can acupuncture and acupressure. For women who have trigger points (small areas of muscle spasm), an injection of local anesthetic into the tender area is very helpful. The anesthesia relaxes the spasm and can often result in long-term relief, even after it wears off. The treatments outlined above may be very helpful for women whose pain is caused by a musculoskeletal problem.

Anne's Persistent Abdominal Pain

Anne is a forty-two-year-old woman who had two years of lower abdominal pain that began shortly after she had a hysterectomy performed for persistent, abnormal bleeding. Since she no longer had her uterus, fallopian tubes, and ovaries, there simply were no pelvic organs present that could possibly cause pain. Her gynecologist had performed a pelvic exam and a sonogram, which were completely normal.

In her quest to be free of pain, she also was evaluated by her internist for intestinal or bladder problems that could cause abdominal pain, but none were found. Anne had reluctantly begun taking pain medications, but now the pain was worse, and the pills were less helpful. Her gynecologist suggested another surgery to determine if scar tissue from the hysterectomy was the cause of the pain. Before agreeing to another surgery, Anne decided to seek a second opinion. When she came into my office, she was emotionally prepared to face a second surgery but wanted to make sure surgery was her best choice.

As we expected, her pelvic examination was entirely normal. However, an area near the side of her previous abdominal incision seemed to be tender. While she was lying down, I gently pushed my finger into all the areas of her abdominal muscles in order to pinpoint the exact area of discomfort. A spot near the left side of her incision was tender when pushed, and this reproduced the pain she felt daily.

It became clear that her pain was from the incision. The most likely cause of this type of pain is muscle spasm or irritation of nerves near the incision. Despite the discomfort the exam had caused her, Anne was elated to find out what seemed to be the cause of her pain. Since the pain was only in the incision, surgery did not seem necessary. That was good news.

I referred Anne to an anesthesiologist in our community who has training in pain management. He began injections of local anesthesia to the area. The first two injections, given about two weeks apart, were only briefly and mildly uncomfortable and provided immediate and enormous relief. Two more injections were given about a month apart, and by the end of this time, Anne was pain free. When I saw Anne a year later for her routine exam, she had been pain free for ten months. The pain has not returned.

What Is the Best Way to Use Pain Medications for Chronic Pelvic Pain?

The most effective medications for managing chronic pain act by preventing the formation of substances called prostaglandins that cause the pain. Called antiprostaglandins, these medications include Advil, Aleve, and ibuprofen and are now available over the counter in low doses.

These medications are most effective for chronic pain relief when taken in small to moderate doses every few hours (see individual instructions), rather than waiting for severe pain to occur. This "scheduled" use of pain medication, which should be started under your doctor's direction, has two major benefits. First, taking the medication on a regular basis prevents the pain from ever getting severe. Second, the reassurance of knowing that the pain will not become severe will free you from the constant worry about it and allow you to focus on your life and work. Worrying about pain truly seems to make it worse, and, not surprisingly, we experience less pain when we are busy and content.

Should Narcotic Medications Be Used for Chronic Pain?

It is not a good idea to use narcotic medications for the relief of chronic pain. Medications such as Percodan, Percocet, codeine, Dilaudid, and Demerol can all be addictive. You need to take these medications in increasing amounts in order to provide continued pain relief. Furthermore, their use may actually cause an increase in pain, because they deplete chemicals in the brain that prevent pain. You will only make your pain worse if you start taking narcotics.

What Other Medications Are Helpful in the Treatment of Chronic Pelvic Pain?

One of the most exciting areas of medicine today is the science of neurobiology, the study of the chemical events that allow the brain to function. For example, a low level of two brain chemicals, serotonin and norepinephrine, has been linked to some forms of depression and also to the perception of pain. And it appears that the inability to produce adequate amounts of brain chemicals is inherited and not under an individual's control. Certain medications that act to increase serotonin and norepinephrine are helpful for some forms of depression and also for people who have chronic pain. While the word *antidepressant* may disturb some women, low doses of these medications can increase serotonin and/or norepinephrine levels in the brain and can help relieve chronic pain, improve sleep, and reduce the depression that often accompanies chronic pain. These medications should be prescribed by a doctor knowledgeable in their use for pain management.

Can Your Attitude About Pain Influence What You Feel?

As noted above, the first order of business if you have pain is to get a thorough medical evaluation. If that evaluation reveals no identifiable or serious problem, then you may feel some degree of reassurance. Not finding an answer is frustrating. But if a proper evaluation has ruled out a condition that might be dangerous, you have received good news. If a minor but not entirely treatable condition is found, there should be some relief in knowing that nothing serious is wrong.

With this reassurance, you should no longer view pain as a signal of bodily danger, and this shift away from focusing on pain may help relieve it. If a person frequently thinks about pain, the focus will be on the negative aspects of his or her life and circumstances. After being pleasantly busy and distracted, we often find ourselves forgetting about any pain or discomfort we had been feeling. Being productive and doing the activities you like to do can lead to a more positive feeling about your life. This may decrease your pain and lead to a feeling of control, something people in pain often say they miss.

This explanation is not meant to negate your true feelings of pain. I respect and understand skepticism about this approach, but a positive attitude does seem to make a difference for people with chronic pain. In studies of women with pelvic pain without any obvious cause, those who were taught the positive approach without surgery felt much better than those who were treated by surgery.

Can Relaxation Methods Be Used to Help Treat Pain?

Your perception of pain is determined by your brain, and this perception is heightened by stress and tension. A number of techniques have been successfully used to help reduce the perception of all types of pain, including pelvic pain, headache, and arthritis. Relaxation techniques that use systematic contraction followed by relaxation of all your muscles are very effective. There is nothing fancy about these techniques, although you will probably need practice before they become effective.

Some of you may remember relaxation techniques from your Lamaze birthing classes. Lie down in a quiet place and start by contracting the muscles in your toes and holding that contraction for a few seconds. Then concentrate on totally relaxing the same muscles. After your toes, you can contract and then relax your calf muscles. By starting at your toes and working your way up your entire body, one part at a time, you can induce a state of total relaxation that will reduce stress. Be sure to spend time contracting your cheek, your forehead, and your neck, since a great deal of muscular tension is often located in the head and neck area. During this time, deep and controlled breathing will also be calming. As you practice this technique, you should gradually be able to achieve total relaxation.

Techniques that divert your attention away from pain also help to reduce pain. Lie down, close your eyes, and imagine you are in a pleasant, beautiful place. This can be very relaxing and refreshing. Like Lamaze techniques, these methods help you focus away from pain and decrease the brain's perception of pain. To make this technique as effective as possible, you will probably have to practice doing it. Transporting yourself mentally to another place may sound easy, but it takes a great deal of focus and concentration. When I need to relax, I always picture myself sitting on a Hawaiian beach, feeling a warm breeze. A pleasant daydream can also reduce tension and stress and help to diminish your perception of pain. Instructional relaxation and visualization tapes are available at many bookstores and health food stores. These techniques are most effective when used either on a regular basis or long before the sensation of pain is strong.

Does Acupuncture Relieve Pelvic Pain?

Acupuncture effectively relieves pelvic pain in some women. The concept of a mind-body connection, long a focal point of many Eastern philosophies, is gaining much attention in Western medicine. The connection of the mind and body during the perception of pain is the perfect example of the complexity of our bodies. As with all types of treatment, if you choose to try acupuncture, you should find a well-trained and respected practitioner. Your doctor may be able to recommend a skilled acupuncturist in your community. Acupuncture provides quick relief for some women; for others the effect is cumulative over a period of time.

Transcutaneous nerve stimulation (TENS) has also been used successfully to treat chronic pain. Using a weak electrical current passed through wires attached to the skin, this technique probably works by stimulating some nerves in order to prevent pain from other areas, just as acupuncture does. Your doctor may be able to refer you to someone with experience in this simple and safe technique.

Can Biofeedback Treat Chronic Pain?

Biofeedback provides pain relief for some women. During biofeedback, your pulse, blood pressure, and muscle tension are monitored continuously through small wires attached to your body. When you are relaxed, your blood pressure, pulse, and muscle tension are at low levels. As you practice relaxing, the monitors report information back to you, usually with a sound signal that lowers its tone as you become more relaxed. In this way, successful relaxation is "fed back" to you, and you learn how to bring about this relaxed state by yourself at any time, without the monitors. Biofeedback is best taught by a psychologist skilled in this technique.

Lila's Difficult Problem

Lila is a twenty-five-year-old woman who came to see me for a *fifth* opinion. For the past two years she had undergone a series of evaluations, tests, procedures, and surgeries all of which had failed to help her chronic pelvic pain. When the pain had started two years ago, Lila had been seen by a gynecologist who felt that she most likely had endometriosis. She had recommended a laparoscopy, which was performed the following month. At that time, very mild endometriosis was found and easily treated with a laser. Lila and her doctor were confident that the treatment would end the pain, but the pain did not improve.

Assuming that the pain was the result of a nongynecologic problem, the gynecologist suggested that Lila see an internist for further testing. Blood tests for liver, gall bladder, and kidney problems were done, but revealed nothing abnormal. X rays of the intestines and a sonogram of the liver, gall bladder, and pancreas were also normal. By this time, Lila had become frustrated and went to see another gynecologist. The second gynecologist reviewed Lila's records and wondered whether the endometriosis had come back and recommended another laparoscopy. This was performed, and very mild endometriosis was again discovered and removed with the laser. The laser treatment did nothing to help her chronic pain. She then went to see a gastroenterologist who looked into her intestines with a small telescope called an endoscope. This was also normal. So, four doctors had cared for Lila and none had been able to cure her pain. Lila came to my office expecting that another laparoscopy needed to be done for her endometriosis. After reviewing all of her records, sonograms, and X rays, and after performing a pelvic exam that was normal, I felt that another laparoscopy would probably not be helpful.

I reassured Lila that not only was her examination totally normal, but all the combined previous testing had found only a small amount of endometriosis. Treatment through laparoscopy had failed to make her better. We discussed the process of endometriosis (see chapter 6) and the fact that it would be unlikely to recur to a significant degree in such a short period of time. At this point I suggested that Lila consider measures less drastic than surgery to deal with her pain. She agreed to see a pain-management physician in our community.

He also reviewed all of Lila's records and performed an examination. He agreed that there was no concern about a serious undetected problem and recommended that Lila consider biofeedback and visualization under the direction of a skilled therapist. Exhausted from all the worry and all the running around to different doctors, Lila agreed. After a few sessions to learn to use both biofeedback and visualization techniques, Lila is now pain free on most days. She is able to work and do her normal activities without interruption. And when she feels that the pain is coming back, she has the ability to control it through the relaxation techniques she has learned. She sees me every six months, or more often if needed, and her pelvic examination has remained entirely normal. While it is clear that most of the testing Lila had was needed to eliminate any serious cause of her pain, continuing down that path was going to get her nowhere. Now she is happily back in control of her life.

Should You Have a Hysterectomy for Pelvic Pain?

The use of hysterectomy as an initial treatment of pelvic pain should be discouraged. About 10 percent of hysterectomies in the United States are performed because of pelvic pain, but many of these women do not have long-term relief of their pain following surgery. One study found that 20 percent of women who had a hysterectomy for pelvic pain had no improvement following surgery, and 5 percent said their pain was actually worse.

One reason for the lack of effectiveness of hysterectomy is that some causes of pelvic pain are not gynecologic in the first place. For that reason, hysterectomy to relieve pelvic pain should be reserved for women who clearly have a gynecologic disease that requires hysterectomy. In one study of women with chronic pelvic pain who were fully and properly evaluated for gynecologic, nongynecologic, and psychological causes of their pain, only 5 percent needed to have a hysterectomy.

On the other hand, hysterectomy may be appropriate for some women who do have a significant degree of pain that results from gynecologic causes and who have not responded to other forms of treatment (see chapter 11). Clearly, this procedure is only appropriate for women who do not want to have children. Pain resulting from severe endometriosis that has not responded to medical therapy and adequate laparoscopic treatment by a gynecologist experienced in treating endometriosis may respond to removal of the uterus, fallopian tubes, and ovaries. Pain that results primarily from severe adhesions due to prior infection or previous surgery can usually be treated by laparoscopic surgery. However, if this has already been tried without success, or if the amount of scar tissue would make laparoscopic surgery impossible, then hysterectomy may be considered.

Eighty-five percent of the women operated on for chronic pelvic pain in the Maine Women's Health Study (see page 281) noted more than eight days of pain per month prior to surgery, and 80 percent noted that the pain limited their activity. After surgery, only 13 percent of the women had significant pain. But it is important to note that in the Maine

Women's Health Study, none of the women had tried a multidisciplinary approach to pelvic pain. Had this been available, some of the women might have been spared from having a hysterectomy.

The decision to have a hysterectomy should not be taken lightly. There is more than one treatment option for almost all medical conditions. And none of the possible side effects of hysterectomy are entirely predictable for each individual. It is in your best interest to be educated about the health care decisions you make. Because of the complexity of chronic pain and continuing developments in its treatment, I believe that chronic pelvic pain is one area where a second opinion from someone who specializes in this field is well worth the time and effort.

REFERENCES

Milburn, A., R. Reiter, and A. Rhomburg. 1993. Multidisciplinary approach to chronic pelvic pain. *Obstetrics and Gynecology Clinics of North America* 20:643–61.

Rapkin, A., L. Kames, L. Darke, F. Stampler, and B. Naliboff. 1990. History of physical and sexual abuse in women with chronic pelvic pain. *Obstetrics and Gynecology* 76:92–96.

Reiter, R., and A. Milburn. 1994. Exploring effective treatment for chronic pelvic pain. *Contemporary Ob/Gyn.* March:84–103.

Rosenthal, R. 1993. Psychology of chronic pelvic pain. *Obstetrics and Gynecology Clinics of North America* 20:627–41.

Steege, J., A. Stout, and S. Somkuti. 1993. Chronic pelvic pain in women: toward an integrative model. *Obstetrical and Gynecological Survey* 48:95–110.

8

OVARIAN CANCER AND THE SEARCH FOR EARLY DETECTION

If *cancer* is one of the most dreaded words in the English language, then for most women *ovarian* is the worst adjective to place before *cancer*. Of all the bad news gynecologists deal with, this is the most frightening. Since the death of Gilda Radner, a comedienne who made so many of us laugh, people seem to be much more aware of ovarian cancer. This increase in interest has led to enhanced medical research. Studies are being done on the cause or causes, the treatment, and a means of early detection. For the 5 percent of ovarian cancer patients for whom the cancer may be hereditary, genetic research is evolving to help determine who is actually at risk. While we still feel as if we are groping in the dark with this disease, when I think back to five years ago, I know that we are making strides. This chapter deals with what we now know about the detection, treatment, and prevention of ovarian cancer. If you are anxious and concerned about this disease, I hope that this information allays many of your fears.

How Common Is Ovarian Cancer?

Though frightening, ovarian cancer is a rare disease. Only one out of every 15,000 women will have the disease at the age of thirty. At forty, about the age at which Gilda Radner discovered she had ovarian cancer, only one of every 10,000 women have this disease. At the age of sixty, the average age at which women get ovarian cancer, only one of every 1,500 women will have it. In your entire lifetime, if you live to be ninety years old, you have a 1 in 70 chance of developing ovarian cancer. Compare this with the 1 in 3 chance a woman has of dying of a heart attack by the time she is ninety, or the fact that you are more likely to die in an auto accident and twice as likely to die from colon cancer than you are from ovarian cancer. These statistics are not meant to diminish the human toll from this terrible disease. However, all of the interest and media coverage surrounding ovarian cancer has given the impression that the disease is now more common, that there is an epidemic. In fact, the incidence of ovarian cancer is no greater today than it was twenty-five years ago.

Are Most Growths on the Ovary Cancerous?

No. In fact, if a premenopausal woman has a growth on her ovary, there is over a 90 percent chance that this growth is benign. In postmenopausal women, an ovarian growth has a 70 percent chance of being benign. Therefore, if a growth is found on your ovary, *do not panic*. It will most likely not be cancer. Chapter 4 is devoted to the most common types of benign ovarian cysts.

What Actually Causes Ovarian Cancer?

Like all cancers, ovarian cancer results from the runaway overgrowth of cells. All the cells in our body have the capacity to multiply—that is how cells grow and how the body repairs damaged tissue on a regular basis. Cells contain numerous genes that actually control cell division and growth. Some of the genes promote cell growth, and other genes act to suppress runaway overgrowth of the cells. Chance alterations in these genes called mutations can cause the genes to malfunction and lead to uncontrolled growth of cells. When the normal controls over cell growth are lost, cancer may result. The specific genes responsible for causing ovarian cancer to develop are not yet known. However, current research may someday allow us to predict which women are at risk for ovarian cancer. In the more distant future, gene therapy may allow alteration of these genes within the body, so that we can actually prevent ovarian cancer.

RISK FACTORS FOR OVARIAN CANCER

We know that ovarian cancer is more common in women whose ovaries have continued to produce eggs without interruption over their lifetimes. Every time you ovulate, the surface of the ovary splits open to let the egg out. When the surface cells grow rapidly in order to heal the opening, they become more vulnerable to substances that can cause mutations (carcinogens). To date, the identity of these carcinogens is not certain (see page 202). In order for cancer to develop, it is likely that a number of factors must be present: the presence of a carcinogen, some predisposition to developing abnormal growth of the ovarian cells, and uninterrupted ovulation, which increases the carcinogen's chances of getting into the cell.

Events that prevent ovulation, such as pregnancy, breast-feeding, and taking birth control pills, will decrease your risk of developing ovarian cancer. During pregnancy, your ovaries do not produce any eggs for nine months. The hormonal changes associated with breast-feeding keep the ovaries at rest for a few more months. Birth control pills work by preventing the release of eggs from the ovary. Likewise, the late onset of your periods or early onset of menopause, which result in a decrease in the total number of times you ovulate in your lifetime, will also decrease your risk of getting ovarian cancer. Fewer ovulations lead to fewer vulnerable, healing, rapidly dividing cells and less risk of ovarian cancer.

Genetic factors also appear to play a role in your risk of developing ovarian cancer. Caucasian women have a higher risk than women of African or Asian heritage. And, as discussed on page 199, a strong family history of ovarian cancer may increase your risk.

Can Fertility Drugs Increase Your Risk of Ovarian Cancer?

Some studies have shown an increased risk of ovarian cancer in a small number of women who have used fertility drugs over a prolonged period of time. However, the risk of developing invasive ovarian cancer for women who had taken at least twelve cycles of fertility drugs was only 1.5 percent, compared to the normal risk of 1 percent. The risk of developing a borderline ovarian cancer, which has a survival rate of almost 100 percent, was 3 percent. An unanswered question is whether infertile women have a propensity to develop ovarian cancer, or whether the drugs actually induce cancer in an otherwise healthy woman.

As noted above, the risk of developing ovarian cancer appears to be related to the number of times you ovulate in your lifetime. Fertility drugs work by causing the ovary to produce eggs and ovulate. Therefore, it makes some theoretical sense that taking fertility drugs might increase your risk of ovarian cancer. However, for reasons that are not clear, other studies have shown that infertile women who have *never* taken fertility drugs also have a slightly increased risk of ovarian cancer.

A number of studies are now being conducted to answer these very important questions: Do all infertile women have a slightly higher risk of ovarian cancer? Do fertility drugs account for a higher incidence of ovarian cancer? Does either infertility or taking fertility drugs affect the incidence of ovarian cancer at all? If you have taken or are considering taking fertility drugs, discuss this issue with your doctor, because new developments continue to be published. At present, the risk of developing ovarian cancer because you have taken fertility drugs appears to be extremely small.

Does Your Diet Influence Your Risk of Ovarian Cancer?

A recent study found that women with a high saturated fat intake had a higher risk of developing ovarian cancer. Most American women consume about 30 grams of saturated fat a day in the form of animal fat, milk products, eggs, and cheese. By decreasing the amount of fat you eat by 10 grams a day, you can decrease your risk of ovarian cancer by 20 percent. If your risk of ovarian cancer is that of the general population, about 1 percent, a decrease in dietary fat can lower your risk to 0.8 percent.

In addition, for every extra 10 grams of vegetable fiber you eat a day, your risk of ovarian cancer decreases by about 40 percent, to 0.6 percent. The reasons for this benefit are not known. In any case, this is another good reason to eat reasonably and to include lots of fruits and vegetables in your diet. Also, decreasing fat and increasing fiber in your diet lowers your risk of heart disease, the major killer of women in this country, and of colon cancer.

Factors That Lower Your Risk for Ovarian Cancer

- Have one or more children
- Take birth control pills (for more than one year)
- No family history of ovarian cancer
- Black or Asian heritage
- Late onset of periods (after age twelve)
- Early onset of menopause (before age forty-five)
- Low-fat, high-fiber diet

What Is Your Risk of Ovarian Cancer If Someone in Your Family Has Had It?

The issue of a family history of ovarian cancer has been overstated. Only *5 percent* of women found to have ovarian cancer have inherited this disease. Therefore, the vast majority of women who get ovarian cancer have no family history of it. If someone in your family has had ovarian cancer, your risk will depend on how close the relative is to you, how old they were at the time they developed the disease, and how many of your relatives have had the disease.

If either your mother *or* your sister has had ovarian cancer, then your lifetime risk might increase from 1 percent to about 2 to 4 percent. If one first-degree relative (mother or sister) *and* one second-degree relative (grandmother or aunt) have had ovarian cancer, then your risk might be as high as 3 to 10 percent. However, if *only* one second-degree relative has had ovarian cancer, then your risk is no higher than if no one in your family ever had the disease.

Your risk of developing this disease may be as high as 40 to 50 percent only if *both* your mother and a sister have had ovarian cancer. This situation is extremely rare. Hereditary ovarian cancer also tends to occur at an early age, before fifty. If your relatives were young when they developed ovarian cancer, then a hereditary cause may be more likely. Knowing the specifics of your family history can either alert you to a possible problem or, more likely, be a source of reassurance.

Do Other Types of Cancer in Your Family Affect Your Risk of Ovarian Cancer?

There are a very small number of families who have *multiple* family members with either breast, colon, uterine, or ovarian cancer. The genes that cause these cancers appear to be passed on together. They may be passed on through either your mother's or your father's side of the family. Women in these families are at increased risk of developing any of these cancers, while the men are at increased risk for colon cancer. These family cancer syndromes are extremely rare and can only be determined if you know your family history in detail. For example, one study examined the incidence of family cancer syndromes among women who had a mother or sister with ovarian cancer. Of the 391 women who had enough information about their family to participate in the study, only 19 families (5 percent) appeared to have inheritable ovarian cancer and another 82 families (21 percent) had inheritable multiple cancers. Most of these families showed a prevalence for cancer over two to four generations. The other 74 percent of the women had no basis for inheritable cancer.

What Should You Do If You Have a Strong Family History of Ovarian, Breast, Uterine, and Colon Cancer?

If you are a member of one of the rare families in which a number of relatives have had these types of cancer, then you should consider seeing a genetics counselor. These counselors are trained to take a detailed family history and then are able to calculate what your risk of developing any of these cancers actually is. Your doctor should be able to help you get in touch with the appropriate genetics counselor.

If your family has an increased risk of these cancers, special tests can be performed to evaluate you on a regular basis. Screening tests for ovarian cancer (sonograms and CA-125 blood tests) may make some sense, although their value has not been proven. If you are felt to be at very high risk, you might also consider having your ovaries removed after you have completed your family (see page 208).

An annual scraping of the uterine-lining cells is a relatively simple office procedure that can detect uterine-lining cells in the precancerous stage. Breast exams and annual mammograms should be performed to screen for breast cancer. Screening for colon cancer can be performed by colonoscopy, which enables your doctor to see and remove precancerous polyps before cancer develops.

Discuss all these tests with your doctor. Early detection saves lives. Have the appropriate screening performed if your family history suggests a higher risk. In the not-too-distant future, it is likely that genetic tests will be available that will identify women who are at high risk for these cancers. Appropriate testing and treatment will then be directed specifically to these women in order to decrease their risk of cancer.

Are There Any Medications That Can Decrease Your Risk of Ovarian Cancer?

Believe it or not, birth control pills have been shown to decrease your risk of ovarian cancer. Continuous ovulation during your lifetime increases the risk of ovarian cancer. Birth control pills work by preventing ovulation, and thus decrease your risk. Even taking the pill for just one year will decrease your risk of ovarian cancer by about 10 percent. Taking the pill for five years or more decreases your risk by 50 percent. Many people have had a fear or a distrust of taking birth control pills.

Early studies, performed twenty years ago when the doses of the pill were extremely high, found a slightly increased risk of heart attack for women on the pill. But for women on the low doses of hormone found in the pill today, the risk of a heart attack is less than 1 in 20,000. For comparison, the high levels of estrogen present during pregnancy increase the risk of heart attack to 1 in 10,000 women.

Some women have worried about taking the pill for long periods of time. Many feel that they should give their bodies a "break" by getting off the pill after a few years. The research shows us that this fear is unfounded; the risks of using the pill actually decrease over time. In addition, taking the pill for long stretches may actually offer some health benefits. Besides lowering your risk of ovarian cancer, taking birth control pills decreases your risks for developing benign ovarian cysts, heavy menstrual bleeding and anemia, uterine cancer (by 60 percent), and benign breast cysts.

Unfortunately, the medical community has not gotten these positive facts across to the public. A recent study of women faculty, students, and employees at Yale University found that 80 percent of these women did not know that the pill could decrease the risk of ovarian cancer. Obviously, we need to provide better education in this area. While the pill is clearly not indicated for, or desired by, everyone, it does have a place in women's medical care. If using the pill interests you, ask your doctor about the positive health benefits of oral contraceptives.

Janet and Jessica's Family History of Ovarian Cancer

Janet and Jessica are sisters whose mother recently discovered she had ovarian cancer. They believed their grandmother had died of ovarian cancer. Janet is thirty-three and wants one more child in addition to the two she already has. Jessica is twenty-seven and is not yet married, but looks forward to having a family. We discussed the fact that they were probably at a higher risk of developing ovarian cancer, probably around 25 percent. Since they both wished to get pregnant in the future, I recommended that they take birth control pills until they were ready to get pregnant. Since the pill stops the ovary from ovulating, it decreases the risk of ovarian cancer. So Janet and Jessica have started taking birth control pills in order to decrease their chance of getting the disease. With the knowledge we currently have, it would be reasonable to surgically remove Janet's and Jessica's ovaries after they have completed their families. Perhaps by that time, there will a genetic marker available to tell us exactly who is susceptible to the illness.

Can Some Types of Surgery Decrease Your Risk of Ovarian Cancer?

Surprisingly, both tubal ligation (getting your tubes "tied") and hysterectomy (without removal of the ovaries) have been shown to decrease the risk of subsequently developing ovarian cancer by almost 50 percent. Although the reasons for this decrease are not entirely clear, here is the current thinking. Blocking off the tubes (tubal ligation) and removing the uterus (hysterectomy) both prevent any substances in the vagina from moving up inside the uterus and out the fallopian tubes, where they can land on the ovaries. Although these substances have not been identified, the theory suggests that once they are present on the ovary, they may induce the development of cancer.

One substance that is a possible candidate for inducing ovarian cancer is talc. Talc has sometimes been found in the ovaries of women with ovarian cancer. Presumably it comes from talcum powder used in hygiene products, which may get into the vagina and then end up on the ovary.

While the association between talc and ovarian cancer is still theoretical, if you are using a powder that is labeled as "talcum powder" or "containing talc," it is advisable to switch to another powder. Professionals in the medical field are still at the supposition and educated-guess stage regarding talc and other substances that may be factors in the development of this disease.

DIAGNOSING OVARIAN CANCER

Your ovaries are very small. Before you reach menopause, the ovaries are about the size of a walnut. After menopause, when they have stopped producing eggs, the ovaries shrink to the size of an almond. The ovaries lie deep within your pelvic area and are covered by your intestines, your abdominal muscles, and the body layer that contains fat and skin. Considering the ovaries' small size and their position under this covering, it is understandable that physicians sometimes have a hard time feeling them.

As the ovaries become affected by cancer, they begin to enlarge. Unfortunately, because of their normal small size and position, growth is hard to detect until it is fairly significant. In addition, the early symptoms of ovarian cancer are vague. Bloating, abdominal discomfort, and pelvic cramps are all early symptoms of ovarian cancer. But these are also common complaints experienced by countless numbers of people. Bloating, abdominal discomfort, and pelvic cramps may be attributed to intestinal problems and are sometimes ignored by the patient or her physician. Usually these symptoms go away on their own without any real illness developing. However, you should report any abdominal complaints that persist more than a week or two to your doctor, and you should probably be examined.

What Does "Screening Test" Mean?

Medical tests are usually performed when a person has symptoms of a disease and a specific diagnosis is suspected. In contrast, a screening test is performed in order to detect a disease in people who feel entirely *well*. In order for a screening test to be effective, it must be able to detect the disease in its earliest stages when cure is possible. A screening test must also be relatively easy and inexpensive to perform and be fairly specific for the disease you are attempting to detect. For example, a test that is even 99.6 percent specific for a particular disease will only detect one truly abnormal woman for every ten women who test positive.

A Pap smear is a very effective screening test for cervical cancer. The test is easy and inexpensive to perform and can detect abnormal cervical cells in a precancerous form. These abnormal cells can be easily treated, thus preventing the development of cervical cancer. The goal is to find a screening test just as effective for ovarian cancer.

Is Sonography a Good Screening Test for Ovarian Cancer?

Unfortunately, the answer is no. Sonography is a medical test that uses sound waves bounced off the ovaries to form a picture on a screen, much like the technology used for ship's sonar. This technique was felt to be a promising method to detect growth in the ovaries that might be the beginning of cancer. The hope was that this test would detect ovarian cancer before it had a chance to spread. Unfortunately, the test has a hard time distinguishing between ovarian cancer and benign ovarian cysts. These benign cysts are much more common than ovarian cancer, and most of them do not need to be treated at all (see chapter 4).

A study that illustrates this problem was conducted in England. An ad for free ovarian cancer screening was placed in the paper. Within a short time, 5,700 women agreed to get this free testing. Of the 5,700 women who had a sonogram of their ovaries, 361 had abnormal-appearing ovaries. The 361 women then underwent major abdominal surgery. Three of these women were found to have widely spread ovarian cancer that would have been easily detected by a pelvic exam. And only three women with early ovarian cancer were found and cured. This is wonderful for the three women whose lives were saved by the sonogram. However, 355 women had a major surgery that they did not need. They were subjected to the risks of anesthesia, bleeding, need for transfusion, infection, and injury, in addition to the discomfort of surgery and the time needed for recovery. At this point, for the general population the risk that an abnormal screening sonogram may lead to unnecessary surgery seems to outweigh the benefit.

In addition, it has been calculated that if all 43 million American women over the age of fifty had a pelvic sonogram every year, we might expect to find an abnormality in 2.5 million women. Thirty-seven thousand of these women would be found to have ovarian cancer that otherwise would have not been detected so early. But 2,463,000 women would have had unnecessary surgery. Of those women, 2,500 might be expected to die from the procedure, and 112,500 would have a serious complication. In addition, the cost of the sonograms would be $11.8 *billion* per year. The cost of the unnecessary surgeries would be about $37.5 *billion* per year. For all these reasons, a sonogram is not recommended as a routine screening test for ovarian cancer.

Susan's Abnormal Sonogram

Susan is a fifty-eight-year-old woman who saw her family physician after a few weeks of mild abdominal pain and bloating. She felt no nausea or vomiting and hadn't had diarrhea, constipation, or any fever. The examination of her abdomen was normal, as was a pelvic and rectal exam. Blood tests for infection and liver and gall bladder problems were also normal. Susan and her doctor were both reassured by all this, and she was given a medication to reduce any spasm in the intestines. When the pain and bloating persisted despite the medication, her doctor ordered some X rays of her intestines and a sonogram of her gall bladder and pelvis. All of these tests were also normal, with the exception of a two-inch fluid-filled cyst seen on her left ovary.

Susan came to the office worried that this test indicated ovarian cancer. On examination, I couldn't feel anything abnormal. In addition, there was no tenderness on examination of her uterus, fallopian tubes, or ovaries, and it seemed unlikely that her original complaints of pain and bloating were related to a gynecologic problem at all. But when I reviewed the sonogram, it was clear that a cystic mass was in fact present. Since Susan was postmenopausal, it was unlikely that this represented a simple ovarian cyst, the kind that would disappear by itself. We performed a CA-125 test (see page 206), which was normal. At this point, the suspicion of ovarian cancer was extremely low, but because a mass was present, I recommended surgery to remove it. We performed a laparoscopy (see page 106) the next week. During surgery, it was immediately clear that the mass was not her ovary, but rather her fallopian tube, which was filled with fluid. This probably resulted from a previous infection that had occurred many years before and had never caused any symptoms or problems. In fact, had the sonogram not been performed, no one would have ever known about the "cyst," and she never would have had surgery.

We removed the tube through the laparoscope in order to prevent similar confusion in the future. The pathologist confirmed that this was an old infection that had been cured by the body's defenses long ago. Interestingly, following all the commotion of testing, surgery, and recovery, Susan's pain gradually went away by itself. I do feel that all the right things were done for Susan's problem and that surgery was indicated under the circumstances. However, I think her case illustrates that medical tests are not foolproof and sometimes can lead to other unnecessary tests or procedures. As noted above, the performance of routine yearly sonograms on all women would certainly lead to more situations like Susan's.

What About Doppler Sonography?

Doppler sonography is a special form of sonography that uses sound waves to measure the speed of blood flowing through blood vessels. Blood vessels that form along with cancerous growths have thinner walls than normal blood vessels, which allow blood to flow faster. The speed of the blood flow can be measured, and the likelihood of cancer determined. The theory makes some sense, but unfortunately the results of this technique have not been very promising so far. Some benign ovarian cysts have the rapid flow that we expect from a cancer, and some cancerous cysts have slow blood flow and appear benign. Perhaps with better technology and more experience, the test may become useful, but at present it is still considered experimental.

Is CA-125 a Good Screening Test for Ovarian Cancer?

Cancer cells are different from normal cells, and they produce different chemicals. One of these chemicals has been detected in the bloodstream of women with ovarian cancer to a much greater degree than in normal women. The blood test to detect this chemical is called CA-125, because it was the 125th substance that was tested to look for a marker for ovarian cancer.

Like sonography, the CA-125 test can appear abnormal in women who do not have ovarian cancer. For women who are postmenopausal, ovarian cancer will be found in only about 8 percent of women with an elevated CA-125 level. The test is even less accurate in premenopausal women. Conditions common in young women—endometriosis, fibroids, ovarian cysts, pelvic infections, pregnancy, normal menstrual periods—can make the level of CA-125 go up in the absence of cancer. In addition, the test can be elevated in healthy women of any age for no apparent reason.

Therefore, it is not a good idea to perform this test on all women in an effort to detect ovarian cancer. If abnormal, the result usually scares the patient. The doctor, also worried about the possibility of ovarian cancer, will more often than not recommend surgery that is likely to be unnecessary.

Also, CA-125 levels are normal in 50 percent of women who *do* have early ovarian cancer, precisely the women we would like to find in order to treat them when the disease is curable. Therefore, we do not recommend CA-125 as a screening test for ovarian cancer.

Olivia's Abnormal CA-125 Test

Olivia is a forty-seven-year-old woman with three children. Recently, her aunt (her mother's sister) was diagnosed with ovarian cancer. Olivia's health was excellent, and she felt fine, but she was concerned and afraid and went to see her doctor. When Olivia told her doctor why she was worried about ovarian cancer, the doctor performed a pelvic examination, which was normal, and then ordered a CA-125 test. The test came back abnormal. At the time I saw Olivia, she was very anxious and had been unable to sleep or relax. I explained to her that the CA-125 test was most likely falsely elevated because of its lack of accuracy in premenopausal women. Unfortunately, this did little to reassure her. I performed another pelvic exam, which was completely normal; her ovaries felt fine.

We talked about what to do at this point and decided to try to get more information about her ovaries. Olivia wanted concrete proof that she did not have ovarian cancer. I repeated the CA-125 test and ordered a pelvic sonogram. Usually, I would not have recommended either test, but Olivia was so concerned that I felt if the additional information was reassuring, we might not have to do any surgery. The sonogram came back perfectly normal, but the CA-125 test was still high. Despite long conversations and reassurances based on the medical facts, Olivia wanted an absolute guarantee that she did not have ovarian cancer. Unfortunately, the only guarantee would be the removal of her ovaries and examination of them under the microscope.

Olivia insisted on surgery despite the risks and time needed for recovery. In addition, her insurance company told her they would not pay for the surgery since she did not have a disease to justify an operation. Olivia wanted the surgery despite the expense. We performed a laparoscopic removal of her ovaries as an outpatient. During the operation her ovaries appeared normal, and immediate examination by the pathologist confirmed that no cancer was present. Olivia was so relieved by the pathology report that in the recovery room she said that the ordeal had been worth it. However, I couldn't help but wish that the initial CA-125 test had never been done.

Do Screening Tests Make Sense If You Are at Very High Risk for Developing Ovarian Cancer?

If you have a very strong family history of ovarian cancer, the goal must be early detection. For those few women who have a ten to fifty times greater risk of developing ovarian cancer (see page 199), it is probably worth the risk of having a false-abnormal test result, even if it leads to unnecessary surgery. A number of medical programs have been established that use sonograms and CA-125 blood tests in an attempt to detect ovarian cancer in high-risk women at an early, curable stage and collect information about the effectiveness of these tests. If you are at high risk, you might ask your doctor if a program exists in your community. To date, these programs have found only a few early, curable ovarian cancers. However, this approach is new, and as information continues to be gathered, it is hoped that some methods will be developed that can lead to early detection of ovarian cancer. Women who are at very high risk might consider the removal of their ovaries.

Should You Have Your Ovaries Removed *Before* They Develop Cancer?

The answer to this question depends on your risk of ovarian cancer and on the level of anxiety you feel based on this risk. Remember that very few women, less than 5 percent who get ovarian cancer, inherit this disease. If you have two first-degree relatives (mother or sisters) with ovarian cancer, you may have as high as a 50 percent risk of developing ovarian cancer; therefore, removing your ovaries as soon as you finish having children is recommended. You should also consider having your children at an early age so that your ovaries can be removed before the age when your relatives developed the disease. After surgery, you may begin to take hormone replacement therapy in order to prevent menopausal symptoms and the development of osteoporosis and heart disease.

Women who have one first-degree relative with ovarian cancer and one first-degree relative with either breast, uterine, or colon cancer are considered to have about a 12 percent risk of developing ovarian cancer. They should also consider having their ovaries removed after completing their families. Removal of the ovaries may now be accomplished using laparoscopic techniques. This surgery, using tiny incisions and the guidance of a small telescope, offers the benefits of outpatient surgery and quick recovery.

What Is the Best Way to Check on Your Ovaries?

The best way for women who do not have a strong family history of ovarian cancer to check for the disease is an annual pelvic exam by their doctor. Sonograms or blood tests are not very good at finding early, curable ovarian cancer, and if you get a false-positive result, you may end up submitting to other tests and occasionally surgery (see page 203). In addition to being misleading, high-tech testing is very expensive. In the near future, a better test probably will be available. But for now, see your doctor for a pelvic exam once a year, or at any other time you have symptoms or problems.

What Should Be Done If the Doctor Feels an Abnormal Ovary on Your Examination?

If your ovary feels enlarged at the time of your pelvic examination, further evaluation will depend on your age and the way the ovary feels to your doctor. As noted in chapter 4, most ovarian cysts are benign and need no treatment at all. This is usually true for women who are premenopausal. For postmenopausal women, the majority of cysts are also benign. However, the risk of ovarian cancer increases as a woman ages. Therefore, cysts found in postmenopausal women are a little more cause for concern.

Benign cysts often feel smooth to your doctor and can be moved when your ovaries are examined. Cancer often feels hard, immobile, and irregular. Although the pelvic examination is helpful to determine if a cyst is present, a sonogram is usually required to determine what type of cyst it might be. The patterns that the cells form within the cyst can be seen on the sonogram and may suggest benign or malignant characteristics.

For a postmenopausal woman found to have an ovarian cyst, the CA-125 blood test result can provide additional helpful information. If the CA-125 result is elevated, it should be viewed with concern, and abdominal surgery should be performed. Since neither the sonogram nor the CA-125 test can make a *certain* diagnosis, surgery is needed to remove the ovary so that it may be examined under the microscope.

As noted before, the CA-125 test should *not* be performed in premenopausal women because it is often inaccurate in that age group. Premenopausal women should have a pelvic examination and a sonogram in order to determine whether surgery is necessary.

Evaluation of an Abnormal Ovary

Premenopausal	*Postmenopausal*
Pelvic examination	Pelvic examination
Sonogram	Sonogram
	CA-125

Is Surgery Necessary If Your Ovary Feels Abnormal?

As described in chapter 4, most ovarian cysts in young women go away by themselves, and no treatment is needed. These cysts tend to appear entirely clear and filled with fluid on the sonogram. If the sonogram shows scattered areas of blood within the cyst (endometriosis) or areas of calcium (dermoid cyst), surgery is usually needed because these cysts will not go away by themselves. If the sonogram shows solid areas of tissue mixed with fluid, either a benign ovarian tumor or ovarian cancer may be present and surgery is necessary. Because of the somewhat higher risk of ovarian cancer, surgery should always be considered when an abnormal ovary is found in a postmenopausal woman.

What Kind of Surgery Can Be Done If You Have an Abnormal Ovary?

As noted in chapter 4, some ovarian cysts are benign but may need to be removed in order to prevent twisting, rupture, or continued growth. If the evaluation of a cyst with pelvic examination and sonogram (and CA-125 in postmenopausal women) suggests that the cyst is benign but needs to be removed, laparoscopic surgery is an excellent technique (see page 106). This method has the benefit of a very short hospital stay (usually less than twelve hours) and full recovery within a week or so.

However, if there is any concern based on the examination or sonogram (or CA-125 test in postmenopausal women) that cancer might be present, then the best choice is abdominal surgery. If cancer is found, standard surgery will give your doctor a better opportunity to remove all of the abnormal tissue. Although some gynecologic cancer specialists have been working on techniques to perform cancer surgery through the laparoscope, they are not fully tested and therefore are not yet accepted as common practice. Abdominal surgery for ovarian cancer is still the accepted standard.

Jacqueline's Enlarged Ovary

Jacqueline is a seventy-three-year-old woman who saw her family doctor for a regular checkup. During the pelvic examination, her doctor felt an enlarged ovary on the right side and referred her for further evaluation. I spoke to Jacqueline about making an appointment and found that she was calm and confident about her health. In order to save time, I suggested that she get a pelvic sonogram and CA-125 test before coming to see me at the office. When she came for her appointment, she had the sonogram pictures and blood test results in hand for me to review.

When I examined Jacqueline, I could feel the enlarged ovary. The good news was that it wasn't very big, about two inches in diameter, and it did not feel stuck to her uterus or intestines, which may indicate cancer. After the examination I reviewed the sonogram and was relieved to see that the cyst on her ovary was totally filled with fluid, just like benign cysts. Her CA-125 blood test was normal. All of the tests pointed to a benign cyst, but it would be impossible to exclude cancer until the ovary was removed and examined under the microscope. However, because I felt the risk for ovarian cancer was extremely small, I recommended laparoscopic surgery to shorten her hospital stay and encourage a quick recovery.

Jacqueline was admitted for surgery the next week. Using laparoscopic surgery, we were able to first drain the fluid out of her enlarged ovary and then remove the ovary through a small incision. The ovary was sent immediately to the pathologist, who examined it under a microscope and pronounced it benign. We then removed her other ovary in order to prevent the development of any cysts, or even cancer, in the future. Jacqueline was able to go home the same day and was back to normal activity within ten days.

TREATMENT FOR OVARIAN CANCER

What If Cancer Is Suspected?

If ovarian cancer is suspected based on a pelvic examination, a sonogram, or an elevated CA-125 level in a postmenopausal woman, then abdominal surgery should be performed. The objectives of surgery are, first, to make a definite diagnosis and, second, to remove the cancer if it is found.

Gail's Abnormal Ovarian Cyst

Gail is a forty-six-year-old mother of two teenagers who came to the office for her regular annual examination. I felt that her left ovary was enlarged to about the size of a baseball. This was surprising to her because she had felt absolutely no pain or discomfort, although it is not uncommon to have a cyst without being aware of any pain or pressure.

The fact that I felt something abnormal frightened Gail, and her first thought was that this was cancer. I tried to reassure her that most ovarian cysts are *not* cancer, and a sonogram would be helpful to get a better idea of what we were dealing with. Unfortunately, the sonogram was abnormal, showing what appeared to be solid areas of growth within the ovary—the picture that we sometimes see with ovarian cancer. I became concerned. The good news was that there was no evidence of anything else abnormal on Gail's sonogram or pelvic examination. My thinking was that this growth might not be cancer, but the only way to know was to perform surgery and remove the ovary.

Gail was anxious and wanted the surgery performed as soon as possible. Because of the possibility of cancer, we made a regular abdominal incision. Laparoscopic surgery has not been fully adopted for patients with cancer. At the time of surgery, the first good news was that we did not see any evidence of obvious cancer. Cancer often looks like granular and irregular growths on top of, or embedded in, normal tissue. Gail's ovary was enlarged, but it and the rest of her pelvic organs looked smooth and healthy. Irregular cancer growths sometimes start to weep a clear fluid that collects inside the abdomen (called ascites), and we saw none of this fluid. I immediately started to feel better about Gail's problem.

We removed the ovary and had the pathologist perform a "frozen section" right away. The pathologist examined the ovary and took a small piece of tissue from an area she thought might be abnormal. She then placed the tissue in a special freezer for a few minutes. Once it was frozen, she cut it into extremely thin slices and placed the slices on a slide. The slide was then dipped into a dish of red- and then blue-colored solution that was soaked up by the cells so that they could be more easily seen under the microscope. When she examined the cells, the pathologist confirmed what we had hoped. The ovarian cyst was benign. The frozen section had taken fifteen minutes. After the surgery, Gail and her family were extremely relieved. I shared their relief and happiness, but at the same time I felt frustrated because we do not have a simpler way to make the diagnosis of a *benign* growth that would have avoided the anxiety, fear, and surgery that Gail had endured.

What Kind of Surgery Is Performed If Ovarian Cancer Is Found?

Ovarian cancer tends to spread to the organs right next to the ovary. Therefore, the uterus, the other ovary, and both fallopian tubes should be removed in order to eliminate any cancer cells that may have already spread. In addition, the fat pad surrounding the intestines, called the omentum, should be removed because it hangs directly over the pelvic organs, and cancer cells can easily attach to it. Removing your omentum may irritate your intestines for a few days and delay your ability to eat after surgery (see page 306); otherwise, there are no side effects or long-term consequences. Biopsies of the inner lining of the abdominal cavity will also be taken to determine if the cancer has spread to these areas. Knowing whether the cancer has spread outside the ovary is important. If the cancer has not spread, then usually no further treatment is needed, and the prognosis is excellent. If the cancer has spread, chemotherapy is usually needed.

Can a Woman Who Has Had Ovarian Cancer Get Pregnant?

If ovarian cancer is found in a woman who wants to have children and it appears *entirely* confined to one ovary, your doctor may consider removing just that one ovary in order to preserve your fertility. There is some risk in this choice because you really do not know for sure if the cancer is confined to just that ovary until the entire ovary and other biopsies from the pelvis are examined by the pathologist. The complete pathology report takes about two days. If cancer is unexpectedly found in areas other than just the one ovary, then more surgery will be needed to perform a complete hysterectomy and remove any remaining cancer cells (see page 212). However, if all the other biopsies are normal, you do not need any further surgery and can get pregnant. Follow-up with pelvic exams, CA-125 tests, and sonograms may be suggested until you do get pregnant. Pregnancy has no effect, good or bad, on ovarian cancer. However, most gynecologic oncologists would recommend that you have a complete hysterectomy after you complete your family to eliminate any chance of cancer recurrence.

What Is Chemotherapy Like?

If the cancer cells have spread outside the ovary, chemotherapy is virtually always recommended. The goal of chemotherapy is to bathe any remaining cancer cells in the body with chemicals that are designed to destroy them. The drugs are usually given through an IV directly into the bloodstream over the course of a few hours. This treatment is given once every three to four weeks for a total of six treatments. Chemotherapy interferes with the ways that cells divide, and rapidly growing cells are more vulnerable to this effect. Cancer cells, which grow rapidly, are thus usually killed.

However, blood cells, hair, nails, and the lining cells of the intestinal tract are also all rapidly growing and renewing tissues. As a result, these cells often suffer the effects of the chemotherapy as well. The most common side effect of chemotherapy is nausea and sometimes vomiting. The nausea is often mild, but if it is a problem, relaxation techniques, changes in diet, or taking specific medications can be used to lessen this side effect. Psychologists who have experience working with cancer patients can help you choose remedies for your side effects.

Hair loss is often an anguishing side effect for anyone receiving chemotherapy. There is no physical discomfort, but it is a constant reminder of loss and illness. Some of the new drugs like Taxol will usually cause hair loss, but it is *temporary*, and the hair will grow back entirely once the treatments are finished.

The white blood cell count of most women decreases during chemotherapy, which makes them somewhat more susceptible to infection during the treatments. Care should be taken to avoid contact with people with colds or other infections. This susceptibility is temporary, and the white blood cells return to normal after about three weeks. The most common and bothersome complaint of women on chemotherapy is fatigue. This feeling results from the decrease in the red blood cell count that accompanies chemotherapy. A decrease in the number of red blood cells, which carry oxygen, lowers the ability of cells in your body to produce energy, and the result is fatigue. Women often describe waves of exhaustion that complicate even the smallest task. The exhaustion may last for a few hours or even a day or two. A good diet, regular exercise, and an ample amount of rest will usually help lessen the fatigue. Medications are now available that increase the white blood cell or red blood cell count, and these may be used if needed.

In general, as time goes on during the course of chemotherapy, you may start to feel worn down, both physically and emotionally. However, within a month of finishing chemotherapy, strength and energy start to return. After a few months, most women feel back to normal, have a more positive outlook on life, and are ready to move forward. Excellent books are available for women with ovarian cancer. (See *Choices, After Cancer* in suggested reading.)

Anne's Ovarian Cancer

Anne is a seventy-two-year-old woman who went to see her internist because of abdominal pain and bloating. She had noted these problems for a few months, but they had been getting worse over the past few weeks. Her clothes were getting tighter around her waist despite the fact that her appetite was not very good, and she was eating less. Her internist felt an abnormal area near her ovaries and referred her for evaluation. On examination, it was clear that there was a mass of extra tissue around both of Anne's ovaries, and her abdomen appeared swollen. Ovarian cancer was my first thought, and this had already occurred to Anne. I asked her to have a sonogram and a CA-125 test, both of which came back abnormal. The diagnosis was almost certainly ovarian cancer, and Anne was very upset and frightened.

I asked Anne to see a gynecologic cancer specialist for a consultation because I expected the upcoming surgery to be very difficult. The cancer felt as if it was wrapped around Anne's intestines, and I was concerned we might need to remove a piece of the intestine in order to remove all of the cancer. I expected that the oncologist's expertise would be needed. He agreed with the planned surgery, and we decided to perform it together. Gynecologic oncologists are first trained as obstetrician-gynecologists and then spend an extra two years training to take care of women with cancer of the uterus, fallopian tubes, or ovaries. Much of that extra time is spent learning to perform the difficult surgical procedures sometimes involved in removing cancer. We scheduled her surgery for the next week so that she would be able to make arrangements for someone to care for her ill husband.

At the time of surgery, it was immediately apparent that cancer was present. The ovaries were both covered with abnormal growths that extended up to the intestines and entwined them. It was no wonder that Anne's abdomen was swollen, and her appetite decreased. During four hours of painstaking surgery, we removed the uterus, fallopian tubes, and ovaries and a small portion of the intestine that had been encased in tumor. We also removed the fat pad around the intestine, which also had tumor on it. We could see that some cells were still stuck to areas of the intestines and the inside lining of the abdomen, but they could not be safely removed. Because of the extensive nature of the cancer, Anne was going to need chemotherapy. The goal of surgery was to remove as much cancer as safely possible, and we were able to remove about 99 percent of the cancer cells.

Anne was depressed after surgery, both because of the hard reality of having cancer and because of her slow recovery following a long and difficult surgery. Her family was very supportive and helped her through the next few days. Her husband was able to come to the hospital with one of their children, and this cheered her up a bit. The final pathology report came back two days after surgery. It confirmed what was certain, that cancer was present. But it also showed that the cancer cells did not appear to be very irregular or wildly growing. Because of this, Anne's prognosis was better. This was some good news to soften the bad.

After Anne recovered from surgery, she began treatment with chemotherapy. Other than some fatigue, she tolerated the chemotherapy well. We measured her CA-125 levels regularly, which fell back to normal and have stayed there.

If ovarian cancer reoccurs, it usually does so within the first year or two. For the first few years, Anne had a pelvic examination and CA-125 test every three months. As each year passed (we are now celebrating number ten for Anne), we all became increasingly confident that Anne was one of the fortunate women who have beaten this disease. I still see her every six months for her pelvic examination, and she remains totally healthy and cancer free.

What Are the Cure Rates for Ovarian Cancer?

The most common type of ovarian cancer comes from the epithelial cells that cover the ovaries. Epithelial cancer is responsible for about 90 percent of all ovarian cancers. If it is found early, before it has spread beyond the ovary (stage 1), it is 90 percent curable. The only treatment necessary is removal of the ovary. However, once the cancer spreads outside the pelvic organs, the cure rate drops to around 30 percent despite major surgery and chemotherapy. That is the current predicament with this terrible disease: How can we make a diagnosis early, when the disease is curable? An enormous amount of research is being undertaken to find ways to prevent ovarian cancer from forming, to detect it early if it does occur, and to treat it more effectively. There is reason to believe that many of these goals will be attained in the near future.

Are There Different Kinds of Ovarian Cancer?

The ovary has a number of different kinds of cells within it that can turn into cancer. The cells that are destined to become eggs can form a number of different cancers depending on which type of cell grows abnormally. This group of cancers is called germ cell cancers. These cancers are very rare, accounting for only 5 percent of all ovarian cancers. It is impossible to tell the different types of ovarian cancer before surgery, but the type can be determined by the pathologist when he or she looks at the cells under a microscope. Germ cell cancers tend to occur in younger women, most often before age thirty. Many of these cancers cause early symptoms such as pelvic pain or pressure; therefore, germ cell cancers are often diagnosed before they spread. On a sonogram, germ cell cancers have a different appearance from functional ovarian cysts, which are extremely common in young women, and the diagnosis may be suspected from that test. The good news is that germ cell cancer is extremely curable.

What Are the Cure Rates for Germ Cell Cancer?

One of the major advances in cancer therapy has come in the treatment of germ cell tumors. Previously difficult to treat, almost all of these tumors now can be *cured* with removal of just the affected ovary, followed by appropriate chemotherapy. Many women who have had germ cell cancers get pregnant and live totally normal and healthy lives.

What Is Borderline Ovarian Cancer?

Borderline ovarian cancer is also an overgrowth of abnormal ovarian cells. Borderline cancer doesn't behave like either a cancer or an entirely benign tumor. These tumors usually grow very slowly and do not spread as aggressively as ovarian cancer does. The entire ovary is usually removed, and the prognosis is very good, approaching a 95 percent cure rate following surgery. The diagnosis can be made only by looking at the cells under a microscope, and once it is made, no further treatment is needed. Careful follow-up is still important because sometimes the tumor cells may have been left behind and can slowly grow back. Another surgery may then be necessary.

Can You Take Estrogen Replacement Therapy If You Have Had Ovarian Cancer?

Estrogen replacement therapy is used after menopause to provide estrogen to your body after the ovary has stopped making it. There is good evidence that estrogen *does not* make ovarian cancer any worse. Because your ovaries must be removed if ovarian cancer is found, you will have lost the main source of estrogen in your body. This loss of estrogen may cause bothersome symptoms such as hot flashes, insomnia, and vaginal dryness, especially if you have this surgery before menopause. In addition, estrogen reduces the risk of heart attacks by 50 percent and the risk of osteoporosis by 70 percent, so estrogen therapy may be a good idea.

How Does Ovarian Cancer Affect Your Emotional Health?

I have learned a great deal from the women I know who have had cancer. Most importantly, I have learned what helped them get through it. Many talk about the essential need for emotional support from loved ones. For many women, having someone to complain to, to cry to, or to talk about fears with seems to be a key part of enduring the treatment process. For some, crying is the only thing to do. Other women feel the need to push forward. They may cry at a later time, or not at all. You know yourself best—there is no "right" way to handle dealing with cancer.

It may seem like an inauspicious time to initiate relationships, but there are likely to be others in your community who are also undergoing treatment for ovarian cancer or other forms of cancer. Support groups are sponsored in hospitals, synagogues, and churches. These groups can be enormously helpful in providing support and education. Individual or family therapy may also help you and your family get through these difficult times. Trained mental health professionals who specialize in working with cancer patients can teach you to control symptoms of the disease, deal with side effects of medications, and cope overall.

It is often the case that family and friends rally around someone undergoing cancer treatment. You may want to let them help you. Many women who are accustomed to running a business or a career, a home, and a family find it difficult to be on the "needy" end. Some have told me that initially they turned down offers of homemade dinners or help with transportation, shopping, or baby-sitting. Cancer makes us all feel helpless. Some women felt that by accepting some help they not only eased their own burden but also helped their loved ones cope by allowing *them* to do something.

Women with cancer often mention the need for a sense of humor. Norman Cousins taught us years ago that laughter is often good medicine. Sometimes the trials and tribulations of the entire process lend itself to a sense of humor. The world of doctors, hospitals, and cancer treatment offers a lot of raw material to work with. Look for those moments.

REFERENCES

Biesecker, B., M. Boehnke, K. Calzone, et al. 1993. Genetic counseling for families with inherited susceptibility to breast and ovarian cancer. *Journal of the American Medical Association* 269:1970–74.

Cousins, N. 1979. *Anatomy of an Illness.* (New York: Norton.)

Droegemueller, W. 1994. Screening for ovarian cancer: Hopeful and wishful thinking. *American Journal of Obstetrics and Gynecology* 170:1095–98.

Einhorn, N., K. Sjövall, R. Knapp, et al. 1992. Prospective evaluation of serum CA-125 Levels for early detection of ovarian cancer. *Obstetrics and Gynecology* 80:14–18.

Hankinson, S., G. Colditz, D. Hunter, B. Rosner, and M. Stampfer. 1992. A quantitative assessment of oral contraceptive use and risk of ovarian cancer. *Obstetrics and Gynecology* 80:708–14.

Kerlikowske, K., J. Brown, and D. Grady. 1992. Should women with a familial ovarian cancer undergo prophylactic oophorectomy? *Obstetrics and Gynecology* 80:700–707.

Morra, M., and E. Potts. 1994. *Choices: The New, Most Up-to-Date Sourcebook for Cancer Information.* New York: Avon.

Moyers, B. 1993. *Healing and the Mind.* New York: Doubleday.

Parazzini, F., S. Franceschi, C. Vecchia, and M. Fasoli. 1991. The epidemiology of ovarian cancer. *Gynecologic Oncology* 43:9–23.

Rossing, M., J. Daling, N. Weiss, D. Moore, and S. Self. 1994. Ovarian tumors in a cohort of infertile women. *New England Journal of Medicine* 331:771–76.

Siegel, B. 1989. *Peace, Love and Healing.* New York: Harper and Row.

9

ABNORMAL PAP SMEARS, HPV, CERVICAL DYSPLASIA, AND CERVICAL CANCER

What Is Cervical Dysplasia and Carcinoma in Situ?

During sexual intercourse, viruses or other as-yet-unidentified cancer-causing agents may get into the cells of the cervix and cause them to grow abnormally. This abnormal tissue growth is called *dysplasia*. Early on, dysplastic cells stay within the cervical skin. The skin has no blood or lymph vessels that the abnormal cells can invade and therefore they have no way to leave the cervix and spread to other areas of the body. Because dysplasia is confined to the skin, it is easy to treat.

In the past, the term carcinoma in situ (CIS) was used if the abnormal cells occupied the full thickness of the cervical skin (see fig. 9.1). However, the presence of the word *carcinoma* often implied that the patient had cancer. But CIS is not cancer: It is a severe form of dysplasia, and the abnormal cells remain confined within the skin. CIS cannot spread to other areas of the body. In order to eliminate this confusion, the term carcinoma in situ was replaced with the term high-grade dysplasia (see page 227). However, if high-grade dysplasia is left untreated over a number of years, the cells may eventually break through the skin layer and invade the layer beneath, which has blood and lymph vessels. Then cervical cancer (see page 239) is present.

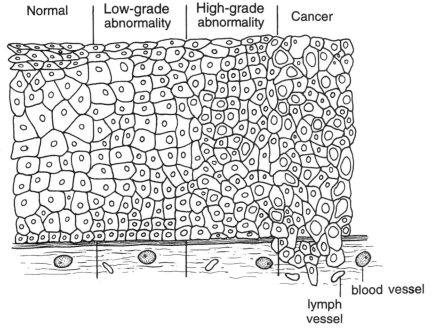

| Normal | Low-grade abnormality | High-grade abnormality | Cancer |

blood vessel

lymph vessel

Fig. 9.1.   Cervical cells

Where Do These Abnormal Cells Develop?

As previously described in chapter 1, the cervix is the opening into the uterus. It can be seen inside the top of the vagina (see fig. 9.2a). The lining cells of the uterus are tall, column-shaped cells, and the cells of the vaginal skin are thin and flat. The area where the lining cells of the uterus meet the cells of the vagina is called the "transformation zone," i.e., the area where one type of cell changes into another type of cell (see fig. 9.2b). The cells near the transformation zone appear to be particularly vulnerable to carcinogens, substances that can cause cancer. The transformation zone is where cervical dysplasia and cancer develop.

What Causes Cervical Dysplasia and Cancer?

The most common cause of abnormal cervical cells known today is a group of viruses called human papillomavirus (HPV). This group of viruses has also been called genital wart virus or condyloma virus. These viruses are very common and have been found in 6 percent of all women. The HPV viruses are actually a group of about seventy similar viruses, and

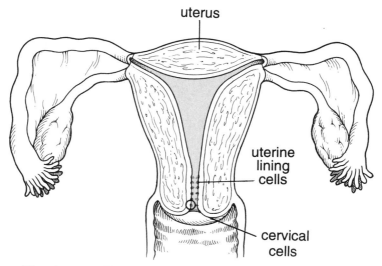

Fig. 9.2a.   The cervix is the opening of the uterus,
found at the top of the vagina.

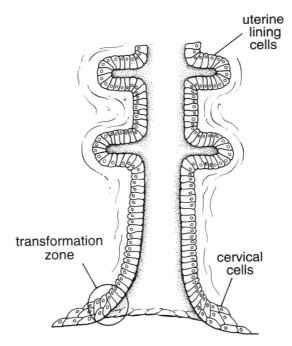

Fig. 9.2b.

about twenty of these can infect the genital skin. If the virus gets into the cells of the vulva, vagina, or cervix, it can alter the normal growth of the cells. A noticeable overgrowth of the skin called condyloma or genital wart may result. These warts can be felt or seen as small raised, rough bumps on the vulva or penis. They are almost always painless but sometimes may cause some itching or irritation. However, if the virus is just present on the cervix, usually no symptoms occur at all, and there is nothing obvious to feel. When there are no symptoms and nothing obvious to feel, the only way to detect whether the virus is present on the cervix is with a Pap smear (see page 226).

The HPV virus is most often found on the skin of men and women who have been infected with it through sexual intercourse. Although virus particles have been found on the underwear of people with the infection, it is unlikely that this source can actually lead to the spread of the infection to another person. If your sexual partner has the virus on his penis, it may enter the skin cells of the cervix (or vagina or vulva) and cause these cells to grow abnormally, progressing to first precancerous and then possibly cancerous cells. Luckily, this process usually takes many years. Yearly Pap smears should detect the changes in the cells long before they become too abnormal and while they are easily treatable. In other words, with the Pap smear we can see cervical abnormalities beginning long before they are actually a threat to your well-being. HPV is probably not the only cause for cervical dysplasia and cervical cancer, but it appears to be the most clearly identified and most common cause.

What Are the Risk Factors for Getting Cervical Dysplasia and Cancer?

Having multiple sexual partners increases the risk of getting cervical dysplasia or cancer. Since the most common cause of cervical cancer is HPV, which is sexually transmitted, the more partners you (and your partner) have had, the greater your risk is of coming into contact with the virus. One more risk factor for HPV is the age at which you begin intercourse. During the hormonal shifts that occur with adolescence, the cervical cells undergo changes that appear to make them more susceptible to infection with the virus. Therefore, intercourse at an early age also increases the risk of getting cervical dysplasia and cancer.

While some cancers are more common in certain families, cervical cancer does not appear to be an inheritable disease. Having a family member with cervical cancer does not increase your risk of getting this disease.

Can Smoking Increase Your Risk of Cervical Dysplasia and Cancer?

The risk of cervical cancer is definitely higher in women who smoke. Your immune system is supposed to remove bacteria, viruses, and abnormal cells from your body every day. Smoking appears to have a detrimental influence on the immune system, making it less effective. If not removed by the immune system, the abnormal cells may develop into cancer cells over a period of many months or years.

In addition, when you smoke, nicotine is absorbed through your lungs into your bloodstream and then is transported to all the cells in your body. Nicotine is broken down by your body into chemicals that are known to cause cancer. The cells of the cervix appear to be especially susceptible to these chemicals. The risk of developing dysplasia of the cervix is three to four times greater for women who have smoked than for women who have never smoked. The risk increases with the amount of smoking, so that the risk of dysplasia is twelve times greater in women who have smoked a pack of cigarettes a day for twelve years. The risk for developing actual cancer of the cervix is two times greater in smokers. If you stop smoking, the risk decreases as time goes on.

Smoking has not been shown to increase your risk of breast or ovarian cancer. However, smoking does cause heart disease. The increase in the mortality rate for women who have heart attacks has directly followed the increase in the number of women who smoke. As a result, women's risk of dying from a heart attack is now close to being the same as that for men of comparable ages. The health risks of smoking are enormous—there are *many* reasons not to smoke.

How Common Is HPV?

HPV is a very common virus, found in about 6 percent of all women. Some studies have found the virus in as many as 20 percent of women college students. However, the presence of the virus does not necessarily lead to problems, because some types of the virus never cause symptoms or abnormalities of the Pap smear. Some women apparently live with the virus without any problems ever developing. In other cases, the virus can be eradicated by the body's own defenses without any treatment at all. Nevertheless, if you have an abnormal Pap smear, you may require some treatment to control the virus.

Fran's Cryotherapy for HPV

Fran is a twenty-five-year-old woman who came to the office for her yearly examination with our nurse-practitioner. On the outside of Fran's vagina, the nurse-practitioner noticed some raised areas that looked like HPV. Fran was unaware of these areas, and they were not tender to touch during the exam. The inside of the vagina was entirely normal, and the cervix appeared clear as well. A Pap smear was taken. In order to determine if the bumps were HPV, the nurse-practitioner injected the area with a very small syringe containing local anesthesia, and a small piece of skin was removed. When the results came back from the lab, they confirmed the presence of HPV. Subsequently, Fran's Pap smear came back entirely normal. Although the abnormal area was small and not causing any problem, we recommended to Fran that the skin be treated. This would prevent any spread of the virus to larger areas of the vagina, or to her partner. In addition, we recommended that Fran's partner be evaluated by his doctor for the presence of the virus (see page 228).

Using a small, very cold metal instrument, the skin was frozen for about three minutes. The procedure, called cryotherapy, caused a stinging sensation for a minute or so. After the treatment was finished, we told Fran to soak in a warm tub twice a day if she had any discomfort. Over time, new skin would replace the skin that was frozen and destroyed. When she returned for her next appointment two weeks later, the only evidence of the freezing was a slightly red tint near the area of the treated skin. We checked her again in two months, and there was no evidence of any of the old virus, or any new virus. Luckily, Fran's regular annual gynecologic exam detected the virus early and prevented the problem from becoming too advanced. However, HPV can sometimes be present but undetected. In addition, reinfection with the virus is possible. Therefore, Fran was advised to continue to have routine Pap smears and checkups in the future.

Are Some Types of HPV Worse Than Others?

It appears so. The different types of HPV differ by small changes in the virus's structure. The viral types are numbered 1 to 70, with new types added as they are discovered. The specific type of HPV can be determined only by sophisticated laboratory testing. We currently know that twenty of the seventy types of HPV are capable of causing the cervical cells to become dysplastic or cancerous. The types of HPV have been grouped together according to their risk of causing cervical dysplasia or cancer. HPV types 16 and 18 are aggressive forms of the virus and are in the high-risk group for causing dysplasia or cancer. These are the most common types of the virus actually found in cervical cancer cells. On the other hand, viral types 6 and 11 do not appear to cause cervical cancer, even if they are left untreated; therefore, they are considered low-risk forms of HPV.

What Are the Symptoms of Cervical Dysplasia or Cancer?

Unfortunately, cervical dysplasia and early cervical cancer do not cause any warning symptoms like pain, irritation, bleeding, or discharge at a time when treatment might be easily accomplished. Later, cervical cancer can destroy the cervical cells to the point that bleeding or constant discharge occurs, but at that point treatment is difficult. This is why early detection of abnormal cells with a Pap smear is so important.

How Do We Diagnose Cervical Dysplasia and Cancer? The Pap Smear

In 1948, a Greek immigrant to the United States named George Papanicolaou discovered that the cells shed from the surface of the cervix could be examined under a microscope to see if they appeared normal. Interestingly, he was not a physician, but was working in a pathology laboratory as a technician when he made this discovery. By examining the size and shape of these cells, he was able to detect cancer of the cervix before it was clinically obvious. Later it was discovered that mildly abnormal cells (dysplasia) that could become cancerous were detectable as well. See chapter 1 for a full description of how the Pap smear is performed. The wonderful thing about the Pap smear is its ability to detect these abnormal cells years before they become cancer, at a time when they can be easily treated. In areas of the world where routine annual Pap smears are extensively used, there has been a dramatic decrease in the rate of death from cervical cancer. The Pap smear is one of the great success stories of modern medicine.

What Does the Pathologist Look For in the Pap Smear?

All cells have two main parts: the inner part or nucleus, which contains DNA, and the outer part, called the cytoplasm, which is the area that produces energy for the cell to function. A normal cell has a small nucleus and a large amount of cytoplasm. When a virus or other carcinogen causes the cell to become abnormal, the DNA in the nucleus starts to grow uncontrollably, enlarging the nucleus so that it crowds out the cytoplasm. This is the abnormality that the pathologist looks for: a large, irregular nucleus and a small amount of cytoplasm (see fig. 9.3).

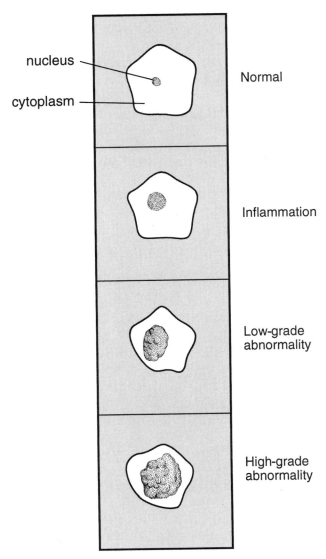

Fig. 9.3.   Cervical cells as seen on the Pap smear

What Do the Pap Smear Results Mean?

The terminology used to describe Pap smear results has changed over the past few years, leading to confusion about what the results of your Pap smear actually mean. Originally, Pap smears were divided into five "classes" based on what the cells looked like to the pathologist. Class I was normal. Class II cells appeared a little irregular to the pathologist, usually representing bacterial infection. Class III and IV Pap smears suggested that dysplastic cells were present, and further testing was needed. Class V usually meant cancer. Unfortunately, this class system led to confusion regarding what "number" Pap smear a woman had and what that really meant. Recently, a new system for Pap smear classification called the Bethesda System has been introduced. The term *low-grade lesion* is now used for cells that appear to be infected with HPV or are only mildly abnormal. The term *high-grade lesion* is used for more abnormal-appearing cells, the type that would have been called class III or IV with the old system. A Pap smear that looks like cancer is now labeled "cancer" rather than class V. The Bethesda System allows the pathologist to actually describe what is seen, rather than just assign a number to the Pap smear result. In that way it is an improvement over the old class system.

Should Your Sexual Partner Be Evaluated for HPV?

If you have HPV, there is about a 60 percent chance that a male sexual partner may have the virus as well. It is therefore probably a good idea for your partner to see a physician familiar with the evaluation of HPV in men. Some family physicians have the expertise to evaluate men for HPV, and most dermatologists and urologists also have been trained to take care of this problem. Evaluation should include the painless application of vinegar to the penis and examination with a magnifying instrument. The vinegar makes the abnormal cells swell, and the magnification is needed because the changes in the skin cells caused by the virus are sometimes not visible to the naked eye. If skin changes are present, treatment is advised in order to prevent the further growth of lesions both for cosmetic reasons and to prevent any further spread of the virus. The effect of the virus on men seems to be less dangerous: Most men with HPV do not develop penile cancer from it. Treatment usually involves removal of the affected area of skin with either a liquid chemical, an electrical instrument, or a freezing instrument. Treatment is usually preceded by a local anesthetic so that discomfort is kept to a minimum.

Condoms play an important part in the prevention of the spread of

HPV. If you have been diagnosed with the virus, you should use condoms during intercourse to prevent any spread of the virus to your partner, in case he does not already have the virus. Some women who have been diagnosed with HPV have found that their partner does not want to be examined for the virus. If that is the case, you should continue to use condoms after you are treated in order to prevent any possible reinfection in the event that he does have the virus. However, it is best for him to be properly evaluated for his own health, as well as for yours. In order to limit any chance of reinfection, the use of condoms should be continued for at least six months after both of you are free of any detectable virus.

TREATMENT

If You Have an Abnormal Pap Smear, Should You Be Treated?

If the cells on your Pap smear appear to be infected with the HPV virus, and these cells exhibit evidence of high-grade dysplastic changes, then treatment is indicated. The treatment options, which are described in the following pages, are aimed at destroying the abnormal cells so that normal cells can grow back in their place.

However, if HPV is found but the Pap smear shows only mildly abnormal cells, then the issue of treatment is controversial. The cervical cells may appear mildly abnormal because they are infected with a low-risk type of virus that will never turn into dysplasia or cancer. We know that about 60 percent of the time mildly abnormal cells will be destroyed by the body's immune system without any treatment at all. For those women, follow-up Pap smears over the next few months or a year will show a return to normal.

On the other hand, sometimes the cells appear mildly abnormal on the Pap smear because they are only in the *early* stages of an infection with a high-risk virus. Over the course of many months or years, it's likely that these cells will become high-grade dysplasia or even cancer of the cervix. There are tests to determine the type of virus (and thus the risk of developing dysplasia or cancer) that you may have, but they are very expensive and are therefore not practical to perform on a regular basis.

Currently, a number of options exist if a mild abnormality is seen on a Pap smear. One option is to repeat the Pap smear every three to six months to see whether the cells go away by themselves. A second option is to test all women with a mildly abnormal Pap smear for the type of virus present and treat only those at high risk of developing a dysplasia or cancer. As noted above, this would be very expensive. The third option is to go ahead and treat everyone with a mild abnormality. These options hinge on cost and the risk of overtreating women who will get better by themselves as opposed to the risk of not treating a small number of women who may eventually require treatment if the abnormal cells get worse. My own feeling is that if you have a mildly abnormal Pap smear, you should consider having repeat Pap smears performed every three months. If the cells appear to be getting more abnormal on the follow-up Pap smears, further evaluation with colposcopy can be performed at that time (see page 231).

The good news is that a quick and cheap HPV typing system has recently been developed and should soon be widely available. With this test, we will be able to easily determine the risk of infected cervical cells developing into a dysplasia or cancer. Then treatment can be performed only when indicated.

Janet's Abnormal Pap Smear

Janet is a twenty-six-year-old woman who has had regular annual Pap smears and pelvic exams, all of which have been normal. At the time of her last examination, her cervix looked healthy, and I expected her Pap smear to come back normal as usual. When the Pap smear results came back, the pathologist had written that the cells appeared to be infected with HPV, but that no other cellular changes were seen. When I called to tell Janet about the results, her first reaction was fear that she might have cancer. When I reassured her that this was clearly not cancer and may not even need any treatment, she felt relieved. We talked about the options, which included repeating the Pap smear every three months versus performing a colposcopy now to evaluate the problem. I encouraged her to wait, but the anxiety was getting to her, and eventually she asked to have the colposcopy. At the time of the colposcopy, her cervix looked entirely normal. No biopsies were needed, and we decided to just repeat the Pap smear in three months. When the Pap smear was repeated, it came back with the same minor abnormality, but the cells were certainly not any worse than before. She agreed to have the Pap repeated again in three months. That Pap smear and all the ones subsequent to it have been normal.

Janet's immune system appears to have eliminated the virus from her body.

What Other Tests Should Be Done If Your Pap Smear Is Abnormal?

The Pap smear is a screening test designed to easily and inexpensively detect women who may have cervical dysplasia or cancer. Like many quick and inexpensive tests, the Pap smear is not 100 percent accurate. If your Pap smear is abnormal, *do not panic!* Most Pap smear labs are very cautious, and it is not uncommon for them to "overread" a Pap smear based on any questionable cells they may see. Some abnormal Pap smears turn out to be the result of mild bacterial infections that can be easily treated with antibiotic creams. Other abnormalities are of the type that can just be followed with regular checkups, with very little risk that any treatment will ever be needed. However, in order to more accurately determine what kind of problem exists, your doctor may want to examine your cervix with a magnifying instrument called a colposcope.

What Is Colposcopy?

The colposcope is essentially a set of binoculars attached to the top of a stand. This instrument allows the doctor to see a magnified view of the blood vessels on the skin covering the cervix. As abnormal cells grow, they push the normal blood vessels of the cervix out of their way. These red blood vessels can be seen as they form unusual patterns on the pale pink background of the skin. The patterns typically change as the cells become more abnormal. Your doctor will look for these patterns to determine whether abnormal cells are present, how abnormal they appear to be, and how large or small an area they involve. Colposcopy is an accurate way to check on the results of the Pap smear. If the cells on your Pap smear were slightly abnormal in appearance and a colposcopy shows that the skin looks normal, then nothing further may need to be done other than to repeat your Pap smear in three months. However, if abnormal patterns are seen through the colposcope, then a cervical biopsy will be needed.

What Is a Cervical Biopsy?

Removal of a small area of the cervix will be performed if necessary. This is called a cervical biopsy. After the tissue is removed, it is sent to a pathologist who examines the cervical cells under a microscope for an accurate diagnosis. A Pap smear evaluates only the cells that can be scraped off the surface of the cervix; the cervical biopsy removes a thicker area that includes many more cells. Therefore, a cervical biopsy is more accurate than a Pap smear.

Looking through the colposcope, your doctor locates the abnormal area by its appearance. He places the biopsy instrument against the cervix and removes the skin cells. The biopsy instrument is long in order to reach the cervix, but the actual piece of skin removed is extremely small, less than one-eighth of an inch wide. The biopsy takes about a second. Some women feel a slight pinching, and other women feel nothing. On very rare occasions, a woman may have a very sensitive cervix, and the biopsy may be painful, but the pain lasts only for a split second and goes right away. If the abnormal cells appear to be growing up inside the canal that leads to the uterine lining, a scraping of these cells may also be performed. This takes about thirty seconds and can cause menstrual-type cramping, which goes away as soon as the scraping is finished.

In order to allow the cervix to heal, you will probably be instructed not to have intercourse or use tampons for two weeks after the biopsy. Any irritation to the cervix before it heals may cause bleeding. If that happens, your gynecologist may need to apply a chemical to the cervix to stop the bleeding. However, the site of the biopsy normally requires no care and heals quickly. Within three to four weeks not even a gynecologist could tell that a biopsy had been taken. The report from the pathologist takes about a week. Treatment will depend on how abnormal the cells look under a microscope and where they are found on the cervix.

TREATMENTS FOR CERVICAL DYSPLASIA

Cryotherapy, LEEP, laser therapy, and cone biopsy have all been used to treat cervical dysplasia with excellent results.

What Is Cryotherapy?

Cryotherapy uses a very cold instrument applied to the cervix to freeze and thus kill the abnormal cells of the cervix. Some normal cells are destroyed as well, but over the following few weeks, new healthy cells grow to replace those that were destroyed. The procedure takes about seven minutes, and most women feel menstrual-type cramps during this time. As soon as the procedure is over, the cramps go away, and there is no further discomfort. For a few weeks following the freezing, the cervix will weep a clear fluid as it heals. This often leads to a clear or yellowish, nonirritating discharge. For the first two weeks after the procedure, intercourse should be avoided so that the cervix can begin to heal. After four to six weeks, the cervix is usually entirely healed.

The good news is that this procedure has a 95 percent cure rate. After cryotherapy, follow-up Pap smears should be taken every three months over the course of the next year to make sure that you are not one of the 5 percent of women who did not get cured. If one of your Pap smears is abnormal again, then the colposcopy is repeated. If needed, you may be retreated with cryotherapy or a different method may be used.

What Is LEEP?

LEEP stands for *l*oop *e*lectrosurgical *e*xcision *p*rocedure. Developed in Europe, it has been frequently performed in the United States since the 1980s. A small wire loop is placed against the cervix, and an electric current is passed through the loop, making it extremely hot. The loop is then able to cut through the cervix in much the same way that a hot knife cuts through butter. The procedure requires special instruments, but it can be performed in the doctor's office and only takes a few minutes to do. Local anesthesia is injected into the cervix, and virtually no discomfort occurs during LEEP. The small portion of the cervix that is removed is then sent to the pathologist for examination. Healing of the cervix occurs over a six-week period, but intercourse can be resumed about three weeks after the procedure, when healing is well on its way. LEEP is both diagnostic and therapeutic: The abnormal cells are removed as treatment, and they are also sent to the lab for diagnosis. LEEP removes more tissue than a regular cervical biopsy, and it is also more expensive. Therefore, we use it only when we think that removing more tissue will be necessary.

Susan's Abnormal Pap and LEEP

Susan is a thirty-three-year-old woman who came in for her annual Pap and pelvic examination. Although she had been treated with cryotherapy ten years earlier for precancerous cells of the cervix, all of her Pap smears since then had come back normal. We were both a little shocked when this Pap smear was read as a high-grade abnormality by the pathologist. While none of the cells looked like cancer, we needed to do a colposcopy to evaluate the cells of the cervix and determine which type of treatment would be needed. Susan came back to the office a week later for her colposcopy. Surprisingly, the outside skin of her cervix looked fairly normal through the colposcope. However, I could not see the area of cells where dysplasia or cancer usually develops, the transformation zone (see page 221). Sometimes after cryotherapy, the healing process can cause the uterine-lining cells to end up higher in the canal of the cervix, where they cannot be seen. This is not dangerous, but it does limit the completeness of the examination.

Because I was not able to see this area of Susan's cervix, I recommended that we remove a portion of the canal of the cervix with the LEEP instrument. Removal would serve two purposes. First, the pathologist could examine the tissue under a microscope and make a final diagnosis of how abnormal the cells appeared to be. Second, no further treatment would likely be needed since the cells would have been removed. Susan agreed. With an extremely small needle, I injected a small amount of anesthetic, mixed with a chemical to help prevent bleeding, into her cervix. The injection did not bother her at all. Next, the wire loop of the LEEP instrument was used to remove a portion of the canal area from her cervix. Because of the anesthetic, Susan felt nothing. I then scraped the cells high up in the remaining cervical canal for the pathologist to check and make sure that no abnormal cells had been left behind. Then I used an instrument shaped like a metal Q-tip to sear a few blood vessels on the cervix in order to stop them from bleeding. The entire procedure took about three minutes.

The pathology report came back about a week later. It showed that the cells were indeed precancerous and had been growing up inside the cervical canal. Fortunately, all the abnormal cells appeared to have been removed, and the scraping of cells from the remaining part of the cervical canal were entirely healthy. The follow-up for Susan included Pap smears every three months for a year, then every six months after that. They have all been fine and no further evaluation or treatment has been necessary.

When Is Laser Surgery Used for Abnormal Cervical Cells?

The medical laser is able to precisely focus high-energy light into a small area, causing intense heat. This heat energy can be used to cut or burn away abnormal cells from the surface of skin. The precision of the laser led to its use in treating the abnormal cells of the cervix. However, this procedure requires a hospital operating room, expensive equipment, and general anesthesia. Recently, LEEP has taken the place of laser procedures because it is performed in the doctor's office, is cheaper and faster, does not require general anesthesia, and is just as effective.

What Is a Cone Biopsy?

A cone biopsy is another procedure to remove the portion of the cervix that contains abnormal cells. The cervical cells are both on the outside skin of the cervix and on the inside lining of the cervix that leads into the uterus. The outside cells are usually easy to see with the colposcope, but the cells inside the canal may not be visible. If your doctor cannot see and properly evaluate these cells, she may need to remove them to make sure all the abnormal cells are eliminated.

A cone biopsy is performed in the hospital, usually with general anesthesia. A scalpel is used to remove a portion of the outside of the cervix as well as the inside canal of the cervix. This portion of the cervix is shaped like a cone, hence the name (see fig. 9.4). Sutures are then placed around the cervix to prevent any bleeding. You may go home the same day. Since there are no abdominal incisions, there is no postoperative discomfort.

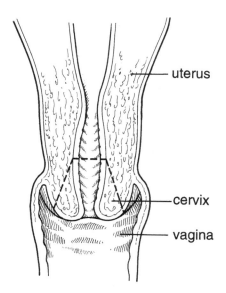

Fig. 9.4.   Portion of the cervix removed during cone biopsy

LEEP is performed in much the same way to accomplish the same results as a cone biopsy. Therefore, because of the ease and rapidity of LEEP, we rarely perform cone biopsies with a scalpel.

Can the Treatment for Cervical Dysplasia Interfere with Fertility or Childbirth?

The healing that follows cryotherapy, laser, LEEP, or scalpel cone biopsy is usually not detrimental to either subsequent fertility or childbirth. However, about 1 percent of women who undergo these procedures have scarring in the cervix that interferes with the ability of sperm to enter the uterus. If this problem occurs, a small tube may be inserted through the cervix and semen may be passed directly into the uterine cavity. This procedure, called intrauterine insemination, is usually successful.

The other problem that may rarely result from treatment for cervical dysplasia is the premature dilation of the cervix during pregnancy. Removal of tissue from the cervix may weaken it, and the weight of the baby may start to stretch the cervix. Since cryotherapy removes no tissue, the risk is very small. Care must be taken with LEEP, laser, or scalpel cone biopsies to remove as little tissue as possible, while still curing the disease. The increased risk of a preterm delivery for a woman who has had one of these procedures is about 5 percent. If you have had treatment for cervical dysplasia, you should tell your obstetrician, so that she can examine your cervix frequently during pregnancy to check for early dilatation.

What Are the Cure Rates for Cervical Dysplasia?

All of the above treatments have virtually the same cure rates, about 95 percent. Therefore, the choice of treatment should depend on the degree of abnormal cells present, the size of the area involved, and the presence or absence of abnormal cells high in the cervical canal. Your doctor will discuss these issues with you and make a recommendation for the best treatment.

Does a Hysterectomy Make Sense for Abnormal Cervical Cells?

If actual cancer is found on the cervical biopsy, then removal of the entire cervix and uterus—a hysterectomy—is usually indicated. The cervix is actually the lower part of the uterus, and one of the first places cervical cancer spreads to is the rest of the uterus. Therefore, hysterectomy is necessary to remove any other cancerous cells that remain after the biopsy. Cervical cancer virtually never spreads to the ovaries, so the ovaries do not need to be removed, especially in young women, and normal hormonal function can continue.

Hysterectomy may also be presented as an option for a woman with a high-grade dysplasia. But since these conditions can be treated by less drastic means, hysterectomy is not indicated unless there are other compelling gynecologic reasons for the procedure. In some situations, the initial removal of abnormal cells may not be complete. For these women, repeated attempts at removal of the cells short of hysterectomy are often warranted. However, sometimes abnormal cells may persist or recur despite appropriate treatments, and hysterectomy may be considered.

Even hysterectomy does not give a 100 percent guarantee that you will never be affected by abnormal cells again. Since abnormal cells usually result from HPV, some virus-infected cells may be left behind in the vagina after the removal of the cervix and uterus. About 5 percent of women who have a hysterectomy for high-grade dysplasia will have the abnormal cells recur in the vagina. If left untreated over many years, these cells can develop into vaginal cancer. These abnormal cells can also be detected with the Pap smear by scraping the top of the vagina with a small spatula. Therefore, it is important to have an annual Pap smear even after you have had a hysterectomy!

Mindy's Three Cone Biopsies

Mindy, now a forty-two-year-old woman, had had an abnormal Pap smear followed by colposcopy and cryotherapy. In the fifteen years since that initial abnormal Pap smear, her Pap had always been entirely normal. I had been her physician for about five years when her annual Pap smear came back with a high-grade abnormality.

Mindy came in for a colposcopy, but I was not able to see all the cervical cells in order to evaluate them. As sometimes happens after cryotherapy, some of the cervical cells had been pushed high into the cervical canal and were now out of view. In order to remove any abnormal cells that were up inside the cervical canal, I recommended a LEEP cone biopsy (see page 233).

The LEEP cone biopsy was done as an office procedure the following week. After removing the canal of the cervix with the LEEP instrument, I usually take a sample of cells from inside the remaining part of the cervix. These cells are sent to the pathologist in order to make sure that no abnormal cells remain above the part of the cervix that was removed. Unfortunately, when the pathology report came back, it showed that abnormal cells still remained high up in Mindy's cervix. I discussed this with Mindy and recommended that we repeat the LEEP procedure in order to remove a piece of the cervical canal even higher up. She agreed.

The second LEEP procedure was also uneventful. However, the pathology report again found very abnormal cells in the portion of the cervix that remained. At this point, both Mindy and I were extremely frustrated. The two LEEP cone biopsies had gone well and had removed enough tissue from the cervix, but both had failed to cure the problem. I was not confident that yet another cone would be any more successful, and I discussed this with Mindy. Since Mindy had completed her family, I suggested that she consider a hysterectomy as a way to completely remove the cervix and eliminate any remaining abnormal cells. However, Mindy felt very strongly that she did not want a hysterectomy. She was afraid that her sexual response and orgasm would be affected if her cervix and uterus were removed. Although this decrease in sexual responsiveness after hysterectomy has not been proved, some women have reported decreased pleasure during orgasm (see page 277). I respected Mindy's desire to avoid the surgery if possible. I discussed the situation with a gynecologic oncologist who agreed that one more chance of removing the cells would be worth a try. Mindy was delighted with the alternative to hysterectomy but extremely nervous about having yet another procedure.

I recommended that the surgery be performed in the hospital under general anesthesia. This would permit me to take out a large portion of the cervix without having to worry about causing Mindy any pain. I performed the procedure using a laser that enables the surgeon to be very slow and to have precise control over what area to remove. Again I scraped the cells remaining in the cervix. The week of waiting for the pathologist's report was an anxious one. Fortunately, the report on the scraped cells was normal. Mindy was extremely relieved, and so was I. I had been reluctant to perform this third attempt at removing the abnormal cells but was now glad that she had asked me to try again. Mindy recuperated nicely from surgery, and all of her subsequent Pap smears have been normal.

CERVICAL CANCER

Once abnormal cells burrow through the last layer of the skin covering the cervix, cervical cancer is said to exist. Directly below the skin are the blood and lymph vessels that can carry these abnormal cells to other areas of the body. Because these cells may have spread, treatment for cervical cancer needs to be more extensive than for high-grade dysplasia. Cervical cancer affects about fifteen thousand American women each year, and about five thousand women die from it each year. It is most likely to affect women in their late thirties or early sixties, but about 25 percent of women who have cervical cancer are less than thirty years old. In the United States, the number of women who die from this disease has decreased by 70 percent since the development of the Pap smear. With the routine use of Pap smears, cervical cancer should be a preventable disease.

What Is a Radical Hysterectomy?

If cervical cancer is found on a biopsy and if it has already started to burrow into the cells below, there is a chance that the cancer may have started to spread. Lymph nodes are part of your immune system and cleanse the body of abnormal cells. The lymph nodes are linked together by a chain of lymph vessels that follow along the blood vessels in your body. Removal of the uterus and the lymph nodes and surrounding tissue near the uterus is advised for women who have cervical cancer. This procedure is called a radical hysterectomy (see page 271). Surgical removal of the lymph nodes and surrounding tissue will enable the pathologist to tell whether the cancer has already begun to spread. In addition, removing tissue and lymph nodes that contain cancer may prevent further spread of the cancer. If cancer has spread to the lymph nodes, then other therapy in the form of radiation may be needed after surgery.

Can Radiation Therapy Be Used to Treat Cervical Cancer?

For some women with cervical cancer, radiation therapy may be suggested instead of surgery, or it may be needed following surgery. If cervical cancer affects a woman whose advanced age or medical problems makes surgery too risky, radiation may be a safer treatment, and the cure rates are comparable to those of surgery. Radiation uses high levels of X rays to destroy cancer cells. Two types of radiation are used to treat cervical cancer. *Intracavitary radiation* uses a device containing radioactive material that is placed through the cervix and into the uterus. This form of radiation is administered in the hospital, but it works quickly so that the device can be removed and you can return home the same day. *External beam radiation* uses a large machine to aim the radiation at the pelvic area. Administered in an outpatient setting, the radiation is usually given for about twenty minutes a day, five days a week, for six weeks. If cervical cancer is to be treated by radiation alone, both types of radiation must be given. For women who are initially treated with surgery and who are found to have cancer that has spread to the lymph nodes, external beam radiation will be recommended after surgery.

What Are the Side Effects of Radiation?

Radiation frightens most people. The machines that administer radiation are large and imposing. Some fear that the radiation will stay with them and contaminate them; however, this does not happen. Radiation is often an excellent way to treat cancer. It does, nevertheless, have potential side effects. The most common side effect is fatigue, which begins about two weeks after treatment starts and can last for a few months after the treatment has ended. Diarrhea and decreased appetite may also occur, and skin irritation at the site of radiation is not uncommon. The radiation may also affect the skin and lubricating glands of the vagina, and intercourse may become painful. Use of lubricants and gentle self-dilation of the vagina will usually help. Many women with cervical cancer (75 percent in some studies) will notice decreased sexual feelings after either surgery or radiation. Having a healthy and interested partner and counseling with a therapist skilled in this area will often help restore your sexual desire.

What Are the Cure Rates for Cervical Cancer?

As with any cancer, the earlier it is found and treated, the better the cure rate. Due to the extensive use of Pap smear testing, today women are diagnosed with cervical cancer at much earlier stages. At present, the cure rate for early cervical cancer is better than 85 percent. Early detection and treatment have really paid off in the case of cervical cancer. Be sure to get regular Pap smears.

REFERENCES

Andersen, E., and M. Husth. 1992. Cryosurgery for intraepithelial neoplasia: 10-year follow-up. *Gynecologic Oncology* 45:240–42.

Berek, J., and N. Hacker. 1994. *Practical Gynecologic Oncology.* Baltimore: Williams and Wilkins.

Morra, M., and E. Pots. 1994. *Choices: The New, Most Up-to-Date Sourcebook for Cancer Information.* New York: Avon.

Shy, K., J. Chu, M. Mandelson, B. Greer, and D. Figge. 1989. Papanicolaou smear screening and risk of cervical cancer. *Obstetrics and Gynecology* 78:838–43.

Wright, T., and R. Richart. 1990. Role of human papillomavirus in the pathogenesis of genital tract warts and cancer. *Gynecologic Oncology* 37:151–64.

Wright, T., S. Gagnon, R. Richart, and A. Ferenczy. 1992. Treatment of cervical intraepithelial neoplasia using the loop electrosurgical excision procedure. *Obstetrics and Gynecology* 79:173–78.

10

UTERINE BLEEDING, PRECANCER, AND UTERINE CANCER

What Is Uterine Cancer?

The uterus, the organ that prepares each month to provide a home to a developing pregnancy, has two distinct layers. The main body of the uterus is made of muscle, and the inner lining is composed of the cells that are shed monthly as the menstrual period (see fig. 10.1). Uterine cancer develops within the lining cells of the uterus, called the endometrial cells, and not in the uterine muscle. For that reason, uterine cancer is often called endometrial cancer. The terms uterine cancer and endometrial cancer are often used interchangeably.

We do not fully understand the reason why the uterine-lining cells begin to grow in an abnormal and uncontrolled manner. When the cells become abnormal, they first go through a precancerous stage. The good news is that both the precancer and early cancer usually cause abnormal bleeding and are therefore often diagnosed at a time when they are quite easy to cure.

What Is Atypical Hyperplasia?

As the endometrial cells overgrow and become abnormal, they go through a precancerous phase called atypical endometrial hyperplasia. Hyperplasia means overgrowth, and simple hyperplasia is a benign condition. However, if the overgrowth is also associated with changes in the cell that allow it to grow uncontrollably, then a precancerous condition exists. Called atypical hyperplasia, this precancerous condition can be detected by observing irregular and dividing lining cells under a microscope. Further uncontrolled growth leads to endometrial (uterine) cancer, characterized by cells that divide wildly.

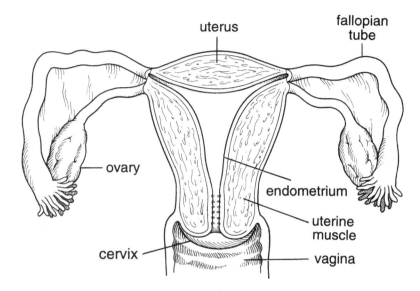

Fig. 10.1.   Endometrium (uterine lining cells)

Is Uterine Cancer Common?

Although uterine cancer is the most common cancer of the female pelvic organs, it is still rare, occurring in only two out of every one thousand women older than fifty. The average age of a woman who has uterine cancer is sixty. It is seen much less frequently in younger women. Only 5 percent of women who develop uterine cancer are under forty years of age, and it is almost unheard of in women under thirty.

What Causes Uterine Cancer?

The actual cause of uterine cancer is not known, but certain things may make a woman more likely to develop it. Imbalances between the two main hormones, estrogen and progesterone, are important factors in this disease.

Estrogen, produced by the ovaries, stimulates the growth of uterine-lining cells. In general terms, an uncontrolled overgrowth of cells is defined as cancer. Therefore, if the cells are exposed to too much estrogen over a long period of time, the precancerous condition called atypical hyperplasia may develop. Further exposure to high levels of estrogen can lead to cancer.

Progesterone, the other main female hormone, which is only produced for the two weeks after ovulation, causes the endometrial cells to stop growing. A lack of progesterone like that found in some women who do not ovulate regularly may allow the cells to grow without this restraint and can also lead to overgrowth and abnormal cells. Even though we don't know the cause of uterine cancer at this time, it appears that long-standing hormonal imbalances are an important element in its development.

Does Being Overweight Increase Your Risk of Uterine Cancer?

We have come to realize that uterine cancer appears more commonly in persistently overweight or obese women. Normally, the cells that compose fat have the ability to convert adrenal hormones, produced in the small adrenal gland above each kidney, into estrogen. The more fat cells you have, the more adrenal hormone is converted into estrogen, thus raising the total amount of estrogen in the bloodstream. Since estrogen stimulates the growth of the endometrial cells, too much estrogen can lead to overgrowth, precancer, or even cancer. Losing weight will decrease this production of extra estrogen and decrease your risk of developing uterine cancer.

Does Frequently Missing Your Period Increase Your Risk of Uterine Cancer?

Women with a history of many missed periods are also at an increased risk of developing uterine cancer. Some amount of estrogen is always produced by the ovary. However, progesterone is produced in the body only after the release of an egg. One of the most common causes of irregular periods is a hormonal imbalance that leads to a failure of ovulation (see page 64). Without ovulation, progesterone is not produced by the ovary. Without the progesterone around to put a brake on cell growth, the lining cells continue to grow unabated. Over many months or years, these cells may overgrow to the point of forming precancer or cancer.

If you are premenopausal and do not have more than a few periods a year, you should discuss your situation with your doctor. Treatment with progesterone tablets is often indicated and is an easy and safe way to stop this overgrowth.

Do Other Medical Conditions Increase Your Risk of Uterine Cancer?

Women who have diabetes or high blood pressure seem to develop uterine cancer more often than women who do not have these medical problems. We do not understand the reasons for this, although diabetes and high blood pressure are more common in overweight people, and being overweight increases your risk of developing uterine cancer.

Does Taking Estrogen Alone for Menopause Increase Your Risk of Uterine Cancer?

Many years ago estrogen *alone* was given to postmenopausal women in order to relieve their hot flashes and other menopausal symptoms. However, in 1975 it was discovered that these women had a higher incidence of uterine cancer. Since we now know that estrogen causes overgrowth of endometrial cells, that increase in uterine cancer can be explained.

If you do not take any hormones after menopause, your risk of developing uterine cancer is two per one thousand women. However, if you take estrogen alone after menopause, your risk of developing endometrial cancer increases to about ten per one thousand women. But if you take progesterone along with the estrogen, your risk decreases to less than one per one thousand women. This decreased risk results from the protective effect that progesterone has on endometrial cells. Therefore, it is recommended that you take progesterone along with estrogen for postmenopausal hormone replacement.

Janet Has Abnormal Bleeding

Janet is a sixty-nine-year-old woman who was referred to me by her family physician because she had begun having vaginal bleeding. When she had entered menopause twenty years ago, she had initially resisted taking estrogen replacement therapy. At the time, this was not uncommon since many women and doctors were skeptical and afraid of hormone replacement. However, severe hot flashes and lack of sleep finally wore her down, and within a year she asked to start estrogen. As was common at that time, estrogen was started alone, without any progesterone.

And for the next twenty years, estrogen alone is what her doctor continued to prescribe, and that is what she took.

The bleeding had started recently, but otherwise she felt fine. Her pelvic examination was entirely normal. Since she had not been taking any progesterone, I knew she was at risk for uterine cancer. Therefore, I recommended that she have a D&C and hysteroscopy to evaluate the cause of the bleeding. As usual, we performed the hysteroscopy first. The hysteroscope is a very small telescope that allows us to see inside the uterus in order to determine what may be the cause of abnormal bleeding. Instead of the normal pale pink, smooth lining of the uterus, a cauliflower-shaped, grayish bleeding area was seen at the top of the uterus. It appeared that a cancer was present (see fig. 10.2).

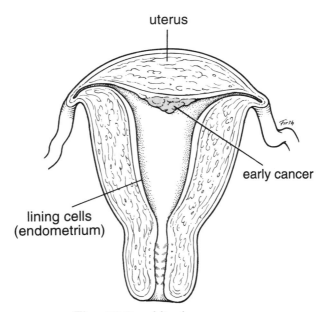

Fig. 10.2.   Uterine cancer

The D&C removed a considerable amount of tissue for the pathologist to examine under a microscope. I told Janet what I suspected, and she was shocked because she had felt entirely well. It is sometimes especially difficult to come to grips with having a major illness when you feel completely well. I explained that this was often the case with uterine cancer. It does not cause pain until it is very far advanced. And, since this was Janet's first episode of bleeding and she had no symptoms and a normal pelvic examination, I was hopeful that the disease was in its early stages and therefore curable.

A week after the D&C, the pathology report confirmed that uterine cancer was present. But the cells appeared to be slow-growing, which suggested an excellent prognosis. For reasons that are not clear, uterine cancer that results from taking estrogen after menopause without any progesterone is usually a slow-growing disease and often is less aggressive than uterine cancer unrelated to estrogen therapy. We scheduled Janet for surgery the next week. In order to remove all of the cancerous cells, removal of her uterus—a hysterectomy—would be necessary. However, the surgery would provide an almost certain cure.

At the time of surgery there was no evidence of any spread of the cancer, and on the morning of her discharge from the hospital, the pathology report from the hysterectomy confirmed that the cancer was the slow-growing type and had not begun to spread. Janet's prognosis was excellent. She was angry about having been given estrogen without progesterone, but was relieved that she would be well.

If you are taking estrogen alone (and you have not had a hysterectomy), you should have some of the lining cells of your uterus removed by your doctor and examined under a microscope. This simple procedure is called an endometrial biopsy (see page 76). If the cells appear normal, then a decision can be made regarding how you should take your hormones. If the cells are abnormal, then you have probably caught the precancer or cancer early, when it is treatable.

Does Taking Tamoxifen for Breast Cancer Increase Your Risk of Uterine Cancer?

Tamoxifen is a medication that is frequently prescribed for post-menopausal women who have had breast cancer. Tamoxifen helps to prevent the recurrence of breast cancer for unknown reasons. However, a possible side effect of the medication is an overgrowth of the endometrial cells of the uterus. In a small number of women taking tamoxifen, precancer or cancer of the uterus may develop.

As a result of this small risk, women who are taking tamoxifen should have an annual endometrial biopsy. This simple test, which takes a few minutes during your annual office visit, uses a thin plastic tube to remove some cells from the uterine lining. By examining the cells under a microscope, the early development of abnormal cells can be monitored. If precancer or cancer is found to be present, hysterectomy may be necessary.

Lillian Takes Tamoxifen

Lillian is a sixty-one-year-old woman who had found a small lump in her breast while doing her monthly self-exam during her morning shower. It was now two years since the lump had been removed and diagnosed as cancer. Luckily, this malignancy was discovered fairly early. There was no spread to her lymph nodes, and she had been told her prognosis was excellent. Her oncologist had placed her on tamoxifen to help decrease her risk of recurrence. For two years, she had been doing well and feeling fine. However, she recently noticed a small amount of vaginal bleeding and was sent to me for further evaluation.

As was expected, her examination was normal. In light of the fact that she was bleeding, and especially because she was taking tamoxifen, I recommended a hysteroscopy and D&C (see page 253), which was performed in the office the following week. The hysteroscopy revealed that an endometrial polyp was present. Polyps are also more common in women taking tamoxifen. I was able to remove it easily, and the pathology report showed that it was benign. With that reassuring news, Lillian was able to continue the tamoxifen as recommended.

Is Uterine Cancer an Inheritable Disease?

Most uterine cancers do not appear to run in families. However, some of the risk factors for uterine cancer, such as diabetes, hypertension, and obesity do run in families and thus may indirectly increase your risk for uterine cancer.

There is also a very small number of families that have a very high incidence of breast, colon, ovarian, and uterine cancers over many generations. This rare syndrome of inheritable cancers is called the Lynch Family Cancer Syndrome, named after Dr. Henry Lynch, who discovered this genetic link. If you are aware of a number of people in your family who have had these cancers, you should consider seeing a genetics counselor who is specially trained to determine your risk of getting a specific disease based on a detailed study of your family history (see page 200). If it is determined that you are at high risk for any of these cancers, appropriate screening tests can be performed for early detection of precancer or cancer. For uterine cancer, an effective screening test is the annual endometrial biopsy.

Does Having Children Decrease Your Risk of Uterine Cancer?

Women who have had a number of full-term pregnancies are at decreased risk of developing uterine cancer. During pregnancy, the placenta normally produces a large amount of progesterone, which relaxes the uterine muscle cells and prevents early labor. When the uterine-lining cells are exposed to this progesterone, any growth, or overgrowth, of these cells is restrained. This small degree of protection from the development of uterine cancer appears to be lifelong.

What Can You Do to Decrease Your Risk of Uterine Cancer?

Interestingly, women who have taken birth control pills for five years or longer have a 60 percent lower risk of getting uterine cancer. All birth control pills contain more progesterone than estrogen. We know that progesterone decreases uterine-lining cell growth. This is apparent to women who have taken the pill because they often notice less menstrual bleeding as a result of this thinner lining. Less cell growth also means a lower risk of overgrowth that might develop to the point of cancer. Another benefit of taking birth control pills is described in chapter 8: The pill decreases the risk of ovarian cancer by 50 percent.

What Are the Symptoms of Uterine Cancer?

Abnormal bleeding is an early sign of uterine cancer, but most women who have abnormal bleeding *do not* have uterine cancer. As discussed in chapter 3, there are lots of other, more likely, nonworrisome causes of abnormal bleeding. But in the rare woman who has developed uterine cancer, the cancer cells often become fragile and are more prone to bleeding.

The bleeding tends to occur irregularly and unpredictably, whenever the cells become fragile enough to break off. Luckily, the blood from these cancer cells can be easily seen as it passes through the cervix and into the vagina. As a result, abnormal cells are often detected at a very early stage, when they are treatable, long before cancer has a chance to spread.

Uterine cancer in its early stages does not cause pain, nausea, vomiting, or other obvious symptoms. Since they feel entirely well, many women are shocked to find that they have uterine cancer. Also, irregular bleeding may last for only a few days and then, as some of the abnormal tissue temporarily heals, may stop for days, weeks, or even months. Therefore, if you have abnormal bleeding, you should see your doctor, even if you otherwise feel fine, and even if the bleeding stops. This is true for women of any age, but is especially true for post-menopausal women, who have a higher incidence of uterine precancer and cancer.

Mary's Uterine Cancer

Mary was a forty-six-year-old woman who had fibroids for a number of years. When she began to have heavy bleeding, she telephoned her doctor, who reassured her that this was the result of her fibroids and nothing to worry about. About six months later she began to have bleeding between her periods, and her doctor asked her to come in for an examination. The pelvic examination showed that her uterus was slightly enlarged from the fibroids but had not changed size in over a year. Again, the doctor told Mary not to worry.

For the next few months, Mary's periods were regular and reasonably normal in flow, and she felt very relieved that the problem had just gone away. However, the following two periods were heavy, and she again began to have bleeding between periods. At this point Mary sought a second opinion and came to me for an examination and consultation. Her pelvic examination showed that her uterus was slightly enlarged from the fibroids, but the history of abnormal bleeding suggested that other tests should be performed to determine whether a cause other than the fibroids might be responsible for the bleeding.

We scheduled a hysteroscopy and D&C in the office (see page 253). During the hysteroscopy, a large amount of extra endometrial tissue was seen, which was an indication of some type of abnormality. A D&C was then performed in order to scrape out the uterine-lining cells for analysis under the microscope. The pathology report from the D&C showed uterine cancer; unfortunately, it appeared to be a fast-growing type. Mary was naturally upset and felt distraught that this problem had likely been with her for a while, but she had been told not to worry about it.

We scheduled surgery, a hysterectomy, for the end of that week. In addition, we planned to remove some lymph nodes near the uterus to make sure the cancer had not begun to spread. Unfortunately, during the surgery, we were dismayed to find many enlarged lymph nodes, which was evidence that the cancer had already spread. We removed the lymph nodes and performed a hysterectomy and sent all the tissue for analysis by a pathologist. As we feared, the lymph nodes were full of cancer. And the uterus contained cancer cells that appeared to be a very fast-growing type.

After the surgery, I joined Mary and her husband to discuss all the implications of these findings. The prognosis was not good since the cancer had already spread to the lymph nodes. Some form of additional treatment would be needed, and I recommended that she see a gynecologic oncologist, a cancer specialist, for further evaluation and treatment. About two weeks later, when she began to feel stronger, Mary went to see the gynecologic oncologist. As soon as she recovered from the surgery, he began to give her high doses of chemotherapy.

Unfortunately, a few months later, a CT scan (a very sensitive X-ray test) showed that the cancer was regrowing—the chemotherapy was not working. The last chance was to place Mary on high doses of progesterone. While this is not expected to cure the cancer, it keeps the cancer controlled for months or even years in some women. A few months later I saw Mary as she was leaving the hospital following one of her frequent follow-up tests. For the first time, she appeared completely discouraged and worn down. The cancer appeared to be winning. A month later, her husband called to tell me that she had passed away.

Cancer is sometimes unpredictable, and Mary's had been fast growing. I cannot help but wonder, though, whether an earlier D&C and earlier detection of the cancer would have saved her life. Both she and her husband had agonized over that question. Mary's fate has reemphasized to me, as a physician, the lesson of never ignoring abnormal bleeding. If your body is signaling you with a symptom, take it seriously and don't ignore it. Make sure your physician does the same.

Does a Pap Smear Detect Uterine Cancer?

Usually not, since this test was designed to detect cervical cancer and was not intended to diagnose uterine cancer. The Pap smear is a scraping of just the cells of the cervix, the lower part of the uterus that connects to the top of the vagina. The uterine-lining cells, called endometrial cells, are way up inside the uterus and are not reached during the Pap smear. Therefore, a normal Pap smear does *not* exclude the possibility of uterine cancer.

On rare occasions, the cells from the uterine lining may fall down into the cervix and can be seen on the Pap smear. Although the occurrence of these cells in the cervix can be normal, the cells may be falling down because they are overgrowing. Full evaluation of the lining cells with a D&C should be done to make sure that no precancer or cancer is present, especially if the cells are found after menopause.

Can a Sonogram Detect Uterine Cancer?

A sonogram, a picture made as a result of bouncing sound waves off parts of the body, can be used to examine the uterus. As uterine-lining cells overgrow, they form a thicker lining that can be visibly detected by sonogram. Unfortunately, the thickened lining of hyperplasia, which is benign, looks exactly the same as atypical hyperplasia (which is precancer) and the same as uterine cancer. Thus, the sonogram cannot make the diagnosis of uterine cancer. If a thick uterine lining is detected on a sonogram, then a D&C should be performed to determine whether abnormal cells are present.

Who Should Be Evaluated for Uterine Cancer?

Any postmenopausal woman who is having abnormal bleeding should be evaluated by her doctor. If you have not have a period for a year or more and then begin to bleed, this is abnormal. If you are taking hormone replacement therapy and bleed at the wrong time, this is abnormal.

Any irregular bleeding that occurs in women after the age of forty should be reported to a doctor. Although it is rare, endometrial or uterine cancer can occur in women before menopause. Very heavy bleeding that requires you to change a tampon or pad every hour or two is also abnormal. If any of these things happen to you, let your doctor know.

How Is the Diagnosis of Uterine Cancer Made?

In order to diagnose uterine cancer, the lining cells of the uterus must be collected so that they can be examined under a microscope. A simple procedure called an endometrial biopsy is one way to collect these cells. It is performed in the doctor's office, takes about one minute, and is essentially painless. A very thin plastic instrument is inserted through your cervix and into the uterine cavity. As the instrument is removed, it uses a gentle suction to scrape off and collect the endometrial cells. These cells are then placed into a bottle and sent to the lab for examination under a microscope.

As an alternative, an office D&C may be suggested to determine the cause of uterine bleeding. The doctor's recommendation for an office D&C rather than an endometrial biopsy will depend on your age, the amount of bleeding you are having, the findings at the time of your examination, and your general medical condition. An office D&C is somewhat more accurate than an endometrial biopsy because it removes more cells for analysis. I think an office D&C is indicated for all women bleeding after menopause, women with very heavy bleeding, or women who have had an endometrial biopsy but have persistent or recurrent bleeding. Also, women who have an enlarged uterus should have a D&C because adequate sampling of the lining cells may be difficult with an endometrial biopsy.

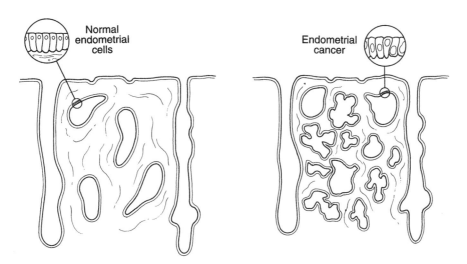

Fig. 10.3.   Uterine lining cells

An office D&C is somewhat more involved than an endometrial biopsy, and mild sedative medication may be necessary. Usually a hysteroscope is first placed through the cervix in order to examine the uterine-lining cells. This helps your doctor see what abnormalities exist and can help identify the area that should be removed for the pathologist. Together, the D&C and hysteroscopy take about five minutes. Discomfort, in the form of menstrual-type cramping, is very mild and is sometimes not experienced at all. If you prefer to have general anesthesia so that you feel nothing, a D&C may also be performed in the hospital. A full description of office D&C and hysteroscopy is found on page 75.

What Does Endometrial Cancer Look Like Under a Microscope?

As normal endometrial cells overgrow, they become more abundant and crowded together. This is called hyperplasia and is not a worrisome condition. In some women, however, in addition to the overgrowth, the individual cells become irregularly shaped, and the nucleus, the part of the cell that contains the genetic material, starts to divide more rapidly than normal. This is called atypical hyperplasia and is considered a precancerous condition. When these cells are even more overgrown and wildly dividing, endometrial cancer is present (see fig. 10.3).

Should You Consider a Second Opinion for the Pathology Results of an Endometrial Biopsy or D&C?

The interpretation of abnormal cells under a microscope is not an exact science, and differences of opinion among pathologists can exist. Pathologists often have areas of expertise, and it is reasonable, especially if there is any question about the findings from a D&C, to have a second opinion from a pathologist experienced in gynecologic pathology. This is something you might discuss with your doctor. In order to get a second opinion, the original glass slides prepared by your doctor's lab can be sent to the second lab, and no new tests or biopsies need to be done. If a diagnosis is not clear, I may rely on a specialty pathologist nearby or sometimes will even send slides to pathologists in other areas of the country for a second opinion.

Is All Uterine Cancer the Same?

The cells that line the uterus are called endometrial cells, and the cancer that results is technically called endometrial cancer. For reasons that are not clear, some of these cells become fast-growing cancers, and some grow much more slowly. The slow-growing cancers are called grade 1 endometrial cancer. Those that grow somewhat more rapidly are grade 2, and very rapidly growing cancers are called grade 3. The slower the growth of the cancer cells, the less likely the cancer will spread and, therefore, the better the chances of cure. There are two other types of cancer of the uterine-lining cells called clear cell cancer and papillary serous cancer. These cancers have the ability to spread very quickly, but fortunately they are very rare.

What Can Be Done If You Have Precancerous Cells of the Uterus?

If a D&C shows precancer (atypical hyperplasia) of the lining cells of the uterus, a number of treatments are available depending on your age and the severity of the abnormal cells. If left untreated, about 30 percent of patients with precancer will develop cancer. The good news is that this is a very slow process, taking an average of seven to ten years. The other good news is that high doses of progesterone can sometimes eliminate the precancerous cells before they get worse. As in every situation involving your health, what you choose to do should be determined by your individual circumstances.

If you are young and want to have children, then you may consider avoiding hysterectomy and attempting treatment with progesterone. Remember that progesterone causes the uterine-lining cells to stop growing, and this is exactly what you want to do with precancerous cells. Progesterone is given in pill form for three months, and then the D&C is repeated. If the abnormal cells have gone away, then careful follow-up, including repeated endometrial biopsies or D&Cs, is in order to make sure the abnormal cells do not reoccur. You may also need to begin treatment for the hormonal imbalance that caused the precancer. However, if the cells are not cured by the progesterone treatment, then you should seriously consider having a hysterectomy in order to prevent the development of uterine cancer.

If you have completed your family and have precancerous cells in your uterus, you should consider having a hysterectomy in order to prevent the development of cancer. Almost all women choose this option, but some choose treatment with progesterone first to see if it will work. If you choose the latter option, you will need another D&C in three months to recheck the lining cells. If the progesterone doesn't work, then a hysterectomy should be performed.

Terry Gets a Second Opinion

Terry is a seventy-five-year-old woman who had recently noticed some vaginal bleeding, which she reported to her doctor. A D&C

was performed, and the pathologist reported that an early cancer was present. Terry was told to have a hysterectomy, but she was unhappy about this recommendation because she wanted to avoid surgery if possible. She sought a second opinion.

When I saw Terry, her pelvic examination was normal. When I read the pathology report, the pathologist had used the words "suggestive of cancer" rather than "cancer." Pathology is not always an exact science, and I felt that the diagnosis may not have been certain. Therefore, I suggested that we have the slides reviewed by another pathologist to determine whether they thought a cancer was truly present. Our pathologist reviewed the same slides, but felt that the cells looked like precancer, not cancer.

Terry's general health was not good, and she wished to avoid surgery if possible. Terry and I discussed the possibility of her taking doses of progesterone for three months. Then we could repeat the D&C to determine if the cells had changed back to normal. While this treatment only had a 25 percent chance of getting rid of the precancerous cells, she was adamant about not having a hysterectomy unless it was absolutely necessary. She was aware that if abnormal cells were still present at the end of three months, a hysterectomy should be performed at that time.

She agreed and began to take the progesterone. In three months she returned for a repeat D&C. This was performed in the office, and the results were back in five days. The pathology report showed that no abnormal cells remained—the progesterone had worked. Just to be safe, I recommended that we repeat the D&C again in six months. And again, the report showed that all the cells were normal. Terry was fortunate and has continued to do well for the past five years.

TREEATMENT FOR UTERINE CANCER

What Happens If Uterine Cancer Is Found?

Uterine cancer is one of the most curable cancers of the body because it is usually found early. If the cancer cells appear to be slow growing based on their appearance under a microscope, and if there is no evidence that the cells have spread at the time of surgery, then the treatment is removal of the uterus. Hysterectomy cures 95 percent of women when the cancer is found early.

In some situations, radiation may also be recommended following hysterectomy. If the cancer appears to be the fast-growing kind based on the appearance of the cells under a microscope, or if there is any evidence of the cells spreading into the muscle wall of the uterus, then radiation is usually needed. The purpose of the radiation is to kill any cells that have already escaped from the uterus and were left behind after the uterus was removed.

Barbara's Cancer Is Detected Early

Barbara is a sixty-seven-year-old woman who went through menopause at age fifty-one. She had decided not to take estrogen and progesterone hormone replacement therapy and had not had any vaginal bleeding since that time. However, one day she noticed a brown discharge and called her primary care doctor. Following her examination, her doctor recommended that a D&C be performed to find out the cause of the bleeding. I performed a D&C and hysteroscopy in the office that week. The results of the D&C showed uterine cancer of the slow-growing kind, grade 1. The cancer had appeared very small at the time of the hysteroscopy and was felt to be very early. Barbara wished to have a quick recovery and requested a laparoscopic hysterectomy (see page 269). Her surgery was scheduled for the following week.

At the time of surgery, the pelvis was inspected with the laparoscope and looked entirely normal. There was no evidence that the cancer had spread. We performed the hysterectomy, and both ovaries were removed as well. Barbara made a quick recovery from the surgery, and was able to leave the hospital the next morning. The final pathology report showed that the cancer had not spread and was, in fact, a grade 1 cancer, the type that grew slowly. Barbara was reassured that she was cured and would not need any radiation. This is our goal—the early detection of uterine cancer.

Should Your Ovaries Be Removed If You Need a Hysterectomy for Uterine Cancer?

If you have slow-growing cancer that has not spread into the muscle wall of the uterus, or outside the uterus, then your ovaries do not have to be removed. Uterine cancer can spread, however, either by traveling through blood and lymph vessels, or by traveling down and out the fallopian tube. Therefore, if the cancer cells appear to be fast growing or the cancer appears to have spread into the uterine muscle or elsewhere, the ovaries should be removed. This will allow the pathologist to confirm that the ovaries do not contain uterine cancer cells. Removal of the ovaries can also prevent the future development of ovarian cancer, and women who have had uterine cancer are at twice the risk of developing ovarian cancer as the general population. Therefore, if you have been found to have uterine cancer of any sort and you have gone through menopause, you should consider having your ovaries removed.

Is Radiation Used to Treat Uterine Cancer?

Radiation may be used in addition to hysterectomy if any factors are discovered that increase the risk that the cancer has spread. Fast-growing cancer cells or cancers that spread into the uterine muscle increase the chance that the cancer has already spread. Sometimes this information can be detected at the time of surgery, but usually the risk of spread can only be known after the pathologist has examined all of the tissue removed. If spread of the cancer is seen, or if the risk of undetected spread is present, then radiation should be considered once healing from the surgery is complete.

The goal of radiation is to kill any remaining cancer cells and prevent regrowth of the cancer. The radiation therapy is administered with a large machine that aims the radiation at the pelvis. It is usually given for about twenty minutes a day, five days a week, for about six weeks. It is not uncomfortable but often leads to fatigue that may last for a few months after the treatments are completed. Diarrhea can occur during the treatments but usually resolves shortly thereafter. While no one looks forward to either surgery, or, if necessary, radiation, the cure rate for uterine cancer is good. Therefore, timely and appropriate treatment should be sought.

If You Have Had Uterine Cancer, Can You Undertake Estrogen Replacement Therapy?

Medical thinking on this question has recently changed, with many doctors believing that the use of estrogen replacement is acceptable after treatment for uterine cancer. We know that if the uterine-lining cells are exposed to prolonged periods of estrogen without the helpful effects of progesterone, the lining cells may be stimulated to overgrow and form precancer and cancer. However, once those cells are removed by hysterectomy, taking estrogen does not appear to have any detrimental effect on the risk of recurrence of the cancer.

Even though recent evidence suggests that taking estrogen after endometrial cancer is probably safe, long-term studies are needed before it can be recommended without reservation. While some women will choose not to take estrogen, others have very bothersome symptoms of menopause or are at risk for heart disease or osteoporosis and may wish to obtain some benefits from estrogen replacement therapy. Progesterone may be taken concurrently with the idea that it may prevent any regrowth of endometrial cancer cells. This is theoretical and has not been scientifically shown to be effective. For now, women who have had uterine cancer should fully discuss this issue with their doctors.

Why Should You Seek Early Medical Evaluation?

For most women who have abnormal bleeding, the cause will not be uterine cancer, but if cancer is present, and they seek care early, it can often be cured. The moral of the uterine cancer story is that the symptom of abnormal bleeding should be checked out quickly. Sometimes we hope that things that scare us will "just go away." The good news is that if we take care of them early, sometimes even bad problems such as uterine cancer will actually "go away" with prompt treatment. Hiding from the possibility of cancer delays treatment and sometimes makes a cure impossible. We all have to fight off the desire to put our heads in the sand. Be aggressive in the maintenance of your good health. If you notice something "new" or "not quite right," let a doctor examine you. Saying to yourself, "Oh, I'm sure it's nothing," is no substitute for the relief you'll feel if there is nothing to worry about or you have caught a problem in time. Early detection and early intervention save lives. Make sure yours is among them.

REFERENCES

Berek, J. and N. Hacker. 1994. *Practical Gynecologic Oncology.* Baltimore: Williams and Wilkins.

Kurman R., P. Kaminsky, and H. Norris. 1985. The behavior of endometrial hyperplasia: A long-term study of "untreated" hyperplasia in 170 patients. *Cancer* 56:403–407.

Lee, R., T. Burke, and R. Park. 1990. Estrogen replacement therapy following treatment for stage 1 endometrial carcinoma. *Gynecologic Oncology* 36:189–91.

Malfetano, J. 1990. Tamoxifen-associated endometrial carcinoma in postmenopausal breast cancer patients. *Gynecologic Oncology* 39:82–84.

Morra, M., and E. Pots. 1994. *Choices: The New, Most Up-to-Date Sourcebook for Cancer Information.* New York: Avon.

Moyers, B. 1993. *Healing and the Mind.* New York: Doubleday.

Siegel, B. *Peace, Love and Healing.* 1989. New York: Harper and Row.

11

HYSTERECTOMY

Hysterectomy, the surgical removal of the uterus, is a procedure surrounded by controversy—and for good reason. Hysterectomy is the second most common major operation performed in the United States today after cesarean section. Approximately 600,000 American women have a hysterectomy every year, at a cost of almost $5 billion. By the age of sixty, one out of every three women in the United States has had a hysterectomy. The controversy about hysterectomy arises from the feeling that many of these procedures are unnecessary.

The percentage of American women who have a hysterectomy is much higher than that of European women. For example, American women are twice as likely to have a hysterectomy as women in England and four times as likely as Swedish women. French doctors almost never perform a hysterectomy for fibroids, which is the most common reason for hysterectomy in the United States. Many factors contribute to these differences, including cultural attitudes, physician training, the availability of elective surgery in a particular country, and the ability to pay for care. However, overall, it appears that the rate of hysterectomy in the United States is high.

There are differences in the rates of hysterectomy between various parts of the United States. Women in the South are 78 percent more likely to have a hysterectomy that women who live in the Northeast, where the rate is the lowest. The rate is also 40 percent higher in the Midwest and

20 percent higher in the West than it is in the Northeast. And while the rate of hysterectomy is lowest in the Northeast, the proportion of hysterectomies performed with an abdominal incision is highest in that region. Vaginal hysterectomy, which is associated with less discomfort and a faster recovery, is most common in the South, where the rate of hysterectomy is highest. The regional differences in the rate of hysterectomy (the number of procedures per 100,000 women in the population) and the type of hysterectomies performed suggest that factors other than good medical care are involved in the decision to have surgery.

The approach to hysterectomy by some physicians has been cavalier. As recently as 1969, an American physician wrote in the medical literature that, after completion of childbearing, the uterus was a useless organ that should be removed to prevent bleeding and the development of cancer. While this opinion clearly has no place in our thinking today, many physicians consider the current rate of hysterectomy to be too high, and doctors continue to disagree among themselves about the appropriateness of the procedure in given situations. The recent medical literature supports the perception of many women that the rate of hysterectomies currently performed is too high. A number of studies have examined the medical appropriateness of hysterectomies. After review of patient records by a panel of expert gynecologists, one study found that 16 percent of the procedures were believed to be unnecessary. Another medical study suggested that the percentage of unnecessary hysterectomies may be as high as 33 percent.

With a justifiable inquiry, women's magazines and books on women's health by both nonmedical authors and physicians have picked up the diatribe against doctors in the name of women's rights. Some describe individual accounts of bad experiences when having a hysterectomy, the insensitive attitude of doctors, or an aftermath of sexual problems and personal struggle. While no doubt some horror stories exist, some of these authors do a disservice to the cause of health education and to those physicians who do provide excellent medical care to women.

For example, one book starts off with a description of a young woman who had a hysterectomy performed without her knowledge. The book goes on to list an extensive array of possible complications from surgery, without any mention of how extremely rare most of those complications are. In my reading of the book, seventeen errors and misstatements of medical facts were made, all of which will alarm women about the care they get.

To compound the disservice done by presenting inaccurate science and medicine, these authors often attempt to dogmatically coerce their readers, in much the same way that they have accused practicing physicians of doing. To these authors, hysterectomy has become a political issue. Some authors state that only 10 percent of hysterectomies are necessary, meaning only those that are performed for cancer. However, if the other 90 percent of hysterectomies are absolutely unnecessary, that leaves little room for women who are truly suffering from gynecologic problems, and who are looking to gain useful and vital information about an often valid way to help themselves.

Symptoms that result from uterine problems, such as severe pain or bleeding, will often respond to medications or other nonsurgical treatment, but sometimes they do not get better. Women with these intractable symptoms that affect their lives may benefit from hysterectomy. As noted later in this chapter, a recent American study done by a female doctor at Harvard found that most women who had a hysterectomy performed for moderate or severe non–life-threatening symptoms were "very satisfied" with the results of surgery. It appears that if you suffer from symptoms such as severe pain or bleeding, hysterectomy can sometimes offer an improvement in the quality of your life. In England, where hysterectomy rates are low, few hysterectomies are performed for these quality-of-life problems. One question often discussed among British physicians is whether it is a good or bad thing that a procedure that can improve lives is not utilized to do so.

American women who have had hysterectomies for symptoms they felt were interfering with their lives have been made to feel guilty that they "gave in." One woman, writing in a column in the *New York Times*, said, "what I find in the feminist literature is a harangue about sexism, ageism, and greed on the part of doctors and pharmaceutical companies, which tells me little or nothing about the surgery I am about to undergo and leaves me feeling guilty for selling out the sisterhood by choosing to have it [hysterectomy]." One of the most important factors in helping you choose appropriate medical care is your comprehensive understanding of the reasons for treatment, the risks, and the potential benefits. This especially applies to hysterectomy.

Unfortunately, as physicians, we sometimes do not explain medical issues very well and often do not discuss the psychological or sexual aspects of hysterectomy at all. A patient education program about the risks and benefits of hysterectomy was introduced into a small town in Switzerland, and the hysterectomy rate was compared to that of a neighboring town that did not have this education program. At the end of the year, the rate of hysterectomies had decreased by 26 percent in the town with the educational program but had increased by 1 percent in the other town. If hysterectomy has been suggested to you as an option for your particular problem, you should carefully weigh the pros and cons, the alternative treatments, and the potential benefits and risks. We have tried to provide you with some of that information. Coupled with the personalized information you have received from your own doctor, we hope you will be able to make a comfortable and informed decision about whether hysterectomy is right for you.

The percentage of women who have had a hysterectomy has actually gone down slightly since 1975, when 725,000 women had a hysterectomy in the United States. However, the total number of women who will have this operation is expected to rise as the baby boom generation enters the ages when hysterectomy is most commonly performed. So, even with a lower rate of surgery, the number of women expected to have a hysterectomy in the year 2005 may approach 825,000. For individual women and our nation as a whole, hysterectomy is an enormous health issue.

What Is a Hysterectomy?

A hysterectomy is a surgical procedure that removes the uterus. The word is derived from *hyster*, the Greek word for uterus, and the word for removal, *ectomy*. It should be noted that the term hysterectomy denotes the removal of *only* the uterus.

Does Hysterectomy Include Removal of the Ovaries and Fallopian Tubes?

By definition, hysterectomy refers to the removal of only the uterus. The Latin word for removal of an ovary is *oophorectomy*. The word for removal of the fallopian tubes is *salpingectomy*. *Bilateral* means on both sides. Therefore, the term bilateral salpingo-oophorectomy means the surgical removal of both tubes and ovaries (see fig 11.1c on page 267). In the past, this procedure has been performed with a hysterectomy about 60 percent of the time. However, for many women it does not need to be done, and the decision about removal of the ovaries should be separate and distinct from that of removal of the uterus (see page 275).

What Are The Most Common Reasons for Performing a Hysterectomy?

The most common reason listed by American gynecologists for performing a hysterectomy is fibroids. This accounts for about 30 percent of all hysterectomies. The symptoms of fibroids that can lead to hysterectomy are pain, pressure, or abnormal bleeding (see chapter 2). Hysterectomies performed because of endometriosis have increased in the past thirty years, and now account for about 19 percent of all hysterectomies. Prolapse, the falling of the pelvic organs into the vagina, is the reason for about 16 percent of all hysterectomies. Atypical endometrial hyperplasia, precancer of the uterine-lining cells, accounts for about 6 percent of hysterectomies. Hysterectomies performed because of cancer of the cervix, uterus, fallopian tubes, or ovaries accounts for about 10 percent of all procedures.

In the past, sterilization was used as a reason for performing hysterectomy. Today, female sterilization can be performed in a safer, quicker, and less expensive way by blocking the fallopian tubes with laparoscopic techniques. Therefore, hysterectomy is not recommended for sterilization. In addition, male sterilization (vasectomy) is even safer, faster, and less expensive than female laparoscopic sterilization.

Should Prevention of Cancer Be a Reason to Have a Hysterectomy?

Some women choose to have a hysterectomy not because they have cancer, but because they are afraid that they might get cancer and want to prevent this from happening. Some doctors are aware of this fear and recommend hysterectomy in order to prevent the formation of cancer. However, the risk of developing uterine cancer is extremely low: Only three women out of a hundred will ever develop this disease. Uterine cancer usually causes symptoms of abnormal bleeding in the early or even precancerous stages, when the disease is curable. Therefore, it does not make any sense to remove the uterus in order to prevent the unlikely future occurrence of uterine cancer.

Removal of the uterus also does not make sense if surgery is needed for the removal of an abnormal ovary. A recent study of women who had surgery to remove an abnormal ovary found that the risk of complications was much lower if just the diseased ovary was removed than if both ovaries and the uterus were also removed simply "because they were there." It also does not make any sense to remove the uterus and ovaries in order to prevent ovarian cancer. In the rare families (see page 200) where the risk of developing ovarian cancer is very high, removal of the ovaries by laparoscopy can be performed as an out-patient procedure; there's no need to perform a major operation in order to also remove the uterus.

It has been calculated that if every woman had her uterus removed at the age of thirty-five just to prevent the development of ovarian, cervical, and uterine cancer, the average increase in life expectancy would be only 2.4 months. And, as noted in chapters 9 and 10, both cervical and uterine cancer are easy to detect at a preinvasive or early stage when they are easily treatable.

TYPES OF HYSTERECTOMY

Total hysterectomy, the operation that is most commonly performed, removes the entire uterus, including the cervix (see fig. 11.1a). *Subtotal hysterectomy* removes only the upper body of the uterus; the cervix is left in place, connected to the top of the vagina (see fig. 11.1b). If the hysterectomy is performed because of cervical cancer, then the cervix must be removed, and total hysterectomy is always performed. The same is true for uterine cancer, since the cancer can spread down the body of the uterus and involve the cervix.

However, if the hysterectomy is performed for uterine fibroids, abnormal bleeding, or pelvic pain, you can have a choice as to whether the cervix should be removed or not. Some women feel that if the cervix is removed, they will have diminished sexual pleasure, while other women do not feel the cervix is part of their sexual enjoyment. This issue is discussed in detail on page 277.

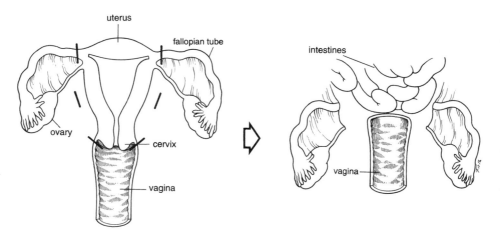

Fig. 11.1a.   Total hysterectomy

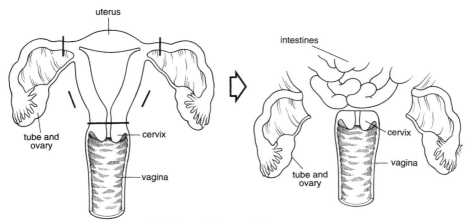

Fig. 11.1b.   Subtotal hysterectomy

If the cervix is not removed, you will need to have annual Pap smears to check for cervical dysplasia and cancer. Even if the cervix is removed, a Pap smear of the vagina should still be done to detect abnormal vaginal cells, but perhaps on a less frequent basis.

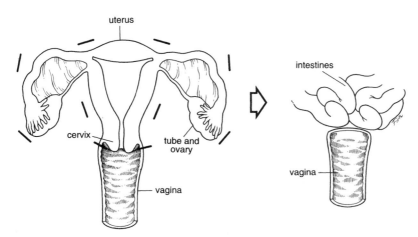

Fig. 11.1c.   Total hysterectomy and bilateral salpingo-oophorectomy

What Are the Different Ways to Perform a Hysterectomy?

There are presently three ways to perform a hysterectomy: abdominal hysterectomy, vaginal hysterectomy, and laparoscopic hysterectomy.

Radical hysterectomy, performed for some types of cervical or uterine cancer, includes the removal of lymph nodes from around the uterus and cervix in addition to the removal of the uterus.

What Is an Abdominal Hysterectomy?

Abdominal hysterectomy removes the uterus through an incision in the abdominal wall and is the type of hysterectomy performed in about 75 percent of women who have the operation in the United States. The abdominal incision may be made either from side to side (bikini incision) (see A in fig. 11.2) or up and down, from the pubic bone to just below the navel (see B in fig. 11.2). After the incision is made in the skin, the abdominal muscles are stretched apart (not cut) so that the abdominal cavity can be seen. This stretching of the muscles causes some of the discomfort that follows abdominal surgery. The operation takes from one to three hours; the hospital stay is from three to five days; and the recovery until normal activity can be resumed is about six weeks.

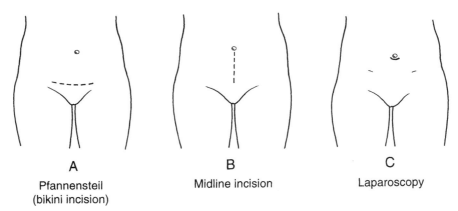

A	B	C
Pfannensteil	Midline incision	Laparoscopy
(bikini incision)		

Fig. 11.2.   Surgical incisions

Abdominal hysterectomy may be utilized because it gives the doctor the ability to see and feel all of the pelvic organs during the operation. It is often used if the doctor expects the operation to be difficult because of scar tissue from previous surgery, previous infection, or endometriosis. It is usually the way a hysterectomy is done if cancer is present, because it allows the doctor to remove all the cancer and inspect and feel inside the abdomen to make sure the cancer has not spread.

Laparoscopic hysterectomy techniques (see page 269) are now being developed to deal with special situations such as scar tissue or fibroids and, in some cases, even cancer. However, because considerable laparoscopic training and skill are needed to do this safely, it is likely that abdominal hysterectomy will have a continued role in the treatment of these problems.

What Is a Vaginal Hysterectomy?

The second most common type of hysterectomy is called vaginal hysterectomy because the surgery is performed through an incision made at the top of the vagina. The blood vessels and other connections of the uterus to the inside of the body are first cut and sutured through the vagina. Once detached, the uterus is removed through the vagina. Since the incision is made only in the vagina, there is no visible scar. The vaginal incision is small and heals quickly and, because the abdominal muscles are not stretched, less discomfort occurs than with abdominal hysterectomy. This procedure takes about one or two hours. The hospital stay lasts from one to three days, and the recovery until normal activity can be resumed is about four weeks.

Vaginal hysterectomy can be used when the uterus is more loosely attached to the inside of the body, as occurs when a woman vaginally delivers her children and with increasing age. As the ligaments that hold the uterus become more relaxed, it can be pulled down into the vagina during the surgery, and the procedure can be performed with good visualization. It is harder to see the uterus during a vaginal hysterectomy; therefore, if scarring to the bowel or bladder is anticipated, abdominal hysterectomy may be performed to avoid inadvertent injury to these areas.

What Is a Laparoscopic Hysterectomy?

Laparoscopic hysterectomy is a new surgical procedure, first performed in 1989, that allows the uterus to be detached from inside the body by laparoscopic instruments while the doctor views the uterus, fallopian tubes, and ovaries through a camera attached to a telescope. After the uterus is detached, it is removed through a small incision at the top of the vagina. One advantage of laparoscopic hysterectomy is that the incisions are smaller (one-half inch) and much less uncomfortable than that of abdominal hysterectomy (see C in fig. 11.2 on page 268). Also, the hospital stay of one day and the ability to resume normal activity in about two weeks are substantially shorter than for abdominal hysterectomy and slightly shorter than for vaginal hysterectomy.

For patients who have known or suspected pelvic scar tissue or endometriosis, laparoscopic surgery allows the surgeon to remove the diseased tissue with the laparoscope before performing a vaginal hysterectomy, thereby reducing the risk that the intestines or bladder might be injured during surgery. For patients who have fibroids that are large and might otherwise be difficult to remove by vaginal hysterectomy, laparoscopic hysterectomy allows the surgeon to detach the blood vessels to the uterus while viewing them through the laparoscope. Then the uterus can be removed through the vagina more easily and with less blood loss.

However, it appears that vaginal hysterectomy is safer and less expensive than laparoscopic hysterectomy. It also has about the same hospital stay and recovery time. Therefore, a laparoscopic hysterectomy should not be performed if a vaginal hysterectomy is possible. However, if an abdominal hysterectomy is needed, laparoscopic hysterectomy may be considered as an alternative.

Laparoscopic hysterectomy is still being studied with regard to its overall risks and benefits. It does require considerable skill and experience on the part of the surgeon. You should ask your doctor what kind of training he or she has gone through and how many procedures he or she has performed with each technique. If your gynecologist is not comfortable or experienced with laparoscopic hysterectomy, then it may be best to have the surgery the way the doctor feels is most appropriate, or you may ask for a referral to someone who is more comfortable performing this procedure.

Caroline Has a Laparoscopic-Assisted Hysterectomy

Caroline, a thirty-four-year-old woman with two young children, had known she had uterine fibroids for one year. While fairly large when initially discovered, the fibroids had recently grown to the size of a large coconut. She had heavy bleeding with her periods, requiring her to change menstrual pads every half hour for two full days. This heavy bleeding had made Caroline weak and irritable. When she had her period, her activity had to be severely limited. Both Caroline and her husband Dan were anxious and worried before the start of her period each month. Dan feared that she would begin to hemorrhage. He was insistent that she get immediate treatment.

Another gynecologist had recommended removal of the fibroids with both the resectoscope and laparoscope. Despite pressure from her husband and the strong recommendation of her gynecologist, Caroline could not commit to the surgery. She was uncertain about wanting more children and thus was ambivalent about a surgery that could compromise her fertility. She was desperate to have the bleeding end, yet wanted some other solution.

Based on my examination, I felt that removal of the fibroids as had been recommended would be extremely difficult, and that repair of the uterus through the laparoscope might not be safe for future childbearing. We discussed the probable need for myomectomy through an abdominal incision (see page 42). Because of the anemia, I recommended that she begin treatment with Lupron to shrink the fibroids (see page 35). In addition, this would stop her periods for the three months she was on the medication. Stopping the heavy bleeding would give her body time to make new blood and correct her anemia. In fact, this was just what happened, and she began to feel stronger and more energetic.

With a return to her usual strength and vitality, Caroline began to devote more time and emotions to her thoughts of having another child. Much to her surprise, she realized that she really did not want any more children after all. By the end of the three months, after careful consideration by herself and with Dan, she decided that she was sure she did not want any more children and requested a hysterectomy. We performed a laparoscopic-assisted hysterectomy, and Caroline had a one-day stay in the hospital and only two weeks to full recovery. She has done well since that time and is happy with the decision she made.

What Is a Radical Hysterectomy?

In addition to the removal of the uterus through an abdominal incision, a radical hysterectomy includes the surgical removal of the lymph nodes and other tissue surrounding the cervix and uterus. Radical hysterectomy is often recommended if a woman is found to have cervical cancer and may also be beneficial in some women with uterine cancer that has spread to the cervix. Lymph nodes are part of your immune system and cleanse the body of abnormal cells. They are linked together by a chain of lymph vessels that follow along the blood vessels in your body. Removal of the lymph nodes and surrounding tissue also aids in the removal of any additional cancer cells. Moreover, the pathologist will be able to tell whether the cancer has already begun to spread, and this information will be helpful in planning further therapy.

After You Have a Hysterectomy, What Do You Look Like Inside?

The small intestines are about twenty feet long and normally curl up around the front and back of the uterus. When the uterus is removed, the intestines move into this spot, so that no "empty space" remains (see fig. 11.1). If your uterus was a relatively normal size before surgery, you will probably not notice any difference in the way your abdomen feels. If you had an enlarged uterus from fibroids, you may feel *less* pressure in your abdomen, as the intestines can now move back to the area where they belong.

The top of the vagina normally attaches directly to the cervix, and both are covered with a continuous layer of skin. If a total hysterectomy is performed, the cervix is cut away from the vagina and the uterus removed. The remaining top portion of the vagina is closed together with dissolvable sutures. Very little of the vagina is removed, but the end result may be a slightly shorter vagina than before surgery. After total hysterectomy, when viewed through a speculum, the cervix is absent and the top of the vagina appears as a continuous, closed layer of skin.

If a subtotal hysterectomy is performed, the attachments of the cervix to the vagina are not cut, and the length of the vagina is not altered. When viewed through a speculum, the cervix and vagina look the same as they did before the hysterectomy.

RISKS OF HYSTERECTOMY

Some books and magazine articles have quoted the risk of having a complication from a hysterectomy as 50 percent. However, this is a distortion of the facts. The majority of these reported "complications" are mild fevers that result from easy-to-treat infections of the incision, the bladder or, rarely, the lungs. Serious complications occur very rarely.

Bleeding that requires transfusion has been reported about 10 percent of the time. However, those statistics were collected before the awareness that HIV could be acquired from blood transfusions. Doctors are now much less likely to give a transfusion for just slight fatigue or mild anemia, as was often done in the past. Therefore, it is likely that the number of transfusions has already declined, but the newer statistics have not yet been reported in the medical journals.

Other risks during hysterectomy include inadvertent injury to the organs near the uterus. The risk of injury to the bladder, ureters, or intestines is about one per one thousand operations. The risk may be higher or lower depending on the reason for your surgery and the technical difficulty that your condition presents.

All operations have risks. But in general, the risk of a serious complication from a hysterectomy is very small. The risk to you will depend on the reason you need surgery, your medical condition, and your age, and the experience of your doctor and anesthesiologist. For women age thirty-five to forty-four, the risk of dying from this procedure is about three per ten thousand women. For women of all ages who are operated on for benign conditions, the risk of dying from a hysterectomy is six per ten thousand women. If a hysterectomy is performed because of cancer, it may be a more difficult operation, and sometimes the initial medical condition of the woman may be worse. For these reasons, the risk of dying from surgery when cancer is present is about thirty-seven per ten thousand women. The Maine Women's Health Study, described in detail on page 281, recently reported that only 1 percent of women in their study who had a hysterectomy had a bleeding complication, 5 percent had a treatable wound or bladder infection, and the total complication rate was 7 percent. Of the four hundred women in that study who had a hysterectomy, none had a serious complication and none died.

Can Hysterectomy Affect Your Bladder Function?

A recent well-conducted study compared bladder symptoms in two groups of women interviewed both before and after they had surgery. One group of women had a D&C performed, while the other group had a total hysterectomy performed. Both groups had an increase in reported frequency of urination, urgency to urinate, and incontinence. Still, there was no difference in symptoms between the two groups, except that the women who had a hysterectomy noted *less* incontinence. Another study precisely measured bladder function before and after hysterectomy and could not detect any adverse change in function after the surgery. Consequently, there is no evidence that hysterectomy leads to bladder problems.

For women who have fibroids pressing against their bladders, frequency of urination or even loss of urine during laughing, coughing, or sneezing can sometimes occur. For these women, hysterectomy may remove the pressure on the bladder and may actually improve bladder function.

Can Removal of the Uterus Increase the Risk of Heart Disease?

In the past, the uterus was not thought to produce any hormones or substances that were medically important. However, a few studies found that women who had only their uterus removed had a 4 percent increased risk of developing coronary artery disease, either in the form of chest pain or an actual heart attack.

It has been discovered recently that the uterus does produce a biochemical called prostacyclin that is able to dilate blood vessels and permit more blood, oxygen, and nutrition to reach the heart. Furthermore, prostacyclin prevents blood from clotting, thus discouraging the blockage of blood vessels to the heart that can result in a heart attack. The theory not yet proven is that prostacyclin produced in the uterus may enhance blood flow to the heart and thus protect your heart. However, this effect on the risk of heart disease would be *very small* compared to exercise, diet, and hereditary factors. Nevertheless, with the presumed increased incidence of heart disease so small, it would take a study of ten thousand women who had a hysterectomy and ten thousand who did not, all of whom were followed until death, in order to prove if an increased incidence of heart disease had, in fact, occurred. Therefore, it is unlikely we will ever know the answer to this question.

Does Removal of the Ovaries Increase the Risk of Heart Disease?

The ovaries produce the main female hormone, estrogen, until the time of menopause. Estrogen has a beneficial effect on your heart and cardiovascular system, and we know that women who have their ovaries removed at an early age, or those who go into early menopause, have a higher risk of having a heart attack later in life. The reasons for this protective effect of estrogen are not entirely clear. However, we do know that estrogen lowers the level of cholesterol in your blood, which reduces the risk of clogged arteries. Estrogen also acts directly on blood vessels to dilate them and allow more blood, oxygen, and nutrition to reach the heart muscle. There are probably other effects of estrogen on the heart that are not yet known. Nevertheless, we do know that the ovaries play a role in the prevention of heart disease.

Therefore, the decision to remove your ovaries during a surgery intended to remove the uterus should be carefully considered as a separate decision, as discussed in detail below. If you need to, or choose to, have your ovaries removed, you should strongly consider taking estrogen replacement after surgery. Replacement estrogen, available in pills, skin patches, or creams, will then continue to provide the protective effect for your heart and blood vessels. To date, no independent beneficial effects of progesterone have been found other than the protection of the uterus from overgrowth or cancer of the uterine-lining cells. Following hysterectomy, this protective effect is not needed; therefore, progesterone does not need to be taken.

If You Need a Hysterectomy, Should You Also Have Your Ovaries Removed?

The answer to this question is controversial and rests on your view of the balance between the benefits of having your own natural supply of estrogen versus your risk of developing ovarian cancer if your ovaries are not removed. Also important are your feelings about having your ovaries removed, regardless of your age.

The following is my opinion about this dilemma. If you need to have a hysterectomy well before menopause for medical reasons, and if you are at no extra risk for developing ovarian cancer, you should strongly consider keeping your ovaries. Retaining your ovaries will provide you with the benefit of having your *own* hormones until you go through menopause. If you are approaching menopause, you might still consider retaining your ovaries. While there is no magic age that can be considered as a cutoff, we often recommend retaining your ovaries if you are younger than age forty-five. Since the average age of menopause is fifty-two, your ovaries will continue to produce your own hormones for five to ten years after a hysterectomy at age forty-five.

However, if you are over the age of fifty and need a hysterectomy, you might consider having your ovaries removed at the same time. At that point, your ovaries may only produce estrogen for a few more years, and removing them will eliminate the 1 percent risk of developing ovarian cancer in your lifetime. For women between the ages of forty-five and fifty, the decision is less well defined and may be more difficult. Personal feelings tend to play a large part in the decision-making process.

Aside from these suggestions, many women wish to retain their ovaries regardless of their age at the time of hysterectomy. Other women who are at a higher risk of developing ovarian cancer or who are just very uneasy about keeping their ovaries may choose to have them removed at the time of hysterectomy, even at a young age. Women tend to make very different decisions based on their particular circumstances, their feelings about hormone replacement therapy, and their fear of ovarian cancer. This decision is yours to make and should be discussed in detail with your doctor.

What Happens to a Woman's Monthly Cycle After Hysterectomy?

After the uterus is removed, menstrual bleeding ceases. But if the ovaries are left in place, the hormones estrogen and progesterone continue to be produced in the normal cyclic fashion. As a result, any breast tenderness and bloating that you may have had prior to your period will likely continue. Some women find that headaches and PMS symptoms are lessened following hysterectomy, presumably because removal of the uterus eliminates prostaglandins and perhaps other substances that possibly cause these symptoms. However, in other women, PMS symptoms are unchanged. The ovaries continue to produce eggs as well. An egg is microscopic and, after it is released during ovulation, it dissolves quickly within the body cavity.

If you have your ovaries removed at the time of a hysterectomy, your body will not have any natural source of estrogen or progesterone, and the monthly changes your body normally experiences will cease. If you choose to take estrogen replacement therapy, the levels of estrogen are constant throughout the month and women will only rarely experience PMS or other cyclical changes.

Can Hysterectomy Lead to Psychological Problems?

Many women fear hysterectomy, and some will delay or avoid surgery even when it is medically necessary. Whether you should or should not have a hysterectomy is a personal decision as well as a medical one. Some women have fears about the actual surgery, discomfort, and possible complications. Some women are concerned about the effect hysterectomy will have on their sexuality, on the way they will feel about their own identity, and the way others (especially their partner, if they have one) will view them. One study found that 16 percent of women had a negative psychological reaction to having had a hysterectomy. The women described feelings of sadness, grief, and lowered self-esteem. Some said that even though they did not want to have more children, the finality of not being able to have more children was upsetting.

Many of the attitudes that a woman brings to the surgery will affect the way she feels about the surgery. Therefore, it is important to give careful thought to whether a hysterectomy is the right thing for you to do. Seeking out an experienced therapist may also be helpful. Balance the possible benefits from surgery, such as the decrease in symptoms, with the way you think you might feel after the surgery.

Can Having a Hysterectomy Lead to Psychological Problems for Your Partner?

Some women may find that their partners have a hard time following hysterectomy. Partners may also experience a sense of loss or sadness that having biological children is no longer possible, and perhaps that middle age has arrived. They may worry about your lack of strength and your need to recover. They may also be afraid of hurting you during sex or be uncertain about how you feel about sex after the operation. These feelings can be found in both heterosexual and lesbian relationships. Anticipating these feelings for both of you and talking about them before, or at least after, surgery will probably go a long way toward resolving these issues. Difficult emotional reactions might be helped by talking to a therapist.

Can Having a Hysterectomy Affect Your Sexuality?

Even in the recent past, sexual problems following hysterectomy were felt to be psychological, simply all in the mind. However, this view is inaccurate, and a better understanding of sexuality has shed new light on this issue. Orgasm is experienced differently by different women. Many women reach orgasm by stimulation of the clitoris, other women by vaginal stimulation, and still others by a combination of the two. Furthermore, uterine contractions occur with orgasm, and this can be an important part of sexual pleasure for some women. Obviously, hysterectomy will eliminate the contractions of the uterus and may change the sexual experience.

Some women also feel that pressure against the cervix during intercourse is pleasurable and is important to their sexual experience. Removal of the cervix may change this sensation and decrease the sense of pleasure. Consequently, subtotal hysterectomy, which removes the body of the uterus but preserves the cervix, may be appropriate for some women. Although this type of hysterectomy has not been proved to be more effective in maintaining an unaltered orgasm, if you feel that cervical sensation has been important to your sexual experience, it is worth discussing with your doctor.

In some women, hysterectomy can result in the formation of scar tissue where the sutures are placed at the top of the vagina. The scar tissue may be less elastic than normal tissue and may lead to discomfort during intercourse. The above problems, however, are not common following hysterectomy. In order to preserve the cervix with a subtotal hysterectomy, an abdominal incision is usually made, resulting in more postoperative discomfort and a longer recovery period. Recently, laparoscopic techniques have been developed to perform subtotal hysterectomy.

On the other hand, if your uterus is causing you to have pain with intercourse, hysterectomy may relieve that pain and make intercourse more pleasurable. One study found that, following removal of the uterus, 75 percent of women noted that sex was better, and only 10 percent of the women felt that it was worse than before surgery. Another study found that the best predictors of sexuality after hysterectomy were the frequency of desire, intercourse, and orgasm prior to the surgery, as well as the woman's attitude toward her partner. And lastly, some women report that hysterectomy eliminates the fear of pregnancy, which actually increases their enjoyment of sex.

Debbie's Problem After Hysterectomy

Debbie is a forty-nine-year-old woman who was seen at a well-known medical clinic for a complete physical. She felt fine and was surprised when the gynecologist at the clinic found uterine fibroids during her pelvic examination. Despite the fact that Debbie lived in another town about two hours away, the doctor recommended that she have surgery immediately. Even though she is a high-level executive used to making quick and weighty decisions, Debbie felt flustered, indecisive, and afraid. Feeling she was already in the best of hands, she chose not to seek a second opinion and had a hysterectomy performed that week. The surgery went well, and she left the hospital five days later feeling relieved that it was over and that she could return to her normal life.

I first saw Debbie a year later. Following the surgery, she had found that intercourse was very uncomfortable. This was very upsetting to her since she and her husband, who had met in high school and been married for thirty years, had an active and wonderful sex life. The discomfort she felt had made intercourse difficult and had strained their relationship. Debbie had returned to see the gynecologist who had performed the surgery, but she had dismissed the problem as psychological, and she had not been of much help to Debbie.

When I examined Debbie, as the speculum was inserted toward the top of her vagina, she moved away in pain. I was able to see an area of scar tissue where the sutures had been placed during the surgery. The area seemed thicker than expected for a year after surgery. On the manual part of the examination, this area was extremely tender to the touch. I reinserted the speculum in order to get a better look at the tender area and was surprised to find an area of raw and unhealed skin at the point of tenderness. This delayed healing is not uncommon and is called granulation tissue, or "proud flesh." It is formed when new blood vessels begin to grow in a wound, but are not covered up by skin when the tissue heals. Sometimes the granulation tissue is found because it starts to bleed, and sometimes, as in Debbie's case, because it is tender.

I felt happy that the problem appeared to be such a simple one, which could be treated by placing a chemical on the affected area to encourage proper healing. This treatment was mildly uncomfortable but took less than a minute. When I saw Debbie three weeks later to check the area, it appeared to have healed well, but it was still uncomfortable. We decided to allow a few more months for the healing to be complete.

Two months later, when I examined the area, it appeared healed, but was slightly thickened from scar tissue, and it was still tender. Debbie was upset, and I was disappointed because what I thought was an easy problem to treat had not gotten better. I felt the next step was an attempt to cut away the scar tissue and repair the vagina in the hospital under anesthesia. I hoped this would allow new tissue to start the healing process over again, this time with more success. Debbie was anxious to try anything and agreed. The surgery was not difficult; the scar tissue was cut away, and the healthy tissue sutured back together. I saw Debbie every few weeks following surgery, and the tissue appeared to be healing fine. About six weeks after surgery, Debbie and her husband had intercourse for the first time in many months. While still mildly uncomfortable, Debbie felt much better than she had since before her hysterectomy had been performed. By the time of her next visit, six months later, Debbie reported no discomfort during intercourse and was back to full enjoyment of sex.

There are a number of lessons to be learned from Debbie's story. First, if you are not sure about what has been recommended to you, there is always time to get a second opinion. Do not rush. Second, if you are having problems after surgery, be evaluated to see if there is a medical, and correctable, reason for how you feel. Even if problems do occur after surgery, many of them can be corrected.

Can Removal of Your Ovaries Affect Your Sexuality?

Many of the inferred effects of "hysterectomy" on sexuality are actually related to the removal of the ovaries and subsequent hormonal deficiency, rather than the removal of the uterus. If the ovaries are removed and no hormonal replacement is started, then sexual enjoyment may be altered. Without estrogen to maintain the health of the vaginal tissue, the vagina may become thinner, drier, and inelastic, often leading to pain with intercourse. Also, estrogen and testosterone, both produced by the ovary, are needed to maintain normal sexual feelings.

Testosterone, the main hormone produced by men, is produced in small amounts by your ovaries, and it increases libido, or sexual desire. Some women will note a decrease in libido after removal of the ovaries, even if they take estrogen replacement. If this happens, you might consider taking testosterone in pill form. In large doses, testosterone can cause side effects such as weight gain, change in the texture or amount of body hair, acne, or oily skin. These side effects can be avoided by taking very small doses. One study found that women who had their ovaries and uterus removed noted a decrease in the frequency of intercourse and orgasm if no hormone replacement was given. But women who subsequently took estrogen had a twofold increase in the frequency of intercourse and orgasm, and women who took both estrogen and testosterone had a sixfold increase. Testosterone may also improve mood, and some women who take testosterone feel better in general, in addition to the return of normal libido.

What Can Be Done If Hysterectomy Has Caused Sexual Problems?

One thing to do is to understand that you are not alone and help is available. First, you should be evaluated physically to make sure your hormone levels are normal or scar tissue hasn't formed to cause your pain. If you feel that your emotions are part of the dilemma, and if you would like to improve your sex life, help is also available. Probably the best place to start is by explaining to your partner how you feel about the change in your sexuality. Hopefully, your partner will not only be understanding but also help you discover different ways of having sexual pleasure. This may be an opportunity to experiment. The goal is for sex to be pleasurable, even if it may feel different.

Psychological counseling, especially sexuality counseling, may also be very helpful. This is a fairly specialized skill, and your doctor may be able to direct you to the appropriate therapist.

BENEFITS OF HYSTERECTOMY

It seems clear that too many hysterectomies are performed in this country every year and that some women could have avoided surgery had they been aware of other alternatives and treatments. However, it is also clear that some women benefit from having a hysterectomy. Not many would argue with the usefulness of removing the uterus for cervical, uterine, or ovarian cancer, where hysterectomy can be lifesaving. But many other women have symptoms that, while not life-threatening, do affect their general physical and emotional health and their ability to perform normal activities. Is there any evidence that a hysterectomy can be of any benefit to these women?

An important study published in 1994, the Maine Women's Health Study, examined how women felt both physically and emotionally before and after hysterectomy. It is the largest study of its kind concerning hysterectomy. More than four hundred women were interviewed before they had a hysterectomy and then followed for a year after their surgery. The study included half of the women who had a hysterectomy in the state of Maine during that time. Likewise, a separate group of 380 women who had similar gynecologic problems but chose not to have a hysterectomy were interviewed. Even though the group of women who chose to have a hysterectomy had somewhat worse symptoms than the women who chose nonsurgical treatment, the large numbers of women interviewed makes the results interesting.

What is especially noteworthy is that the study found that after hysterectomy a substantial number of women had a marked improvement in their symptoms, which included pelvic pain, urinary problems, bleeding, fatigue, and psychological and sexual problems. They also reported a significant improvement in mental health and general health at the end of one year. Many of the women reported a marked improvement in the quality of their lives. Therefore, for some women, especially those who had significant symptoms as a result of gynecologic problems, hysterectomy may be beneficial. The details of the study are outlined below.

Can Hysterectomy Help Relieve Gynecologic Symptoms?

In the Maine study, 93 percent of women reported "some" or "a lot" of discomfort or limitation of their activity before surgery. The reasons for hysterectomy included fibroids, endometriosis, heavy bleeding, prolapse, and chronic pelvic pain. The women studied noted significant symptoms that had a substantial negative effect on the quality of their lives. After hysterectomy, the vast majority of these women noted an improvement in their symptoms. For example, of the 85 percent of women who had pelvic pain "frequently" before surgery, only 13 percent complained of this problem after surgery. While 70 percent of the women had pain with intercourse before surgery, only 30 percent had this problem after hysterectomy. And while 60 percent of the women had diminished enjoyment of sex before surgery, only 15 percent complained of this after surgery. Therefore, the Maine study showed that hysterectomy may be helpful for women who are significantly affected by gynecologic symptoms.

Can Hysterectomy Improve the Way You Feel?

In the Maine study, 72 percent of women felt "much better" and another 16 percent felt a "little better" after they had a hysterectomy performed. Only 3 percent of the women interviewed felt worse than they did before surgery. Remember that most of these women had a significant degree of symptoms before surgery, and therefore would be expected to benefit more from surgery than someone with only mild symptoms. Also, despite some other accounts to the contrary, only 3 percent of the women had a negative feeling about themselves as women as a result of having their uterus removed.

Can Hysterectomy Improve Quality of Life?

Women entering the Maine study had lower scores in tests of their quality of life than the general population, but had improved scores equal to those of the general population after their hysterectomies. This improved quality of life was expressed as less pelvic and back pain, less pain with intercourse, less abdominal swelling, and less fatigue. Significant improvement in activity, general health, and mental health was also seen in women who had a hysterectomy. The Maine study found that the women who had a hysterectomy were much more able to go where they wanted, do things for fun and recreation, and work after surgery than they had been able to do before surgery.

Jane's Hysterectomy

Jane is a forty-four-year-old woman who had known that she had uterine fibroids for about three years. They had never caused her any problems until recently, when she noted fairly constantly abdominal pressure and discomfort during intercourse. When she was examined, I noted the fibroids to be larger than they had been before. Since the symptoms were not severe, Jane decided to be re-examined in three months to see if the fibroids continued to grow.

At the follow-up visit, the fibroids were the same size, but Jane felt more disturbed by the symptoms they were causing. She no longer wanted to have intercourse and found herself in pain and irritable almost every day. She asked about the possible treatments. We discussed the possibility of no treatment until menopause, when the fibroids would most certainly shrink. But Jane felt that this was too far off. The second option was to perform a myomectomy, which involves removing the fibroids, but leaving the uterus. Since the fibroids were large, the myomectomy would need to be performed through an abdominal incision. (At the time, another option possible today, myoma coagulation, had not yet been developed [see page 49].) The last option was hysterectomy, which would also require an abdominal incision. Jane felt that if she was going to go through an abdominal incision and the needed recovery, she probably ought to have her uterus removed, so that she would not have to deal with fibroids in the future. But Jane was concerned about hysterectomy because she had heard that the surgery might affect her sexuality. After a long discussion about the risks and benefits of each option, Jane decided to think about it and wait a little longer.

Three months later, Jane was ready to do something about her fibroids. The constant pressure was interfering with her job and daily activities, and intercourse was totally unenjoyable. We went over the options again, and Jane was fairly certain that she wanted a hysterectomy but was still worried about the effect it might have on her sexuality. We discussed the possibility of performing a subtotal hysterectomy and leaving the cervix in place, but after much thought, she decided to have a total hysterectomy without the removal of her tubes or ovaries.

The surgery went well, as did her recovery. At her appointment six months after her hysterectomy, I asked Jane how she was doing. She said she no longer had discomfort during the day, and the pain with intercourse had totally disappeared. Intercourse was now totally enjoyable. She was surprised at how much discomfort she had learned to live with and was relieved that it was over. She felt certain that the hysterectomy had been the right thing for her to do.

Can Medication Relieve Pelvic Pain or Bleeding?

The second part of the Maine Women's Study was an evaluation of the symptoms of women who chose to be treated with medication for their problems. These women were then compared to women who chose to have a hysterectomy for similar problems. For many of the women, medication was effective and allowed them to avoid surgery. The two groups of women were not entirely similar because the women who chose surgery had worse symptoms than those who chose medication. But the authors of the study felt the results were valuable because there were significant similarities between the two large groups of women.

The study reported that of the 85 percent of women who complained of significant pelvic pain before treatment with medication, 50 percent still had this problem after treatment. For women who had a hysterectomy, 95 percent complained of pain before surgery, but only 3 percent had pain after the hysterectomy. For women who had pain from fibroids, 50 percent were better following medication, while 85 percent reported feeling better after hysterectomy. For women who had abnormal bleeding, 60 percent were better following medication while, as would be expected, 100 percent of women had no problems with bleeding following their hysterectomy.

The study found that more women in the hysterectomy group were satisfied with the relief of symptoms they achieved and were ten times more likely to have a positive feeling about how they felt following hysterectomy than for those who chose medication.

Although the results of this study should be interpreted with care, it does appear that hysterectomy may provide relief for women who have a *significant* degree of symptoms, especially if other treatment has failed. As new developments come along, the need for hysterectomy should decrease. However, hysterectomy does appear to have a place in the appropriate treatment of some medical problems.

Will Hysterectomy Become a Less Common Operation?

New treatments for fibroids and abnormal bleeding, two of the most common reasons for hysterectomy, should decrease the need for the surgery. Recent studies of women with fibroids have shown that the medical risks of no treatment, even with large fibroids, have been overstated in the past. Therefore, for many of these women, no treatment may be needed. If treatment is necessary, myomectomy by either hysteroscopy, laparoscopy, or abdominal surgery can often be used to remove fibroids and alleviate symptoms without removing the uterus (see page 41). Myoma coagulation, a new procedure described on page 49, uses a laparoscopic technique to destroy fibroids without removing them at all. To date, the early results have been promising. Medications used to shrink fibroids have been developed but are only effective in the short term because of their solely temporary benefit, their side effects, and their expense. However, it is likely that in the near future these problems will be worked out, and medication alone may be available to treat fibroids.

Abnormal bleeding may now be treated by endometrial ablation with 90 percent of women reporting excellent results, allowing them to avoid hysterectomy (see page 78). Endometriosis, the third most common reason for hysterectomy, may be treated by medical therapy, although the side effects and expense of the medications limit its use at the present time. Laparoscopic techniques short of hysterectomy may also be used to alleviate pelvic pain associated with endometriosis (see page 164). Hysterectomy, for most of these conditions, should be a last resort, not the first one.

Mary's Fibroids

Mary is a forty-seven-year-old woman who had known that she had fibroids for about five years. At first, the fibroids had been small and she was not bothered by them at all. After a few years, they began to grow little by little, until they were the size of a four-month pregnancy. She had been told by a number of doctors over the past few years that surgery would be necessary. However, Mary was afraid of surgery, afraid of being in a hospital, and afraid of any of the possible risks to her health. She had wanted to avoid surgery if at all possible. She had been very active, playing tennis and exercising regularly, and while the fibroids had slowed her down a bit, she was still able to do these things.

I was the fourth doctor to see Mary for her fibroids. At the time she had started to have heavy and irregular bleeding, but otherwise she felt fairly well. Her examination showed that the fibroids had not grown any further. In order to make sure that there was no reason for the abnormal bleeding other than the fibroids, I recommended that she have a D&C and hysteroscopy (see page 75) in the office. Mary was relieved that she did not have to go to the hospital and agreed. The procedure went well, and no abnormal cells were found, suggesting that the bleeding was from the fibroids. In addition, based on a blood test (hematocrit) done prior to the D&C, Mary was not at all anemic. Therefore, the amount of blood she was losing did not seem to be harming her.

In the weeks following the procedure, Mary and I had two long discussions about her options. These included follow-up with pelvic examinations to monitor any further growth of the fibroids, myomectomy to remove the fibroids, myoma coagulation to shrink the fibroids, or hysterectomy. Mary once again chose the option of careful follow-up with pelvic examinations every three months. I felt totally comfortable with her decision. There was nothing wrong with her medically, and she was able to live with the fibroids comfortably enough to do the things she wanted to do.

Now, two years later, Mary continues to do well and has avoided surgery. We are both aiming toward her menopause when the fibroids will be expected to shrink down to about half their present size (even if she chooses to start hormone replacement therapy). Mary is totally comfortable with her decision, and, for her, it is clearly the right one.

QUESTIONS TO ASK YOUR DOCTOR

It is important for you to understand why your doctor has suggested a hysterectomy as treatment for your gynecologic problem. The best way to help you make a decision as to whether the procedure is right for you is to ask your doctor the right questions.

The most common reasons for surgery are pain, bleeding, or symptoms from fibroids. You know the reason you went to see the doctor in the first place. The first question that you should ask is, "What exactly is causing my pain?" Sometimes the reason will not be entirely clear to the doctor. In particular, the cause of pelvic pain may originate in the intestines or the bladder and not in the uterus. You should ask if there are other tests that can be done to make the diagnosis more apparent. The decision whether to have these tests should be yours, and should be balanced with their side effects and cost. For example, laparoscopy can help to make a diagnosis of the cause of pelvic pain, but you may or may not want to go through an operation to have an exact diagnosis made.

Once a diagnosis, or probable diagnosis, has been established, you should also ask what the consequences to your health will be if you do not have surgery, either at all or at this time. For non–life-threatening problems, one option is always to do nothing. However, doing nothing often means more frequent visits to your doctor to monitor your problem.

The next question to ask the doctor is "What are the nonsurgical alternative therapies available to treat my condition?" For every condition, there are usually alternatives of varying degrees of effectiveness. As described throughout this book, medications, pain management, even homeopathics or other alternative therapies may sometimes be tried to alleviate symptoms. But again, I would advise you to continue to see your doctor regularly in order to detect any changes in your condition.

You should also ask about your doctor's experience doing the operation that has been proposed. You should feel comfortable with the number of procedures he or she has performed for problems *like yours*. If the doctor's experience is limited, you may ask who the assistant is going to be, and how much experience the assistant has had. Additional training and experience must be acquired before some of the newer procedures, such as endometrial ablation, laparoscopic surgery, or laparoscopic hysterectomy, can be safely performed. Some hospitals have strict requirements for training before a doctor is allowed to perform these operations, while other hospitals have no such requirements. Therefore, it is important for you to ask about surgical training and experience.

Should You Get a Second Opinion?

You should also ask your doctor whether a second opinion would be a good idea. Most doctors will welcome the idea of a second opinion. If they have done a complete job on the diagnosis and on the explanation of the problem to you, then they should feel confident about the range of options they have suggested to you. In addition, no doctor knows everything, and your doctor may welcome any other new ideas about your problem. Other thoughts on second opinions are discussed on page 292.

What Is Right for You?

The decision to have a hysterectomy should not be taken lightly. There are medical conditions that require treatment—cancer, prolonged heavy bleeding to the point of severe anemia, or incapacitating pain. However, as outlined throughout this book, all medical conditions have more than one option for treatment. Medicine is an evolving art as well as a science. Recently, with more open attitudes toward women's opinions and feelings, and with the advent of new technology, doctors have been looking for new medical treatments for gynecologic symptoms in order to avoid hysterectomy. As outlined above, there are possible side effects of hysterectomy, none of which are entirely predictable for each individual. But, for some women, hysterectomy will be the right treatment.

As with most decisions, you should carefully consider the pros and cons of hysterectomy as they relate to *your particular* medical situation and emotional well-being. On one hand, you should weigh the degree of discomfort that your gynecologic problem presents to you, the ways in which it interferes with your health, both emotionally and physically. On the other hand, weigh the potential risks of the operation, including the possible physical and emotional side effects of having a hysterectomy. There are women who happily choose to live with fibroids the size of a five-month pregnancy despite the fact that they have some daily discomfort and look pregnant. Other women choose surgery for small fibroids because they are distressed by symptoms or by worry and don't wish to live with the problems any longer.

The universal indications for hysterectomy have not been defined. Ultimately, the final decision about the appropriateness of a hysterectomy, or any type of surgery or medical care, should be made by each woman herself. That is what this book is about.

REFERENCES

Arnot, B. 1993. Finding the right health care can mean the difference between life and death. *Good Housekeeping* 216:58–61.

Bachman, G. Hysterectomy: A critical review. 1990. *Journal of Reproductive Medicine* 35:839–62.

Carlson, K., B. Miller, and F. Fowler. 1994. The Maine women's health study: I. Outcomes of hysterectomy. *Obstetrics and Gynecology* 83:556–65.

Carlson, K., B. Miller, and F. Fowler. 1994. The Maine' women's health study: II. Outcomes of nonsurgical management of leiomyomas, abnormal bleeding, and chronic pelvic pain. *Obstetrics and Gynecology* 83:566–72.

Centerwall, B. 1981. Premenopausal hysterectomy and cardiovascular disease. *American Journal of Obstetrics and Gynecology* 139:58–61.

Coulter, A., K. McPherson, and M. Vessey. 1988. Do British women undergo too many or too few hysterectomies? *Social Science and Medicine* 27:987–94.

Dranov, P. 1990. An unkind cut. *American Health* 9:36–42.

Gambone, J., R. Reiter, and J. Lench. 1992. Short-term outcome of incidental hysterectomy at the time of adnexectomy for benign disease. *Journal of Women's Health* 1:97–200.

Griffith-Jones, M., G. Jarvis, and H. McNamara. 1991. Adverse urinary symptoms after total abdominal hysterectomy—fact or fiction? *British Journal of Urology* 67:295–97.

Gross, J. 1994. Our bodies, but my hysterectomy. *New York Times*, June 26, 1994.

Helstrom, L., P. Lundberg, D. Sorbom, and T. Backstrom. 1993. Sexuality after hysterectomy: A factor analysis of women's lives before and after subtotal hysterectomy. *Obstetrics and Gynecology* 81:357–62.

Langer, R., M. Neuman, R. Ron-el, A. Golan, I. Bukovsky, and E. Caspi. 1989. The effect of total abdominal hysterectomy on bladder function in asymptomatic women. *Obstetrics and Gynecology* 74:205–7.

Ryan, M., L. Dennerstein, and R. Pepperell. 1989. Psychological aspects of hysterectomy: A prospective study. *British Journal of Psychology* 154:516–22.

Wilcox, L., L. Koonin, R. Pokras, L. Strauss, Z. Xia, and H. Peterson. 1994. Hysterectomy in the United States, 1988–1990. *Obstetrics and Gynecology* 83:549–55.

12

IF YOU ARE FACING SURGERY

In some situations surgery may be recommended by your physician. Although many people around the world walk into hospitals each day to face an operation, very few of us can do it without at least some fear. It is always a step that requires a great deal of thought and consideration since it involves some discomfort, some risk, and some disruption of one's life.

I strongly feel that the decision to have surgery is always up to the patient. It is your body and your life not your doctor's. Do everything you can to understand your condition and the surgical and medical options available to treat it. Take charge of your medical care by educating yourself. Knowledge is often a good antidote to anxiety. Any medical problem, particularly one that seems to be pointing toward surgery, is anxiety producing. You will begin your own healing and recovery by taking charge of the decisions that need to be made.

DECISIONS BEFORE SURGERY

What Should Happen During the Doctor's Consultation?

When one of my patients needs surgery, I like to set up a consultation visit to discuss all the available options, even the ones I may not feel are entirely appropriate for that particular woman. The role of a physician at this point is to provide information so that you can make decisions in order to get well. Diagrams or photographs of anatomy and surgical procedures are always a part of my consultation visit. Most of us are not familiar enough with anatomy or medical terminology to get a genuine understanding of a problem or the surgical options from just a verbal explanation. Being able to visualize the problem through diagrams or photos helps to make all the options and procedures clear. During this long talk together, we discuss the risks and benefits of each possible solution to the problem.

We also talk about the recovery period after surgery and predict, as best we can, how long it will take to get back to work and normal activities. People seem most comfortable with decisions made when all information available is understood and carefully considered. If you know and understand the whole story, your head and your heart will lead you to the best decision. The notion of physician as educator and the patient as an active participant in the decision process is one that is very important to me. When this relationship works well, I feel comfortable that the patient will make a decision that is right for her. I have been told by my patients that these appointments are worth their weight in gold when choices need to be made.

Should You Bring Someone to the Doctor's Office?

If I needed surgery, I would not want to be alone at the time decisions were being discussed or made. I have found it very helpful for the woman facing surgery to have a family member or friend accompany her to the consultation visit. You will often feel calmer with a loved one near, and you will be better able to take in the information discussed. Sometimes your companion is able to listen when you are too anxious to do so or will simply pick up something you missed. Often your companion is able to hear the optimism and reassurance in the words spoken when you may only be able to hear your own fear. Having another person hear the information at least insures that there will be someone knowledgeable for you to talk to after the appointment is over. Having a loving, trusted, and informed companion on the ride home may be the nicest gift you could give yourself.

After all the options, both surgical and nonsurgical, are presented and understood, I will then make some recommendations based on my best medical judgment. Often women will ask, "What would you do if you were me?" I always find this a difficult question to answer because so many nonmedical factors need to be considered. Ask yourself: How much discomfort am I in because of this condition? Can I or should I tolerate it? Can I afford, both emotionally and physically, not to have surgery? Can I afford the time off work to recuperate if I do have surgery? What are my emotions about my condition? How do I feel about having surgery? How will my choice affect my family? These are questions only you can answer. If medically appropriate, I always like to offer at least two possible treatment options. This helps to insure the possibility that each woman will have a choice that she feels comfortable with.

When Should You Make a Decision About Surgery?

I don't think any decision should be made about surgery at the initial consultation visit. You should think about the information and options for a while in a relaxed environment. Be sure to call the doctor back with any questions that you may not have thought of before, or for questions that were not completely answered during the visit. Almost all women call me back within a few days with a few more questions. This is your body; do not be afraid to ask questions.

Should You Get a Second Opinion?

If surgery has been recommended to you, I think a second opinion is an excellent idea. Very few things in medicine are black or white, and there is a lot of room for differences of opinion. A number of possibilities exist after a second opinion. First, the physician you see for the second opinion may give you the exact same options as your original gynecologist. This may put your mind at ease in that you will feel sure that nothing has been overlooked. Second, the new physician may bring up other options that are available to you or give you more information to think about. On occasion, the physician giving the second opinion may disagree with what you have been told or even disagree with the diagnosis. For my patients who seek a second opinion, I always ask them to call and talk to me about the results of that consultation. This allows me to answer any new questions and respond to any suggestions the other physician has offered. I never feel offended if a patient wants a second opinion. Many of my colleagues and I encourage seeking second opinions, particularly when the patient is unsure of what is best for her. This is your body and your health. Do not be afraid to get another opinion.

Who Should You Go to for a Second Opinion?

It is probably *not* a good idea to ask your gynecologist who you should see for a second opinion. Despite a high degree of honesty in the profession, your doctor may refer you to someone she knows well, who may be less likely to disagree with the diagnosis or proposed treatment. There are a number of good sources available to you to suggest the name of a doctor for your second opinion. Your family doctor or internist will know other gynecologists in the community who are knowledgeable, honest, and provide good care. Another possibility is to call the gynecology floor of your local hospital. The head nurse may be able to suggest doctors for you who have experience with your particular problem. Nurses have a unique vantage point since they see physicians interact with and care for patients and also know how each doctor's patients do following surgery. Nurses are a good source for a physician referral. You may also consider calling a teaching hospital near you and asking for a faculty member with expertise in your area of concern.

I do think, however, that you should tell your gynecologist that you are going to get a second opinion. This will maintain the trust and honesty in your relationship. You should also consider telling him who the doctor will be. There may be doctors in the community who are well known but who may not have knowledge about the specific procedure or problem you are faced with. This will give your gynecologist an opportunity to voice any concerns about the doctor you have chosen. This need not dissuade you from using that doctor for a second opinion, but you will at least be prepared for any differences of opinion.

What If You Decide Surgery Is Right for You?

If you decide to have surgery, another visit should be set up with your doctor to go over the specific details of the procedure you are to have performed. Again, it is nice to have someone accompany you. Once a decision has been made, we go over a paper called the informed consent. If properly done, filling out this form allows for a frank discussion of what you should expect from surgery. It allows the doctor and patient to go over the details of the operation to be performed, the specific risks of the procedure, the alternatives to the surgery, and the possible consequences if the surgery is not performed. Basically, this is the time when you will hear all the risks and possible complications during and after your surgery. This is difficult and may feel as if it's the last thing you want to hear, but ultimately it is quite helpful to you. I see this form as part of my job as an educator. I choose to fill out the form by hand in the patient's presence and make it specific for each woman's situation. Doctors are certainly not trying to erode your confidence at this point, but we are legally and morally bound to tell you about all the things that could happen. Most people's emotional reaction to this form is fear, which is understandable. Just remember to be sure and hear the optimism in your doctor's message. This is another opportunity for you to inform and educate yourself. Learning as much as you can will help, not hurt, you. And your doctor should be available to answer any questions related to the risks of the procedure.

How Do You Schedule Surgery?

The next step is to schedule the surgery based on the urgency of the problem, your schedule, the availability of your family or friends who may be helping you out after surgery, your doctor's schedule, and the availability of the hospital operating room. In our office, we have a person who sits down with the patient and helps them through this process. Scheduling the date of surgery, blood donation appointments (see below), lab test appointments, and appointments with a primary care doctor can all be arranged at this time. We like to write all this information down so that you can refer to it later.

Planning can go a long way toward reducing anxiety. We also tell our patients to stop taking any products containing aspirin for the two weeks before surgery, since they can lead to more bleeding during the operation. You will also be instructed to not eat or drink anything for at least eight hours prior to your surgery. Anything in your stomach at the time of the operation could cause vomiting and aspiration of food into your lungs—a serious problem. And last, but certainly not least, if you smoke, you should stop at least a few weeks before surgery to allow your lungs to clear and reduce your risk of breathing problems after surgery.

Should You Donate Your Own Blood Before Surgery?

If time and circumstances allow, we like to have a woman donate her own blood before surgery. While the need for transfusion is usually small, it is always better to have your own blood (called autologous blood) available if needed. This reduces the risk of AIDS from one unit per two hundred thousand of donated blood to essentially zero. The risk of getting hepatitis from donated blood is 0.1 percent. Giving blood is very much like having a blood test taken. A needle is inserted into a vein in your arm and attached to a plastic bag. You may be asked to open and close your fist to help pump the blood out of the vein. The entire procedure takes about forty-five minutes, and there is no discomfort other than the initial stick of the needle.

If you are going to donate your own blood, you will be advised to take iron pills to build up your blood prior to donating the first pint of blood. Sometimes iron pills can cause stomach upset, but taking them with food often prevents this from happening. The iron should be continued until after you have surgery. First, one pint of blood is taken, and then another pint is taken a week later. After another week to allow you to rebuild your blood, surgery can be performed. If you are able to wait, having your own completely safe blood available to you is well worth it in the event that you need it. For some procedures the risk of needing a transfusion is so low that you may not want to donate your own blood. You should discuss this issue with your doctor.

What Other Tests May Be Needed Before Surgery?

A few days prior to your surgery, blood tests will be performed to check your blood count. Depending on your age and medical history, other tests—an EKG to check your heart, a chest X ray to check your lungs, other blood tests to check the kidneys or liver, or a blood sugar to check for diabetes—may be needed to be sure that all bodily functions are strong. These test results are reviewed by your doctor and anesthesiologist prior to surgery.

If you have had problems with your heart or lungs before, your doctor may want you to set up an appointment with an anesthesiologist before your surgery so that these problems may be discussed and any further tests or preparations ordered ahead of time.

What Should You Do to Prepare for Surgery?

You may also find that this time prior to surgery can be useful to get ready in other ways. If you can, take care of any business that may cause you anxiety. Make arrangements for child care, pay your bills, and get someone to water plants and take care of your pets. Also, it's a good idea to inquire about disability benefits at work so that you know in advance how much time off you will be allowed and how much money you will receive. Try to tie up loose ends at home and at work. This taking care of details will give you peace of mind during your hospital stay and recovery period.

If you have the luxury of free time before your scheduled surgery, use it to be nice to yourself and to stay in a positive frame of mind—visit friends and family, write letters, listen to music, see a movie. Concentrate on building up your confidence and optimism. Picture yourself getting well and getting strong. Try to keep your attitude about your surgery and your health positive and healing. Know that there are good times and good health in front of you. Enter the hospital as confidently and as peacefully as you can. A positive outlook can aid in your recovery.

AT THE HOSPITAL

What Happens When You Get to the Hospital?

Hospitals are generally large places with lots of rules and red tape. I hope that you will be met by friendly and helpful staff when you arrive for admission. A smile from a staff member can go a long way toward making you feel welcome and safe. That smile and courteous help in filling out forms cannot, of course, be guaranteed. Here is another instance where taking a trusted companion with you can help insure your comfort. He or she can do any running around that needs to be done, can help listen to instructions, and can give you the much needed smile that a harried clerk may not manage.

You are usually asked to go to the hospital two to three hours before surgery. Generally, you go to the admitting office where admission and insurance forms will need to be filled out. You should remember to pack your insurance information the night before so that it will be readily available. You should also be sure to leave all your valuables at home. Hospitals usually have a place to store valuables, but it is better not to have to worry about them. You will then be escorted to your room in the preoperative area, which is usually right near the operating room.

If you didn't believe you were going to have an operation before, the reality begins to hit about now. You will be asked to get undressed and put on a hospital gown. Many people begin to feel as if they are sick the moment they don this particularly unattractive piece of clothing. Contrary to popular belief, the gown was not designed to humiliate you and keep you uncomfortable. It is completely functional for surgery in that it is easy to put on and take off and gives the doctors and nurses quick access to you. But since the back of the garment usually leaves parts of your body exposed, it is not especially pleasant for you to wear.

The nurses will ask you about the reason you are in the hospital, your allergies to any medications, and any other medical problems you may have. You may be asked some of these questions repeatedly by a number of nurses or doctors during the time prior to your surgery. You will also need to sign another surgical consent form for the hospital, much like the one you signed in the doctor's office. Be reassured this is all for your safety in order to eliminate any confusion or mistakes. Because of these safety systems, I have never seen a case of mistaken identity occur.

Do You Need an IV?

Prior to surgery, a small needle is inserted into one of the veins of your arm, and a plastic tube is attached to the needle. A bag of fluid is attached to this tube and run into your vein. This IV, which means intravenous, provides you with the necessary water, salt, and sugar during the operation. It also provides access to your bloodstream for your anesthesia and any other medications you might need. While having an IV started is not fun, there is only minimal discomfort associated with inserting the needle and no discomfort thereafter.

Will You Need an Enema?

Before some types of surgeries, an enema is given to clean out your intestines. This empties the lower intestine and keeps it away from the uterus, fallopian tubes, and ovaries so that the surgeon can see the pelvic area more clearly. Discuss the need for an enema with your doctor. If it is necessary, some women prefer to give themselves one in the privacy of their own home before going to the hospital.

When Do You See the Anesthesiologist?

On the day of surgery, your anesthesiologist will visit you and review your medical history and allergies to any medications and discuss your options for anesthesia. The type of anesthesia used will depend on the type of surgery, the expected length of the surgery, your medical condition, your preference, and the comfort and experience of the anesthesiologist with different techniques. This is the time to ask any questions and express any preferences regarding anesthesia that you may have. By this time you are usually ready to get the surgery over with. The anesthesiologist will usually have some kind and comforting words for you and often will also give you some medications to help you relax before taking you into the operating room.

Is It Normal to Be Nervous About Anesthesia?

Over the years, as I have listened to people's concerns regarding surgery, it seems to me that one of the issues that causes a great deal of anxiety is the idea of general anesthesia, or being "put to sleep." The loss of control inherent in being put to sleep is a very powerful notion. We all try to retain as much control as we can over our own lives. Once again, education and a positive attitude can help to allay your fears and give you more of a sense of control. Anesthesia, like most fields in modern medicine, has made great strides in providing safe and effective care. Your anesthesiologist is a highly trained specialist, skilled in providing a safe and painless experience. Complications are extremely rare. In some cases, there will be anesthesia options available to you. Following is a brief overview of what we can do to insure that your surgery is safe and pain free.

What Is General Anesthesia?

General anesthesia is actually a combination of liquid medication injected into your IV to induce sleep, plus the administration of a medication that you breathe to keep you asleep. Initially, a clear plastic mask will be placed over your face to give you oxygen. This may feel a little confining, and the rubber may smell funny, but it is not at all uncomfortable. At this point, a medication is given in the IV that will put you to sleep. It takes less than a minute, and most patients do not find this unpleasant. I usually stay with my patients as soon as they are brought into the operating room. You will probably not know anyone else in the room, and I think the presence of your surgeon is comforting. I like to talk to my patients to help them relax. When they are falling asleep, I will tell them to think about something pleasant—a trip to Hawaii or the Caribbean. As they drift off to sleep I tell them, "Everything will be fine—we'll take good care of you." Besides making the experience more pleasant, there is even some evidence that this encouragement will actually help you recover faster.

After you are asleep, the anesthesia gas will be passed either through a mask over your mouth and nose or a tube placed through your mouth into your windpipe. The gas then seeps through your lungs and dissolves into the bloodstream. This dissolved gas reaches your brain and, in ways that are not totally understood, keeps you comfortably asleep for the duration of the operation. You will not feel any of the surgery.

What Is Epidural Anesthesia?

We feel physical pain because our nerves transmit this sensation from the site of the pain up to our brains. Nerves communicate with each other by sending chemical signals to the next nerve along the line. The brain soon gets the message, and we know that we're hurting. Local anesthetic, like the type your dentist uses, works by preventing the release of these chemical signals. When this happens, the nerves can't relay the message up to the brain to tell it that you hurt and you do not feel the pain.

Epidural anesthesia uses the same principle. After local anesthesia is placed in the skin, a small needle is guided into your back. A small plastic tube is placed through this needle into a space right outside your spinal cord. The needle is removed, but the plastic tube is left in place outside the spinal cord. Liquid local anesthetic that numbs the pain-sensing nerves and the motor (movement) nerves of your spinal cord is then dripped through the tube. The anesthetic prevents these nerves from sending the brain any pain signals. At the same time, the anesthetic prevents the nerves from making your muscles move. As the anesthetic begins to work, you may feel warmth and tingling in your legs and feet and then, within about fifteen minutes, you will be unable to feel or move anything from your abdomen to your toes. Because the numbing medication is confined to a localized area, your brain remains awake and alert, and you are able to breathe on your own. You are also able to speak, hear, and answer questions. In addition to the epidural anesthesia, some patients choose to have valium or another type of sedative given through the IV to help them relax during the surgery.

For abdominal surgery, some women prefer epidural anesthesia because they are concerned about the sense of losing control during general anesthesia. Others may prefer general anesthesia, since they may not want to "be awake" during the operation.

Are There Advantages to Epidural Anesthesia?

An advantage of epidural anesthesia is that it blocks the brain's perception of the initial pain signals from surgery. Even though you are asleep during general anesthesia, the nerves in your skin and body are able to send signals to your brain that are perceived subconsciously. It appears that these signals program the brain to be more sensitive to pain and, after you wake up, you may feel more postoperative pain. If these initial signals are blocked before you are operated on, which epidural anesthesia does, postoperative pain seems to be diminished. Some studies have shown that patients who have epidural anesthesia have less pain following surgery than those given general anesthesia.

Why Must General Anesthesia Be Used for Laparoscopic Surgery?

If your operation is being performed with the laparoscope, general anesthesia is almost always used. During laparoscopy, carbon dioxide gas is put into your abdomen to form a bubble. This bubble pushes the intestines away from the uterus, fallopian tubes, and ovaries so that the pelvic area can be seen and the surgery can be performed. But the bubble of gas also pushes the intestines into the upper abdomen and against the diaphragms, the muscles that push and pull on your lungs, allowing you to breathe. Let's say you wanted to remain conscious during laparoscopic surgery and requested an epidural or spinal anesthesia. As the gas was pumped into your abdomen to enable us to do the surgery, you would begin to feel the pressure on your diaphragm. You would soon feel as if you were unable to breathe. Needless to say, this would be terrifying. Also, you might inadvertently move around in an attempt to breathe more deeply, and this could be dangerous in the middle of your surgery. For this reason, when you have laparoscopic surgery, general anesthesia is more pleasant and safer.

What Type of Anesthesia Can Be Used for Abdominal Surgery?

Most abdominal surgery, other than laparoscopy, can be performed with either general or epidural anesthesia. You should discuss the options with your surgeon prior to the day of surgery. On the day of surgery, and while you are still alert, your anesthesiologist will also discuss the appropriate choice of anesthesia with you based on your medical situation and your own preferences.

When Do You Go to the Operating Room?

About fifteen minutes before surgery, you will be wheeled on a gurney (a bed on wheels) to the operating suite. Some hospitals kindly allow your family to accompany you to the door of your operating room. You will then be wheeled to the hallway outside the operating room. For some people, this causes some anxiety because strangers (surgeons, orderlies, and nurses) may be walking by as they go about their business. Hopefully, the relaxing medications you have been given should be working pretty well by now. Besides making you relaxed, you may also feel a little light-headed and have a dry mouth. These are normal side effects of the medication and are nothing to worry about.

Before being taken into the operating room you will be checked in by the nurse. They will ask you some seemingly ridiculous questions such as your name, what is wrong with you, what operation is to be performed on what part of your body. These questions avoid the wrong patient ending up in the wrong operating room or with the wrong operation. Again, in my eighteen years of practice, I have never seen an error made.

What Happens in the Operating Room?

Next you will be wheeled into the operating room. An operating room looks like it does in the movies, but it is always a little intimidating when it's real, and you are the patient. Large lights are on the ceiling, and the room looks sterile and impersonal. It usually feels cool because the rooms are kept at around 65°F. During surgery you will be covered with sterile sheets; the surgeons will be wearing sterile gowns, and everyone will be under hot lights. If the room is kept warm, the surgeons tend to sweat and fatigue easily, so the room is kept cool.

You will be helped over to the operating table, and a few small stick-on pads and wires will be put on your chest to monitor your heartbeat. More relaxing medication is given in the IV, which usually feels very pleasant and reduces much of the anxiety you may be feeling. Again, you may feel a little light-headed, but it's not bothersome. Some patients anticipate feeling uncomfortable and have a fear of losing control in the operating room. I find that quiet conversation with my patient goes a long way to avoid this fear. At this point, the anesthesia is given as described previously.

Are There Better Ways of Starting Anesthesia?

The hospitals in England have a better way of starting general anesthesia. Patients are admitted to a small room next to the operating room where they are prepared for surgery, and the medications are given. The family can be present until just before surgery. After the family leaves, the patient is given anesthesia in this comfortable and now familiar room and then wheeled, while asleep, into the operating room. The patient never sees the starkness of the operating room. This certainly seems a more humane way to take care of someone facing an operation.

What Is a Bladder Catheter For?

After you are anesthetized, a small rubber tube called a catheter is often placed in your bladder to allow urine to drain during surgery. This keeps the bladder from pushing on the uterus, fallopian tubes, and ovaries during surgery and also prevents the bladder from overstretching with urine during surgery. If you are leaving the hospital the same day, the catheter is usually removed before you wake up. If you are staying in the hospital, it is usually left in overnight so that you don't have to get out of your bed to urinate during the night. The catheter may cause a sensation of pressure, but it is not painful. If you feel alert and well enough to get out of bed and go to the bathroom by yourself you may ask to have the catheter removed right away. But most patients would rather not have to get up at night and choose to leave the catheter in until the morning. After the catheter is removed you may notice some mild discomfort when you urinate. This sensation results from stretching and irritation of the urethra (the tube through which the urine leaves the bladder) by the catheter. This irritation is not worrisome, and the feeling will go away in a day or two. If the irritation gets worse rather than better, let your doctor know so that your urine can be tested to check for a bladder infection. If so, the infection can be easily treated with antibiotics.

What Other Preparations Are Made in the Operating Room?

After you are asleep or sedated, your abdomen and vagina are washed with iodine to remove bacteria from the operative area. If you are allergic to iodine, let the nurses know, and they will use a different solution. Before the surgery actually begins, sterile paper sheets are placed over your body to keep bacteria away from the surgical area and reduce the risk of infection. Now the operation can begin.

What Is Everyone Doing During Surgery?

During the operation, the doctors and nurses often talk to one another to ask for instruments or to describe what is happening. Many anesthesiologists will play music during surgery. I find the music relaxing and am always glad when an anesthesiologist plays a tape or CD. There is evidence that the patient actually "hears" the music and that this is soothing and helps the recovery process. In the movies, you probably have seen doctors and nurses talking casually about sports or the weather during surgery. This does happen, but generally only during the more routine, easy parts of the surgery. When the operation gets to a more difficult part where concentration and complete attention is necessary, most surgeons and operating room staffs get very quiet. They know they have an enormously serious job to do and concentrate on their area of responsibility. Once the difficult portion of the surgery is finished and we know that the patient is doing well, the mood in the room relaxes again.

During the entire surgery the anesthesiologist will monitor your heartbeat, your breathing, and the amount of blood lost and will advise the surgeon if anything appears abnormal. The different types of surgery and techniques are described in the other chapters of this book.

What Happens Immediately After Surgery?

If you have had general anesthesia, the anesthesiologist will begin to decrease the amount of anesthesia just before the end of the operation so that you will start to wake up just after the surgery is over. You will be fairly groggy and won't remember much of what happens at this point. If you have had an epidural anesthetic, you will be fairly awake and alert but will be unable to move your legs. Next, you will be taken to a recovery room nearby, and the nurses will take your blood pressure, pulse, and temperature (with a sensor placed on your skin). The anesthesiologist will tell the nurses the type of operation you have had, any problems that may have occurred during surgery, any medical problems you may also have, and any problems they should look out for. The nurses then take over your care and will call your doctor or anesthesiologist with any problems or questions.

How Will You Feel Immediately After Surgery?

When you are in the recovery room, you will slowly start to awaken and be able to talk to the nurses taking care of you. It will probably be an hour before you feel fairly alert and able to stay awake without dozing off. Depending on the extent of surgery, you may begin to feel some soreness or pain at this point, and pain medication will be given to you if you need it. General anesthesia can make you queasy, and if you have any nausea or vomiting, medication can be given to relieve the feeling. You may also feel cold or get the chills, and the nurses will bring you some warm blankets. This part of recovery is not pleasant because you feel somewhat disoriented, possibly nauseous, possibly in pain. The recovery room nurses will be helpful and reassuring during this time.

When you are awake, alert, and your heart and breathing are stable, you will be wheeled in your bed to your room. The nurse on your floor will get a status report on your surgery and condition. You will have your blood pressure, pulse, and temperature taken on a regular basis, and you will be given medication for pain and nausea as needed. At this point, you will probably be annoyed from having been poked and prodded when you don't feel well. Please understand, though, that your condition right after surgery is very important and needs to be watched closely, at least hourly, for the first few hours. If you need something, ring the bell that is provided at the side of your bed in order to call for a nurse.

How Soon Can You See Your Family and Friends?

Your family will be asked to wait in the surgery waiting room or hospital lobby during your surgery. After you have been transferred to the recovery room and all the nurses' orders have been written, I usually go out to talk to family and friends to tell them how you are doing. It is a good idea to tell your doctor ahead of time what, if any, information should be told to whom. Certain information may be appropriate for some of the people close to you but not for all. It is also helpful for your doctor to have one main person to communicate with, who then can pass the information on to others.

Following most procedures, you will stay in the recovery room for about two hours and then be moved to a hospital room. At this point, your family and friends are welcome to be with you. They should be prepared for you to look a little pale and you may be too groggy to talk much, but at least you may be heartened by being together. In some situations, the nurses or doctors may ask your visitors to leave the room for a while so that they may care for you. Certain hospitals may also have visiting hours or limit the number of visitors that may be in your room at one time. These rules are good to know before your surgery so that everyone can plan accordingly. It is probably a good idea to limit your visitors early on because you will find even short visits to be quite tiring.

Is There Anything New for Postoperative Pain Relief?

The first few days after surgery are the hardest, and research is always being done in an effort to ease postoperative pain and soreness. The standard method of giving pain medication is by injection. This is done when you request something to reduce the pain. With injections given this way, the amount of pain reliever in your system is very high initially and then wears off to almost nothing. The high initial dose of injected medication is often sedating and makes a person groggy. Many of us won't like this feeling and will put off the next dose of medication until we are in pain just to avoid feeling useless and groggy.

However, if you wait too long and develop severe pain, your brain becomes sensitized to the pain, and it will take more medication to stop it. Also, after the first time or two of feeling pain, you may begin to anticipate its return with each passing hour. Many people find themselves anxiously awaiting their next shot. This anxiety and tension actually increase the pain, and higher doses are needed for pain control. Thus, the whole process becomes ineffective.

A recent and quite effective innovation is called patient-controlled analgesia (PCA). With this method, a small pump is attached to the IV you already have. The pump contains pain medication that is allowed to go into your system at a very controlled, slow, and steady rate. With a constant *low* level of medication continuously bathing the area of your brain that perceives pain, you do not develop significant pain. Because the doses are so small, the total amount of medication necessary per day is much smaller than with shots. You will not feel as groggy, and the pain relief is much better.

Since we each feel pain as individually as we feel pleasure, you may need to adjust your medication dose at times. There will be a small button located at your bedside that can be pushed to give you a little extra dose of medication if needed. To make sure that no one uses the extra doses so much that they endanger themselves, the entire pump is under the watchful eye of a computer programmed per your doctor's instructions. The computer only allows a predetermined small dose of medication to be given during a predetermined time interval. Extra pushing of the button does nothing. If you feel you need more medication, tell your doctor, and the pump can be reprogrammed.

Some women have been concerned that the pump might malfunction and cause a large dose of medicine to be given by mistake. In millions of uses of this pump, that has been reported to have happened only once. That is not a statistic worth worrying about. If your hospital offers PCA, discuss this form of pain relief with your doctor.

What Is Epidural Morphine?

If you have had epidural anesthesia, you may have the option, following the completion of surgery, of having a small dose of morphine injected through the plastic tube that was placed in your back. Although the exact mechanism of its action is unknown, this small dose of morphine can often provide excellent pain relief for the next twenty-four hours without any need for additional medication. Some patients, however, experience bothersome nausea or itching as a side effect of the epidural morphine. If so, other medication can be given to relieve these symptoms. If you are going to have an epidural anesthetic, you can discuss this type of postoperative pain relief with your anesthesiologist before your surgery.

When Will You Use Oral Pain Medication?

If you have had PCA, you will be switched to pain medication in pill form once you feel better, which is generally in about two days. If you have had epidural morphine, the pain relief lasts for about twenty-four hours, and pain pills can be started at that time. These pills should be taken regularly every few hours while you are awake in order to prevent the pain from becoming bothersome. Don't wait until the pain is severe before taking the medication because you will then require higher doses, and the pills will not work as well. Studies have shown that patients who wait too long to take pain medication because they want to avoid taking too much, end up taking a greater amount of medication in order to relieve the stronger pain.

Generally people find that by the time they go home, pain medication is only needed rarely. I usually send people home with a mild medication that can be taken for soreness or discomfort. It is a great feeling to know that you are feeling better and stronger each day as the pain medication becomes a thing of the past.

How Soon Can You Eat After Surgery?

If you have had major surgery, you usually will not be allowed to eat until the next morning. Most of my patients have not cared much about this, since the surgery and anesthesia may cause nausea. In addition, most women find themselves sleeping a great deal right after surgery and are not usually very hungry. Every morning after surgery, your doctor will listen to your abdomen with a stethoscope. If she hears gurgling, this signifies that the intestines have recovered from surgery and you will be able to start drinking liquids. Usually, this happens the first morning after surgery. If your intestines sound quiet, you are not yet ready to digest food. And if you eat too soon, nausea and vomiting may result. At this point, you have had enough discomfort and aggravation, and the last thing you'd want is to feel nauseous or to start to vomit. You will feel stronger as the days pass. Once your intestines recover, they will begin to push gas through the rectum. By then you will be able to eat and digest regular food.

What Activities Will You Be Able to Do in the Hospital?

The morning after major abdominal surgery, you will be able to get up out of bed and sit in a chair next to the bed. You should also be able to walk, with some assistance, to the bathroom. You may be sore, and the incision may be uncomfortable, so you should start out slowly until your body tells you how much you can do. By the second day, most women are up and around for short walks down the hall. You will probably find this tiring, but it is important to walk and keep your circulation going. By the third day, most women are able to get up periodically, walk for about fifteen minutes at a time, and take a shower.

RECOVERY

How Is Recovery Different If You Have Laparoscopic or Other Outpatient Surgery?

Most outpatient surgical procedures require less recovery time. Often if a catheter was placed in your bladder during surgery, it will be removed before you wake up. Once you are alert, and your heartbeat and breathing are fine, you will be helped out of bed and asked to go to the bathroom. The nurses will want to see that you can walk and will want to know that you can urinate by yourself before they let you go home. If you can't urinate because of the anesthesia or irritation from the catheter, they may want you to stay longer. You will be allowed to drink water when you feel ready and will be allowed to eat if you are able. Once you are stable, totally alert, and able to urinate, you will be allowed to go home. If you plan or need to stay overnight, you will be moved to a regular room in the hospital.

What Activities Will You Be Able to Do at Home?

If needed, you will be given pain medication to take at home. For the first week or so, physical activity should be limited to walking to meals or to the bathroom and to short walks (fifteen minutes) inside or outside. Because an abdominal incision needs six weeks to heal fully, you should not lift, exercise, have intercourse, or do anything that puts stress on your incision for that time. Walking is fine, and stairs are okay but should be taken slowly. As you feel stronger, you can increase your walking. When you feel up to it, probably after a few weeks, you can go outside to visit friends, eat, shop, or see a movie.

You will feel exhausted after surgery, and too much activity will actually make you feel sore. Most women need to sleep a good part of each day, and the simplest activity will leave you winded. The fatigue will not harm you, so do not let it worry you. Your body has undergone an enormous stress and needs time to recuperate. You will return to a good energy level in about six weeks. Some women need more time, others less. Just give yourself adequate time and care.

It is a good idea to arrange for help with shopping and meals before you go to the hospital. That way you will not need to worry about this right after surgery. For the first week or so you should let friends and family help you.

When Can You Return to Normal Activity After Laparoscopic Surgery?

Most patients recover quickly following laparoscopic surgery because the incisions are small and cause little discomfort. There also tends to be less irritation to the inside of your abdominal cavity than with major abdominal incisions, so you will be able to eat a few hours after surgery. You should be able to be up and around by the morning after surgery. Discomfort is usually minimal, and oral pain medication should be adequate for relief. Depending on the type of surgery performed, you may be able to return to work and exercise and activity within a week or two.

What Should You Watch Out for at Home?

After surgery you can expect some discomfort, some occasional lightheadedness, some vaginal spotting or light bleeding, and some occasional queasiness. Most doctors will instruct you to call them if you notice an increase in pain, vomiting, persistent nausea, temperature over 100.4°F., heavy vaginal bleeding, or a feeling of faintness that persists for more than a few minutes.

When Will You See Your Doctor After You Go Home?

Most physicians will want to see you back in the office at two weeks and at six weeks after your surgery. At your two-week visit, your incision will be checked, and you may have a pelvic exam to make sure that there is no infection and that healing is proceeding normally. This visit also gives you an opportunity to ask your doctor any questions that have come up about your activity, stamina, emotional well-being, return to work, and so on. Usually after this visit, you can slowly increase your activity. If all is well, I usually will let women drive a car following the two-week visit. Prior to this, you may become weak or light-headed while driving, and that might be dangerous.

At your six-week postoperative visit, a full pelvic examination is performed to see if your healing is complete. None of this should be uncomfortable. If all is back to normal, you should be able to resume full activity at this point, including a return to work. Of course, each patient and situation is different, and all of the above should be discussed with your doctor.

HOW YOU CAN BE SURE TO GET GOOD CARE

We have tried to provide you with descriptive and intelligent coverage of gynecologic problems and state-of-the-art information regarding a range of solutions. We have focused on the common gynecologic problems that are sometimes difficult to understand and often not adequately covered during doctor's visits or in magazines. We want to foster an empowering, compassionate view of the doctor-patient partnership, something we believe is vital to good care. It is in your best interest to be educated about the health care decisions you make. If you need more information, seek it out. Read more; get a second or third opinion. Ask all the questions you need to, until you feel comfortable with the answers. Seek out information about possible alternatives. When it comes time to make any decisions, you will then have the peace of mind that you have done your homework and are making the right choice for you.

INDEX

PLUME **DUTTON**

HELP YOURSELF—TO BETTER HEALTH

☐ **HEALTHY FOR LIFE** *The Scientific Breakthrough Program for Looking, Feeling, and Staying Healthy Without Deprivation* **by Dr. Richard F. Heller and Dr. Rachael F. Heller.** This groundbreaking book links a single basic physical imbalance—known as hyperinsulemia or simply Profactor-H, which is tied to the carbohydrate-rich foods you eat—to nine of this country's top killer diseases. Now, the Profactor-H Program offers a simple, no-measuring, no-counting plan that allows you to enjoy all the foods you need and love every day. (937331—$24.95)

☐ **STAY YOUNG THE MELATONIN WAY** *The natural plan for better sex, better sleep, better health, and longer life* **by Stephen J. Bock, M.D. and Michael Boyette.** For centuries, scientists have sought to unlock the secret of aging. Now new medical breakthroughs have focused on the role of melatonin, our natural "timekeeper" and drop for drop one of the most powerful hormones in the body. (275253—$10.95)

☐ **THE COMPLETE GUIDE TO MASSAGE** *A Step-by-Step Approach to Total Body Relaxation* **by Susan Mumford.** This handsome, full-color illustrated guide to the sensuous pleasures and benefits of massage takes you step-by-step through the art and power of massage—from beginning strokes to full-body advanced techniques. (275180—$16.95)

☐ **THE BODY SHOP BOOK** *Skin, Hair and Body Care.* **Introduction by Anita Roddick.** This book collects, for the first time in one place, everything The Body Shop has learned about the whys, wheres, and how-tos of skin, hair, and body care from the top of your head to the tips of your toes. The lively text is enhanced by easy-to-follow diagrams and charts that are full of problem-solving advice. (939504—$26.95)

Prices slightly higher in Canada.